Nanotherapeutics: From Laboratory to Clinic

Nanotherapeutics: From Laboratory to Clinic

Editor

Lino Messana

scitus academics

Nanotherapeutics: From Laboratory to Clinic
Edited by **Lino Messana**

ISBN: 978-1-68117-693-2
Library of Congress Control Number: 2016958864

www.scitusacademics.com

Notice

Printed in United States of America on Acid Free Paper

Preface

Over the last two decades, significant progress has been made in the field of nanomedicine, resulting in a number of products, including therapeutics and imaging agents, enabling more effective and less toxic therapeutic and diagnostic interventions Nanomedicine is a combination of nanotechnology and medicine and it provide new direction in medical diagnosis, monitering and treatment at the level of single molecules or molecular assemblies at the "nano" scale of about 100nm or less. Nanomedicine is the application of nanoscale technologies to the practice of medicine. It is used for diagnosis, prevention and treatment of disease and to gain increased understanding of underlying disease mechanisms. Presently nanomedicine involves detection of particles, drug delivery system, emulsions, and carriers for delivering vaccines: and biomaterials with unusual properties and improved biocompatibility. The application of nanotechnology in areas of drug delivery and therapy is intended to have a great impact on public health. Nanoparticles and nanodevices e.g. nanobiosensors and nanobiochips are being used to improve drug discovery and development. Drug targeting by using nanoparticle should reduce systemic toxicity, encapsulation and nanocarriers protect drugs from metabolism and from excretion. Drug diffusion through pore is a novel method of administering antiangiogenic and antioxidant drugs in the treatment of proliferative vascular disease.

Nanotherapeutics: From Laboratory to Clinic focuses on nanomedicine products related to drug delivery and therapy i.e. nanotherapeutics. This book provides up-to-date research material in the area of nanotherapeutics. Its content is clear and instructive and imitates recent information in pharmaceutics. It should be of a valuable tool for all types of readers, including students, research scientists, pharmacists from the industry and practitioners from hospitals who want to develop their familiarity about nanomedicine. We discuss the regulatory pathway and initiatives endeavoring to ensure the safe and timely clinical translation of emerging nanotherapeutics. From this concise book, readers will gain an insight into the basics of nanoparticle preparation and find a more detailed account of what is therapeutically feasible by using nanoparticle approaches.

Nanotechnology represents a cluster of technologies with different characteristic and applications. Nanomedicine related solicitations are under development and this is a long process of converting nanomedicine in to commercially viable products. The crucial goal of nanotherapeutics is comprehensive monitoring repair and improvement of all human biologic system. There is great concern over the environmental and health risk with the use of nanomedicine. The protection and maintenance of health information of the patients is the ethical issue and ensuring privacy is of greatest importance while using nanomedicine.

Table of Contents

Chapter 1

Nanotherapeutics Using an HIV-1 Poly A and Transactivator of the HIV-1 LTR-(TAR-) Specific siRNA

Supriya D. Mahajan,[1] Ravikumar Aalinkeel,[1] Jessica L. Reynolds,[1] Bindukumar Nair,[1] Donald E. Sykes,[1] Wing-Cheung Law,[2] Hong Ding,[2] Earl J. Bergey,[2] Paras N. Prasad,[2] and Stanley A. Schwartz[1]

[1]Division of Allergy, Immunology, and Rheumatology, Department of Medicine, University at Buffalo, The State University of New York, 640 Ellicott Street, Room 444 Innovation Center, Buffalo, NY 14203, USA
[2]Institute for Lasers, Photonics and Biophotonics, University at Buffalo, The State University of New York, Buffalo, NY 14260, USA

ABSTRACT

HIV-1 replication can be efficiently inhibited by intracellular expression of an siRNA targeting the viral RNA. We used a well-validated siRNA (si510) which targets the poly A/TAR (transactivator of the HIV-1 LTR) site and suppresses viral replication. Nanotechnology holds much potential for impact in the field of HIV-1 therapeutics, and nanoparticles such as quantum rods (QRs) can be easily functionalized to incorporate siRNA forming stable nanoplexes that can be used for gene silencing. We evaluated the efficacy of the QR-si510 HIV-1 siRNA nanoplex in suppressing viral replication in the HIV-1-infected monocytic cell line THP-1 by measuring p24 antigen levels and gene expression levels of HIV-1 LTR. Our results suggest that the QR-si510 HIV-1 siRNA nanoplex is not only effective in delivering siRNA, but also in suppressing HIV-1 viral replication for a longer time period. HIV-1 nanotherapeutics can thus enhance systemic bioavailability and offer multifunctionality.

1. INTRODUCTION

Treatment of human immunodeficiency virus type 1 (HIV-1) disease with highly active antiretroviral therapy (HAART) has enormous clinical benefits; however, there exists the problem of continuing emergence of drug resistance, treatment adherence and serious risk of toxicities, with the prospect of life-long antiretroviral treatment, additionally viral reservoirs persist in several sequestered sites such as the central nervous system (CNS) and testis. Therefore, developing strategies that treat HIV infection and eliminate persistent viral reservoirs are needed and gene therapy approaches such as RNA interference (RNAi) have emerged as a therapeutic possibility for the elimination of HIV-1 [1–3].

RNAi works either through binding with HIV-1 to inhibit provirus integration into cellular genome or with mRNA products to inhibit genes that play a vital role in HIV-1 infectivity by knocking down the virulence capacity of the virus [2, 3]. RNAi is a highly potent mechanism of posttranscriptional gene silencing which is mediated by sequence-specific siRNAs, which can effectively down regulate expression of either a cellular RNA target molecules by selective degradation of mRNAs [4–6]. Viral replication can be successfully inhibited using siRNA; however, designing a functional siRNA that targets a highly divergent virus can be challenging [1–5]. Recently, a very elegant and comprehensive study by Naito et al. analyzed several promising siRNA sequences of near full length HIV-1 group M strains from the Los Alamos sequence database and selected a set of optimal antiviral siRNA [7, 8]. Delivery of optimal amounts of these synthetic antiviral siRNAs by transfection into cultured cells can effectively inhibit HIV-1 infections; however, the antiHIV-1 effects of these delivery methods are transient due to the degradation and dilution of siRNAs during cell division.

A major hurdle limiting the use of the gene silencing technology is the lack of methods to safely and efficiently deliver siRNA molecules to target cells/tissues. In the free form, siRNA molecules have a very short half life in physiological conditions, owing to their vulnerability for degradation by endogeneous nucleases. Therefore, they need macromolecular carriers (vectors) that will not only protect them from degradation in the biological milieu, but also steer them to desired cells/tissues as well as facilitate their cellular entry. Nanoparticle surfaces can be easily modified to incorporate cationic charges, which will facilitate their stable electrostatic complexation with anionic genetic materials such as siRNA, for the purpose of targeted gene delivery/silencing [9–11]. HIV-1 nanotherapeutics can increase drug solubility, enhance systemic bioavailability, and at the same time offer multifunctionality.

In the current study, we have used a synthetic siRNA (si510) described by Naito et al. [7, 8] which is a highly effective siRNA against divergent HIV-1 strains which targets the poly A/TAR (transactivator of the HIV-1 LTR) site and successfully targets viral transcripts and achieves effective viral inhibition. HIV-1 TAR RNA is the binding site of the viral protein Tat, the transactivator of the HIV-1 LTR (long terminal repeat). It is present at the 5′ end of all HIV-1 spliced and unspliced mRNAs in the nucleus as well as in the cytoplasm. A TAR-specific RNA will affect the viral and cellular binding factors thereby decreasing virion production and effectively inhibit viral replication [12]. HIV-1 contains duplicated long terminal repeat (LTR) sequences flanking the proviral genome. These LTRs contain identical poly(A) (polyadenylation) signals, which are both transcribed into RNA, to allow efficient viral expression [12]. Thus the si510 siRNA that targets both the poly A/TAR can effectively suppress viral replication. Naito et al. reported that the siRNA transfections using the si510 sequence that were done in their study were done using a commercially available reagent Lipofectamine (Invitrogen, CA) and that this transfection was transient in nature and that the percentage decrease in viral replication was >90%, 48 hours posttransfection [7]. The goal of the current investigation to evaluate if complexing the si510 siRNA to a nanoparticle such as a quantum rod (QR) would effectively suppress viral replication for a extended period of time. In addition to efficacy, the dose and time kinetics of this siRNA nanoplex was evaluated in the HIV-1-infected monocytic cell line THP-1. We believe that the results of this study will attest to the fact that nanotechnology can play a pivotal role in HIV-1 therapeutics.

2. METHODS

2.1. Study Design

Following synthesis and characterization of the nanoplexes (QR-si510 siRNA complex), we evaluated their uptake in vitro cultured monolayers of an HIV-1-infected monocytic cell line THP-1 using confocal imaging. THP-1 cells were treated with various concentrations of the si510 siRNA ranging from 5 nM to 100 nM over a range of time periods from 6 hr to 1 week posttransfection and the antiviral efficacy the nanoplexes was tested. Two independent methods were used to evaluate antiviral effects: (1) the measurement of p24 antigen levels using a commercially available p24 ELISA assay and (2) quantitating HIV-1 LTR-R/U5 gene expression using quantitative real-time PCR.

2.2. Synthesis and Aqueous Dispersion of the QRs Terminated with Carboxyl Groups

The formation of the Cadmium (Cd) Selelinum (Se) CdSe core nanocrystals, and thin layer of Zinc Sulfide (ZnS) shell (<1.5 nm) is grown over the nanocrystal core. CdS/ZnS graded shell on CdSe QRs in organic media was carried out as described by Yong et al. [13]. To form the nanocrystal core, 6 mmol cadmium oxide (CdO) was dissolved in 10 mL of oleic acid at 280°C, producing a homogeneous reaction mixture of cadmium complex. Then, a solution of selenium (Se) precursor was injected into the reaction mixture. The Se : Cd molar ratio was 1 : 3. The length of reaction time following the injection determines the final size of the nanocrystals. The CdSe nanocrystals were then purified by precipitation from the reaction mixture with ethanol followed by centrifugation. For the growth of a ZnS shell over the CdSe cores, the CdSe cores were dispersed in 5 g of TOPO at 250°C. A mixture of diethylzinc (Et_2Zn) and hexamethyldisilathiane ($(TMS)_2S$) (Zn : S = 1 : 1 molar ratio) were mixed with Trioctylphosphine (TOP) and the solution precursor was added dropwise into the CdSe core nanocrystals reaction mixture at 250°C. After ~20 minutes of heating, the heating mantle was removed, and then the reaction mixture was air cooled to room temperature. Following their synthesis, the CdSe/CdS/ZnS QRs were dispersed in aqueous media by coating with mercaptosuccinic acid (MSA). Briefly, 3 mmol of MSA was dissolved in 10 mL of chloroform under vigorous stirring. After stirring for 10 to 15 minutes, 2 mL of concentrated (~40 mg/mL chloroform) CdSe/CdS/ZnS QR dispersion was added into this mixture. This solution was stirred overnight at room temperature. The QRs were separated from the surfactant solution by addition of ethanol and centrifugation. The red-brownish precipitate was redispersed in 10 mL HPLC water and the solution was further filtered using a syringe filter with a pore diameter of 0.45 μm. The QRs have relatively good colloidal stability and no precipitation was observed after several months of storage [13–15].

2.3. Physical Characterization of QRs

The physical properties of the nanoplex were established using transmission electron microscopy (TEM), dynamic light scattering (DLS), spectrophotometry and spectrofluorimetry. TEM was used to determine the particle size and size distribution. The aqueous dispersion of the nanoparticles was drop cast on a TEM copper grid (electron microscopy sciences, Inc.) and visualized using a JEOL JEM 2020 electron microscope. DLS measurements were carried out using a Brookhaven 90Plus particle size analyzer, with a scattering angle of 90°. UV-vis absorption spectra were recorded using a Shimadzu UV-3101 PC spectrophotometer, using a quartz cuvette with 1 cm path length. Fluorescence spectra were recorded on a Fluorolog-3 (Jobin Yvon, Longjumeau, France) spectrofluorimeter.

2.4. Cell Viability Measurement Using an MTT (3-(4,5-Dimethylthiazol-2-yl)-2,5-Diphenyltetrazolium Bromide, a Tetrazole) Assay

MTT cell proliferation assay measures the reduction of a tetrazolium component (MTT) into an insoluble formazan product by the mitochondria of viable cells. The MTT assay is a quantitative, sensitive detection of cell proliferation since it measures the growth rate of cells by virtue of a linear relationship between cell activity and absorbance. Typically 10,000 cells suspended in 100 µL of media were incubated with 10 µL of MTT reagent (Cat # 30-1010 K; ATCC) for approximately 3 hours, followed by addition of a detergent solution to lyse the cells and solubilize the colored crystals. Colorimetric detection was done at a wavelength of 570 nm. The amount of color produced is directly proportional to the number of viable cells.

2.5. Determination of the Delivery of Nanoplexes into THP-1 Cells

Nanoplexes (QD-siRNA) are discrete spheres, having a mean size of 15–20 nm. They are sufficiently small to diffuse into cells by endocytosis and favor nucleic acid transfer and release from the endosome across the nuclear membrane. Nanoplex suspensions are prepared by adding 5–100 nM si510 siRNA/10 ul volume to 20 µL of QR solution suspended in a total of 200 µL of serum-free media to permit complex formation for 15 min at room temperature followed by addition of the nanoplex to the THP-1 cells plated in 35 mm glass bottom culture plates. Commercial transfection reagent, Lipofectamine (Invitrogen, Carlsbad, CA) is used as a control and used according to the manufacturer's protocol. Cells are cultured in an incubator (VWR Scientific, model 2400) at 37°C in a humidified atmosphere of 5% CO_2 for a period ranging from 12 hr to 1 week posttransfection.

2.6. Imaging of Nanoparticles

A Nikon Eclipse TE2000 microscope equipped with the Nuance GNIR imaging system (Cambridge Research & Instrumentation Inc., Cambridge, MA) was employed for cell imaging. This imaging system is capable of multispectral (wavelength-resolved) imaging in the range of 500–950 nm. Custom-designed filter cubes, with corresponding dichroic and emission filters acquired from Omega Optical, were used to cut off the excitation light and obtain high contrast fluorescence images. Additionally, a water-immersion objective lens (Nikon, Fluor 60X, NA1.0) is used for cell imaging.

2.7. Cell Line

Monocytic THP-1 cells (American Type Culture Collection [ATCC], Manassas, VA); were maintained at 37°C, under 5% CO_2 in RPMI 1640 medium supplemented with 10% (v/v) heat-inactivated fetal bovine serum (FBS) (Sigma, St.Louis, MO), penicillin (100 units/mL), streptomycin (100 mg/mL), and L-glutamine (2 mM). THP-1 cells are cultured as a single-cell suspension cultures and were split at a ratio of 1 : 4 once a week.

2.8. HIV-1 Infection of THP-1

Undifferentiated THP-1 cells are susceptible to infection by T-tropic human immunodeficiency virus type 1 (HIV-1) isolates that use the coreceptor CXCR4 (X4 strains). Undifferentiated THP-1 (cells/mL) were infected for 3 hours with HIV-1_{IIIB} (NIH AIDS Research and Reference Reagent Program) at a concentration of $10^{3.0}$ $TCID_{50}$/mL cells, equivalent to 10 ng viral isolate/mL of culture media. Following that, the infected cells were washed with Hanks buffered saline, reconstituted in RPMI media (fortified with 10% FBS) and incubated at 37°C/5% CO_2 for 7 days. Levels of p24 in the culture supernatants were measured using a commercially available p24 ELISA kit (Zeptometrix, Buffalo, NY) 7 days postinfection. These infected THP-1 cells were then washed and reconstituted in fresh culture medium and used for evaluating the antiHIV-1 efficacy of the nanoplexes.

2.9. p24 ELISA

HIV-1 infection was monitored by the viral p24 level in harvested cell culture supernatants, using enzyme-linked immunosorbent assay (ELISA) plates obtained from a commercial vendor (Zeptometrix Buffalo, NY). The results are expressed in pg/mL as the mean and standard deviation (SD) of duplicate determinations from two wells.

2.10. Real-Time Quantitative PCR (Q-PCR)

Cytoplasmic RNA was extracted by an acid guanidinium-thiocyanate-phenol-chloroform method using Trizol reagent (Invitrogen, Carlsbad, CA) [16]. The amount of RNA was quantified using a Nano-Drop ND-1000 spectrophotometer (Nano-Drop, Wilmington, DE) and the isolated RNA was stored at −80°C until used. The LTR-R/U5 region represents early stages of reverse transcription of HIV-1. Following conversion of RNA to cDNA using reverse transcription, relative abundance of mRNA species was quantified by real-time quantitative PCR using the LTR/RU5-specific primers and the Brilliant SYBR green QPCR master mix (Stratagene Inc, La Jolla, CA; Cat# 600548-51). The followings are the primer sequences used for LTR/RU5 (Forward primer 5′-TCTCTCTGGTTAGACCAGATCTG-3′ and Reverse primer 5′-ACTGCTAGAGATTTTCCACACTG-3′). Relative expression of mRNA species was calculated using the comparative C_T method [17]. All data were controlled for quantity of RNA input by performing measurements on an endogenous reference gene, β-actin. In addition, results obtained on RNA from treated samples were normalized to results obtained on RNA from the control, untreated sample. Results were expressed as transcript accumulation index (TAI) [17, 18]. This calculation assumes that all PCR reactions are taking place with 100% efficiency.

3. RESULTS

3.1. Characterization of the Nanoplexes

The physical properties of the nanoparticle formulations are usually established using the following techniques: (a) dynamic light scattering to estimate the hydrodynamic diameter and surface charge of the aqueous dispersed nanoparticles, (b) transmission electron microscopy (TEM) to determine particle size and size distribution, and (c) evaluation of the spectral properties of the fluorescent nanomaterials using simple spectrophotometry and spectrofluorimetry. Figure 1 shows the size-distribution of the QR-siRNA nanoplex via TEM and DLS measurements. TEM image (Figure 1(a)) shows the rods with average length and diameter of 15 nm. Figure 1(b) shows the absorption and emission spectra of the free siRNA and the siRNA bound to the QR with the QR emission wavelength around ~620 nm. Transmission electron microscopy (TEM) images of nanoplexes show that they remain as individual particles with a diameter of ~15–20 nm (Figure 1(a)). It can be visualized from the TEM that siRNA complexation did not cause any aggregation of the QRs. The concentration of these positively charged QRs was approximately 0.1 mg/mL and the optimal concentration of QR that was used to conjugate with the si510 HIV-1 siRNA to form a nanoplex was 200 pg.

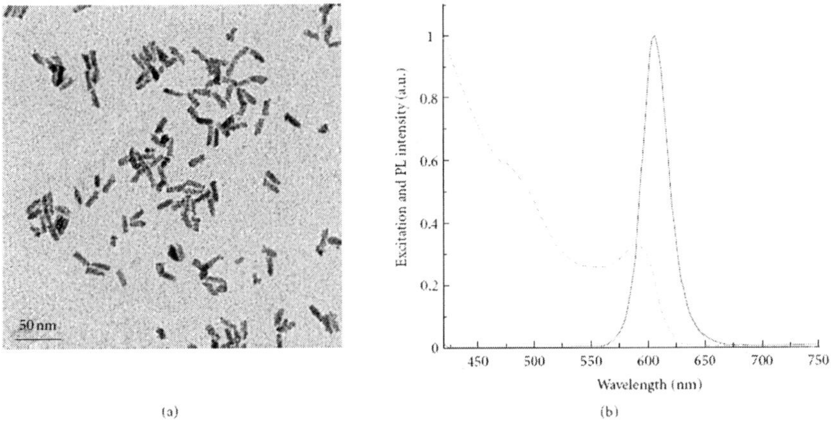

Figure 1. QR-si510 siRNA nanoplex characterization: Representative figures of (a) Transmission electron microscope image of nanoplexes showing that the average diameter of the nanoplex is ~15–20 nm (bar scale = 50 nm). No aggregation was observed after nanoplex formation. (b) Absorption (red line) and Emission spectra (green line) of QR-si510 siRNA nanoplexes.

3.2. Effect of the QR-si510 HIV-1siRNA Nanoplex on Cell Viability in THP-1 Cells

An MTT assay was done to evaluate the effect of the nanoplexes on cell viability of the THP-1 cells. Cell viability was also tested in the THP-1 cells prior to being infected by HIV-1 as well as after 7 days post infection and over 99% viability was observed in cells prior to be treated with the nanoplexes. THP-1 cell viability was measured after treatment with the nanoplexes at 12, 24, 96 hr, and upto 1 week posttransfection using the maximum dose (100 nM) of QR-si510 HIV-1 siRNA. Our results (Figure 2) show greater than 90% viability in THP-1 cells treated with QR-si510 HIV-1 siRNA nanoplexes and under all treatment conditions for up to 1 week. These results demonstrate that the QR-mediated delivery of siRNA did not produce any appreciable cytotoxicity in THP-1 cells.

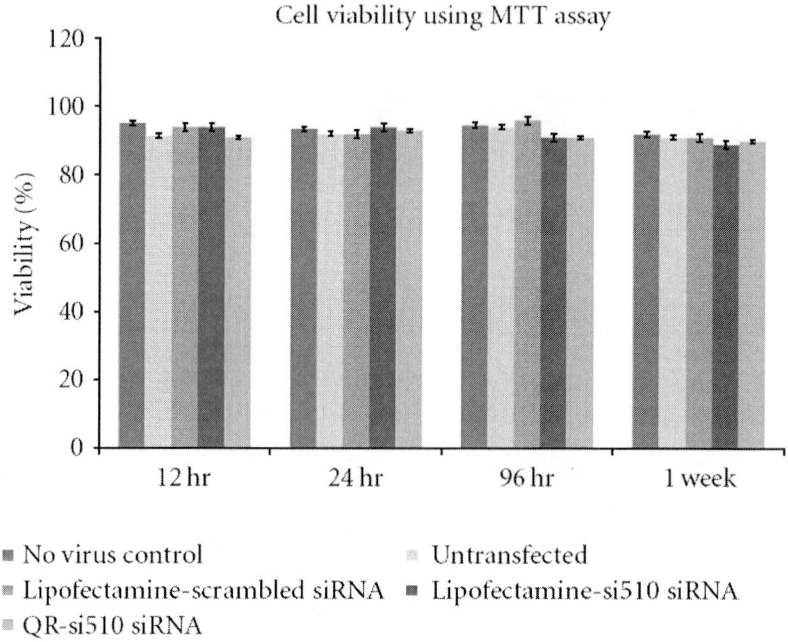

Figure 2. The time-dependent cytotoxicity of QR-si510 siRNA nanoplex on THP-1 cells using the MTT assay. Our results show absence of any toxicity in THP-1 monocytic cultures treated with lipofectamine transfected scrambled siRNA, Lipofectamine transfected si510 HIV-1 siRNA and the QR-si510 siRNA nanoplex as compared to the untransfected control over a 12 hr to 1 week time period. The concentration of both the scrambled siRNA and the si510 HIV-1 siRNA were 10 nM. Also included in the MTT assay were THP-1 cells not treated with the HIV-1 virus (no virus control). The results shown are mean ± SD of 3 separate experiments.

3.3. Effect of the QR-si510 HIV-1siRNA Nanoplex on HIV-1 Replication

The ultimate goal of our studies was to evaluate the nanoplex uptake by the THP-1 cells and examine the efficacy of the nanoplex in inhibiting HIV-1 viral replication by measuring the antiviral activity in the cells and culture supernatants. To determine the nanoplex uptake by the THP-1 and the dose and time kinetics of the nanoplex THP-1 cells were treated with various concentrations of the si510 HIV-1siRNA ranging from 5 nM to 100 nM over a range of time periods from 6 hr to 1 week posttransfection and the antiviral efficacy the nanoplexes was tested. At the end of the incubation period, the THP-1 cells and culture supernatants were harvested and the antiviral activity was measured using the p24 ELISA assay, as well as gene expression of HIV-1 LTR was quantitated in the RNA extracted from the THP-1 cells using real-time PCR.

The results of our dose response experiments (Figure 3) show a significant decrease in HIV-1 p24 production in HIV-1-infected THP-1 cells transfected with the QR-si510 HIV-1siRNA nanoplexes as compared to HIV-1-infected THP-1 cells transfected with a commercially available transfection reagent Lipofectamine (Invitrogen, Carlsbad, CA). No significant differences in p24 levels was observed when THP-1 cells were treated with different concentration of si510 HIV-1siRNA which ranged from 5 nM to 100 nM. Comparisons between the untransfected control and the QR-si510 HIV-1 siRNA nanoplex transfected THP-1 cells show a significant decrease in p24 production. The p24 levels in cells treated with 5, 10, 40, 80, and 100 nM concentrations of si510 HIV-1 siRNA were 159 ± 9.6 pg/mL, 111 ± 10.9 pg/mL, 102 ± 11.3 pg/mL, 89 ± 8.3 pg/mL and 91 ± 9.6 pg/mL, respectively, that corresponded to a 79.05% decrease (), 84.63% decrease (), 85.65% decrease (), 88.15% decrease () and 87.69% decrease () in viral replication as measured by p24 production. While the concentrations of the si510 HIV-1 siRNA varies from 5–100 nM, the QR concentration in the nanoplexes was constant and was 200 pg. In our time kinetics experiments we used the optimal 10 nM concentration of si510 HIV-1 siRNA. Comparisons between the untransfected control and the QR-si510 HIV-1 siRNA nanoplex transfected THP-1 cells at 12, 24, 48, 96 and 1 week posttransfection showed a significant decrease in p24 production as early as 12 hrs posttransfection (Figure 4). The p24 levels in THP-1 cells at 12, 24, 48, 96 hr, and 1 week posttransfection were 114 ± 10.5 pg/mL, 122 ± 11.2 pg/mL, 76 ± 9.4 pg/mL, 72 ± 8.7 pg/mL and 64 ± 6.3 pg/mL, respectively, and corresponded to a 85.33% decrease (), 83.93% decrease (), 90.04% decrease (), 89.79% decrease () and 91.00% decrease () in viral replication as measured by p24 production. The QR concentration in the nanoplex was 200 pg. The results of our time kinetics experiments show that 48 hrs posttransfection, a 90% suppression of viral replication was observed (Figure 3) and this suppression was observed even 1 week posttransfection. The 48 hr time point was determined to be the optimal time for transfection with the nanoplex, as a 90% decrease in p24 production was observed at that time point.

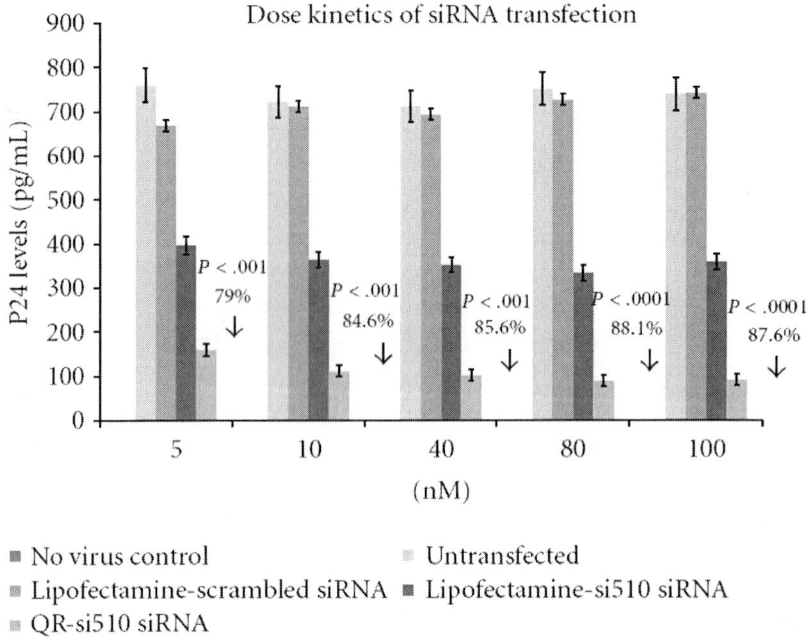

Figure 3: The dose-dependent kinetics of QR-si510 siRNA nanoplex on HIV-1-infected THP-1 cells. THP-1 monocytic cultures were treated with lipofectamine transfected scrambled siRNA (5–100 nM), Lipofectamine transfected si510 HIV-1 siRNA (5–100 nM) and the QR-si510 siRNA (5–100 nM) nanoplex for a 48 hr time period and the p24 production was measured in the supernatants at the end of the incubation period using a commercially available p24 ELISA kit. Untransfected HIV-1-infected THP-1 and the non-HIV-1-infected THP-1 cells (nonvirus control) were the experimental controls. The lipofectamine was used as per manufacturer's protocol. Our results show that 10 nM of the QR-si510 HIV-1siRNA nanoplex was optimal in achieving almost 85% suppression of viral replication. The results shown are mean ± SD of 3 separate experiments.

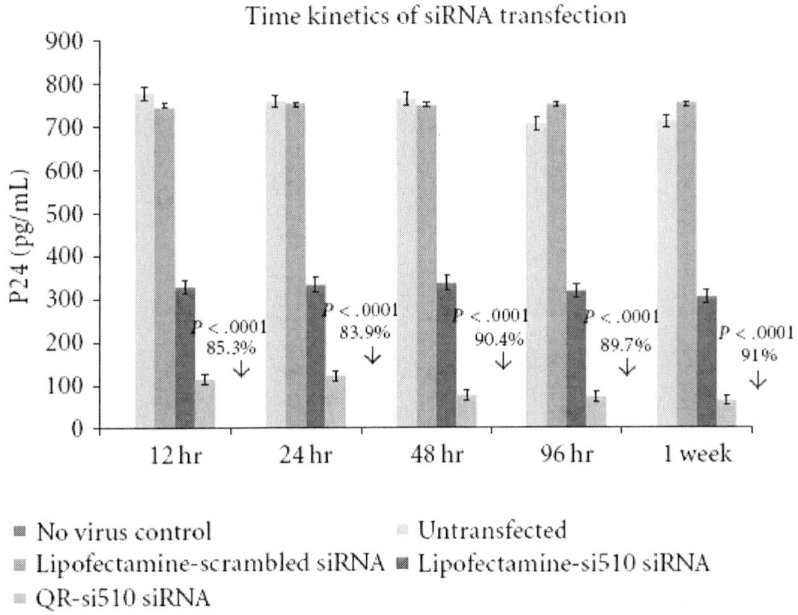

Figure 4. The dose-dependent kinetics of QR-si510 siRNA nanoplex on HIV-1-infected THP-1 cells. THP-1 monocytic cultures were treated with lipofectamine transfected scrambled siRNA (10 nM), Lipofectamine transfected si510 HIV-1 siRNA (10 nM) and the QR-si510 siRNA (10 nM) nanoplex for time period ranging from 12 hr to 1 week posttransfection. At the end of the incubation period, the p24 production was measured in the supernatants using a commercially available p24 ELISA kit. Untransfected HIV-1-infected THP-1 and the non-HIV-1-infected THP-1 cells (nonvirus control) were the experimental controls. The concentration of both the scrambled siRNA and the si510 HIV-1 siRNA were 10 nM and the lipofectamine was used as per manufacturer's protocol. Our results showed that 90% suppression of viral replication was observed 48 hr posttransfection and that further this suppression was observed even 1 week posttransfection. The results shown are mean ± SD of 3 separate experiments.

Additional experiments to determine changes in viral replication by measuring HIV-1 LTR gene expression using real-time PCR were done using 10 nM concentration of the QR-si510 HIV-1 siRNA nanoplex at various time points ranging from 12 hr to 1 week posttransfection. The

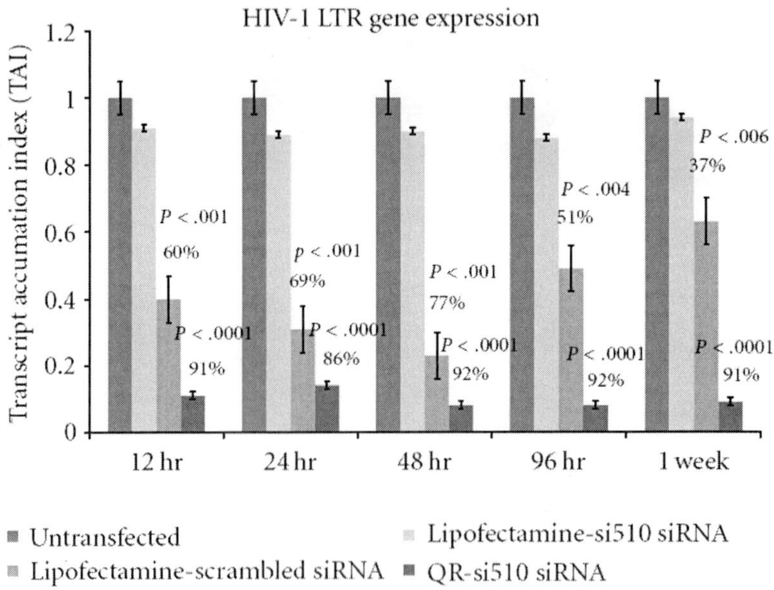

Figure 5. Effect of QR-si510 siRNA nanoplex on LTR/RU5 gene expression in HIV-1-infected THP-1 cells. THP-1 monocytic cultures were treated with lipofectamine transfected scrambled siRNA (10 nM), Lipofectamine transfected si510 HIV-1 siRNA (10 nM) and the QR-si510 siRNA (10 nM) nanoplex for time period ranging from 12 hr to 1 week posttransfection. At the end of the incubation period, RNA was extracted, reverse transcribed and the LTR/RU5 gene expression quantitated using Q-PCR. Our results show a significant decrease in HIV-1 LTR gene expression in HIV-1-infected THP-1 cells treated with the 10 nM QR-si510 HIV-1siRNA nanoplex at 12, 24, 48, 96 hr, and 1 week posttransfection as compared to the untransfected THP-1 cells and the scrambled control. The results shown are mean ± SD of 3 separate experiments done in duplicate.

results of our HIV-1 LTR gene expression studies show a significant decrease in HIV-1 LTR gene expression in THP-1 cells treated with the 10 nM QR-si510 HIV-1siRNA nanoplex at 12, 24, 48, 96 hr, and 1 week posttransfection as compared to the untransfected THP-1 cells and also the scrambled control. The percentage decrease in HIV-1 LTR gene expression was 91% (TAI = 0.11 ± 0.02 versus 0.91 ± 0.05, ()), 86% (TAI = 0.14 ± 0.06 versus 0.89 ± 0.03 ()), 92% (TAI = 0.08 ± 0.03 versus 0.90 ± 0.07 ()), 92% (TAI = 0.08 ± 0.05 versus 0.88 ± 0.03 ()), and 91% (TAI = 0.09 ± 0.04 versus 0.94 ± 0.08 ()) as compared to the scrambled control (Figure 5). The percentage decrease in HIV-1 LTR gene expression in THP-1 cells treated with the 10 nM of si510 HIV-1siRNA transfected with Lipofectamine at 12, 24, 48, 96 hr, and 1 week posttransfection were 60% (TAI = 0.40 ± 0.09 versus 0.91 ± 0.05, ()), 69% (TAI = 0.31 ± 0.07 versus 0.89 ± 0.03 ()), 77% (TAI = 0.23 ± 0.05 versus 0.90 ± 0.07 ()), 51% (TAI = 0.49 ± 0.11 versus 0.88 ± 0.03 ()), and 37% (TAI = 0.63 ± 0.06 versus 0.94 ± 0.08 ()), respectively, as compared to the scrambled control. These results confirm that the QR nanoparticles are a more effective than the commercially available transfection agent lipofectamine in not only delivering siRNA but also suppressing HIV-1 viral replication for a prolonged period of time.

3.4. Imaging of Nanoparticles

The cellular uptake of the QR-siRNA nanoplexes was studied using confocal microscopy. Figure 6(a) shows the confocal microscopic imaging and the local spectra of THP-1 cells treated with functional QR-si510 HIV-1siRNA nanoplexes. Confocal microscopy images were obtained with laser excitation at 405 nm. Figure 6(a)shows the representative local spectra obtained from different points in the confocal images from cells. The red labeling of THP-1 cells confirms the fluorescence signal is localized to the QR si510 HIV-1siRNA nanoplexes which is evident from the sharp emission spectra peaking around 625 nm. Additionally, it is important to note that the cellular autofluorescence which is normally located around 500 nm shows no interference with the emission from QRs. Our results show uptake of the QR-si510 HIV-1siRNA nanoplexes by the THP-1 cells at 12, 48, 96 hr, and 1 week posttransfection (Figure 6(b) (A)–(J)).

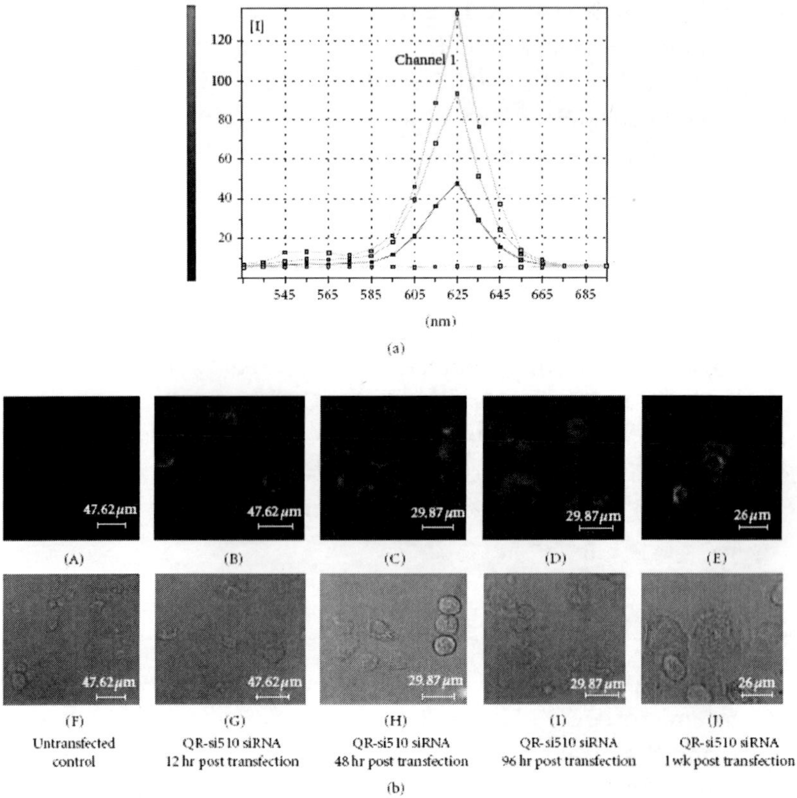

Figure 6. Confocal images of THP-1 cells treated QR-si510 siRNA nanoplexes: THP-1 cells were treated with QR-si510 siRNA nanoplexes for 12, 48, 96 hr, and up to 1 week and uptake of the nanoplexes was observed using confocal microscopy. (a) Representative local emission spectra confirms that the fluorescence signal in the THP-1 cells is localized to the QR si510 HIV-1siRNA nanoplexes, evident from the sharp emission spectra peak of 625 nm. (b) (A–J): Parallel Fluorescence and transmission images showing fluorescence (red) staining indicating QR-si510 siRNA nanoplex uptake by THP-1 cells.

3.5. Statistical Analysis

An Independent -test or one-way ANOVA was applied to compare changes between transfected and untransfected groups. Comparison among the means was performed with the post hoc Bonferroni analysis test using the PRISM statistical analysis software (GraphPad Software,

Inc. La Jolla, CA). The quantitative data are presented as mean ± SD unless specified otherwise. Statistical significance was considered at .

4. DISCUSSION

Developing strategies that treat HIV infection and eliminate persistent viral reservoirs are needed and gene therapy approaches such as RNA interference (RNAi) have emerged as a therapeutic possibility for the elimination of HIV-1 [19]. The RNAi pathway generates small interfering RNA (siRNA) from either long double stranded stretches of RNA or RNA hairpins, respectively, and this siRNA then guides an effector complex to a homologous sequence of mRNA and regulates suppression of gene expression. We choose an siRNA that targets the HIV-1 TAR element since the presence of TAR is important for activation of viral transcription by the HIV-1 Tat protein. Recently, Naito et al. did an exhaustive comprehensive computational analysis where they validated the functionality of several siRNA's that targeted multiple subtypes of HIV-1 and the highly conserved regions of the HIV-genome [7, 8]. They identified several highly effective siRNA's that have a potential to target >90% of HIV-1 strains, we choose an siRNA sequence from their list of highly effective siRNA's called si510 which targets the TAR/poly A region of the HIV-1 LTR.

The use of semiconductor nanocrystals (NCs) or so-called quantum dots (QDs)/quantum rods (QRs) as luminescence probes for numerous biological and biomedical applications has become an area of intense research over the last decade [9–11, 20]. QRs offer several advantages over organic dyes, including increased brightness, stability against photobleaching, broad absorption spectra, and a tunable and narrow emission spectrum [9, 10]. As a result, they have demonstrated the potential to dramatically outperform conventional organic dyes in imaging of cellular and subcellular structures and in a variety of bioassays [9, 10, 13, 20]. More importantly, the surface of the QRs can be easily functionalized to incorporate biologicals such as siRNAs, antibodies, peptides, and proteins [20]. Furthermore, the size of these nanobioconjugates under physiological condition are typically less than 50 nm, making these QR-based nanoparticles ideal candidates for in vitro and in vivo studies and applications [14, 15, 21].

In this investigation, we evaluate the specificity and efficiency of QRs as nonviral gene nanocarriers for the si510 HIV-1 siRNA that targets the TAR/poly A region of the HIV-1 LTR thereby suppressing HIV-1 viral replication. We validated the process of complexing the si510 HIV-1 siRNA to a quantum rod (QR) and examined the efficacy, the dose and time kinetics of this QR-si510 HIV-1 siRNA nanoplex in suppressing viral replication in the HIV-1-infected monocytic cell line THP-1.

Figure 1 showed the size-distribution of the QR-si510 HIV-1siRNA nanoplex via TEM and DLS measurements. Our TEM images of the nanoplexes show that the nanoplexes have a diameter of ~20 nm (Figure 1(a)) and that no aggregation of the QRs is observed demonstrating the colloidal stability of the nanoplex. The QR's we synthesized are positively charged and concentration of these positively charged QRs was approximately 0.1 mg/mL. The concentration of QR in the QR-si510 HIV-1 siRNA nanoplex was 200pg; however, the concentration of the siRNA within the nanoplex ranged from 5 nM to 100 nM. Our data suggest that as little as 10 nM quantity of the QR-si510 HIV-1siRNA nanoplex was optimal in achieving almost 85% suppression of viral replication (Figure 3).

The optimal amount of QR available for complexation with the siRNA was determined based on our previous studies using QR that were synthesized based on similar methodologies and had similar charged and concentration as determined by their Optical density (OD) measurements [14, 15, 21]. The results of our time kinetics experiments showed that 90% suppression of viral replication was observed 48 hr posttransfection and further this suppression was observed even 1 week posttransfection (Figure 4). Comparisons between lipofectamine and the QR's indicate that the QR's are superior to lipofectamine in not only delivering siRNA thereby suppressing HIV-1 viral replication as indicated by the significant decrease in p24 levels and by the significant decrease in HIV-1 LTR gene expression (Figure 5), but also that they are able to prolong the viral suppression for a extended period of time possibly due to the slow release of siRNA into the cells. Further, our imaging studies (Figure 6) show significant uptake of the QR-si510 HIV-1siRNA nanoplexes by the THP-1 and localization of these nanoplex within the cell was observed even 1 week posttransfection. Additionally, it is important to emphasize that no significant cell toxicity was observed when the THP-1 cells were treated with the nanoplexes and >95% viability was observed even 1 week posttreatment (Figure 2).

Gene therapy techniques such as siRNA possess great potential in HIV-1 therapeutics; however, they must overcome the key obstacle of reaching the interior of the HIV-1-infected cells. Nanoparticles have the potential to be a successful delivery vector for antiHIV-1 siRNA, anti-HIV drugs since these nanoparticles can be modified to improve the stability of the drug/genetic material in the biological environment; and have the capacity to mediate the biodistribution of active compounds; the ability to load, transport, target, and release their therapeutic payloads and can facilitate transport of these therapeutic payloads across the blood-brain barrier (BBB). Thus, the QR-si510 HIV-1 siRNA nanoplexes provide an advantage over current therapeutic options, with respect to delivery and release of genetic material to a specific cell. These studies indicate that the nanoplex consisting of QR-si510 HIV-1 siRNA is both safe and effective in suppressing viral replication, thus confirming that nanotechnology will play a significant role in future HIV-1 therapeutics.

ACKNOWLEDGMENTS

This study was supported by Grants from the National Institute of Health (RO1CA119397 (PNP); NIAID-RO1LM009726-01 (SAS), NIDA K01 DA024577 (JR), NIDA-1R21DA030108-01 (SM)), the John R. Oishei, and the Kaleida Health Foundations.

REFERENCES

1. L. B. Ludwig, “RNA silencing and HIV: a hypothesis for the etiology of the severe combined immunodeficiency induced by the virus,” Retrovirology, vol. 5, article 79, 2008.

2. R. M. Surabhi and R. B. Gaynor, “RNA interference directed against viral and cellular targets inhibits human immunodeficiency virus type 1 replication,” Journal of Virology, vol. 76, no. 24, pp. 12963–12973, 2002.

3. K. Ui-Tei, Y. Naito, and K. Saigo, “Essential notes regarding the design of functional siRNAs for efficient mammalian RNAi,” Journal of Biomedicine and Biotechnology, vol. 2006, Article ID 65052, 8 pages, 2006.

4. S. Bannwarth and A. Gatignol, "HIV-1 TAR RNA: the target of molecular interactions between the virus and its host," Current HIV Research, vol. 3, no. 1, pp. 61–71, 2005.

5. R. J. Pomerantz, "RNA interference meets HIV-1: will silence be golden?" Nature Medicine, vol. 8, no. 7, pp. 659–660, 2002.

6. S. Hwang, N. Tamilarasu, K. Ryan et al., "Inhibition of gene expression in human cells through small molecule-RNA interactions," Proceedings of the National Academy of Sciences of the United States of America, vol. 96, no. 23, pp. 12997–13002, 1999.

7. Y. Naito, K. Nohtomi, T. Onogi et al., "Optimal design and validation of antiviral siRNA for targeting HIV-1," Retrovirology, vol. 4, article 80, 2007.

8. Y. Naito, K. Ui-Tei, T. Nishikawa, Y. Takebe, and K. Saigo, "siVirus: web-based antiviral siRNA design software for highly divergent viral sequences," Nucleic Acids Research, vol. 34, pp. W448–W450, 2006.

9. P. N. Prasad, Introduction in Biophotonics, John Wiley & Sons, New York, NY, USA, 2003.

10. P. N. Prasad, Nanophotonics, John Wiley & Sons, New York, NY, USA, 2004.

11. J. Qian, K. T. Yong, I. Roy et al., "Imaging pancreatic cancer using surface-functionalized quantum dots,"Journal of Physical Chemistry B, vol. 111, no. 25, pp. 6969–6972, 2007.

12. J. Park, P. E. Nadeau, and A. Mergia, "Activity of TAR in inducible inhibition of HIV replication by foamy virus vector expressing siRNAs under the control of HIV LTR," Virus Research, vol. 140, no. 1-2, pp. 112–120, 2009.

13. K. T. Yong, J. Qian, I. Roy et al., "Quantum rod bioconjugates as targeted probes for confocal and two-photon fluorescence imaging of cancer cells," Nano Letters, vol. 7, no. 3, pp. 761–765, 2007.

14. G. Xu, K. T. Yong, I. Roy et al., "Bioconjugated quantum rods as targeted probes for efficient transmigration across an in vitro blood-brain barrier," Bioconjugate Chemistry, vol. 19, no. 6, pp. 1179–1185, 2008.

15. A. Bonoiu, S. D. Mahajan, L. Ye et al., "MMP-9 gene silencing by a quantum dot-siRNA nanoplex delivery to maintain the integrity of the blood brain barrier," Brain Research, vol. 1282, pp. 142–155, 2009.

16. P. Chomczynski and N. Sacchi, "Single-step method of RNA isolation by acid guanidinium thiocyanate-phenol-chloroform extraction," Analytical Biochemistry, vol. 162, no. 1, pp. 156–159, 1987.

17. S. A. Bustin, "Quantification of mRNA using real-time reverse transcription PCR (RT-PCR): trends and problems," Journal of Molecular Endocrinology, vol. 29, no. 1, pp. 23–39, 2002.

18. A. Radonić, S. Thulke, I. M. Mackay, O. Landt, W. Siegert, and A. Nitsche, "Guideline to reference gene selection for quantitative real-time PCR," Biochemical and Biophysical Research Communications, vol. 313, no. 4, pp. 856–862, 2004.

19. Y. Bennasser, M. L. Yeung, M. Benkirane, and K. T. Jeang, "RNA interference and HIV-1: hits and misses," Current Opinion in HIV and AIDS, vol. 1, no. 3, pp. 208–211, 2006.

20. X. Michalet, F. F. Pinaud, L. A. Bentolila et al., "Quantum dots for live cells, in vivo imaging, and diagnostics," Science, vol. 307, no. 5709, pp. 538–544, 2005.

21. S. D. Mahajan, I. Roy, G. Xu et al., "Enhancing the delivery of anti retroviral drug "saquinavir" across the blood brain barrier using nanoparticles," Current HIV Research, vol. 8, no. 5, pp. 396–404, 2010.

Chapter 2

Nanotherapeutics in Cancer Prevention, Diagnosis and Treatment

Samaya R Krishnan[1] and Suraj K George[2]

[1] Dept. of Cellular and Structural Biology, University of Texas Health Science Center at San Antonio, San Antonio, Texas, USA

[2] Dept. of Hematopathology, Division of Pathology and Laboratory Medicine, The University of Texas MD Anderson Cancer Center, Houston, Texas, USA

1. INTRODUCTION

Definitions of nanotechnology vary widely. Some scientists restrict the definition to work with molecules and devices between 1 and 100nm, while others widen these parameters to 1-1000nm. Kostoff believes that nanotechnology is best defined by the capacity to artificially construct and manipulate structures at nanoscale, and nanoscale's novel properties [1].

Drug loaded nanoparticles are widely utilized in the treatment of a number of diseases, such as metabolic disorders, autoimmune diseases, inflammatory disorders, neurodegenerative diseases and cancer. For instance, nanomedicines have been extremely useful in improving the efficacy of small molecule drug delivery across the blood-brain barrier for the treatment of CNS diseases [2]. In addition, nanoparticles serve as artificial oxygen carriers that can act as a substitute for blood, saving the lives of those in dire need of transfusion [3]. Although liposome-encapsulated formulations of Doxorubicin were being widely administered as early as the 1990's, nanotherapeutics is still viewed as a new and emerging field. The current chapter will focus on the progress made using nanoparticles in cancer prevention, diagnosis and treatment. This is certainly an area of rapid progression, with current nanotherapeutics for cancer encompassing a vast array of nanomaterials and nanodevices [4, 5]. But some critics believe that nanotechnology has not fulfilled its early promise and have expressed concern that progress and investment in the laboratory has not been mirrored by comparable progress or significant clinical success in cancer treatment [5, 6], a concern echoed in the title of Vendito and Szoka Jr's 2013 review: 'Cancer nanomedicines: So many papers and so few drugs!' [7]

However, much investment, research and development into nanotechnology diagnostics, therapies, devices, biosensors, and microfluidics continues to provide advances in the prevention, diagnosis and treatment of cancer [4]. Many scientists believe that nanoparticles are the future of diagnosis and drug delivery [8] with the potential to overcome many of the obstacles that cancer presents.

2. OBSTACLES IN CANCER DIAGNOSIS AND TREATMENT

2.1. Late Stage Diagnosis

Late detection and diagnosis of cancer remains one of the fundamental causes of low survival rates [9,10], so developing a test that detects clinically apparent cancer before symptoms appear is obviously an important goal [9]. The traditional biomedical imaging tools of magnetic resonance imaging, ultrasound and positron emission tomography have several limitations in the diagnosis of cancer, including an inadequate imaging period, a risk of renal toxicity and an inability to detect tumor cells smaller than 1cm [6, 11]. Improvements in PET, CT and MRI, through the use of small molecule imaging agents, such as 2-deoxy-2-(^{18}F) fluoro-D-glucose [FDG], iodinated small molecules and chelated gadolinium respectively, are routinely used in the diagnosis of cancer. However, poor stability, rapid clearance and low signal intensity have limited the use of these techniques and prompted more research into the use of nanoparticles as a diagnostic tool [12].

2.2. Challenges In Targeting, Transport And Delivery Of Treatment

Chemotherapy's perennial problem has always been that, due to challenges presented by its targeting, transport and delivery, a pharmacologically active concentration in tumor cells is often only achieved at the expense of what Couvrer terms 'massive contamination of the rest of the body' [13]. This toxicity can result in the use of suboptimal and/or intermittent dosing, to allow the body to rest, or in some cases to forgo chemotherapy altogether [14].

Many traditional chemotherapeutics have poor stability and aqueous solubility. Due to this limitation, many drugs, despite significant biological activity, are disregarded at early stages of drug screening in the laboratory. In addition, distribution of some drugs is too general, with only a small fraction of drugs reaching the cancer site; injected agents are often cleared by the monocytes and macrophages of the reticuloendothelial system (RES) [15]. To be successful, a therapeutically sufficient quantity of the drug, still in a viable state, must survive clearing and be delivered to different regions of tumors via blood vessels, cross the vessel wall and then finally penetrate through the interstitial space to reach the target [16], where unpredictable blood flow and often abnormal vasculature in tumors, particularly in necrotic and semi-necrotic regions, can make accurate delivery even more difficult [17, 18].

Other than conventional chemotherapeutic drugs, biological molecules, such as antibodies and nucleic acids, are being widely explored for the treatment of different diseases, including cancer. Nucleic acid drugs, such as aptamers, anti-sense DNA/RNA, and small-interfering RNA, have shown great promise in the treatment of cancer. However, these drugs are greatly limited by serum nucleases, opsonization and clearance by macrophages and clearance by the renal system. Some of the nucleic acid therapeutics, such as stable nucleic-acid–lipid particle (SNALP), have used nanocarriers to effectively overcome the above mentioned barriers and are being used in the treatment of cancer [19].

2.3. Chemoresistance

Chemoresistance, a major cause of cancer treatment failure, is linked to cancer stem cells (CSC). CSCs possess unique properties, such as quiescence, mesenchymal morphology, increased DNA repair ability, overexpression of antiapoptotic proteins, drug efflux transporters and detoxifying enzymes [20]. These properties, together with the favorable tumor microenvironment and hypoxic stability, mean that they often escape elimination by current radio and chemotherapies. Having survived through chemotherapy, they can give rise to metastases and recurrent tumors which then increase in malignancy and resistance [20].

Chemoresistance can be divided into two types: intrinsic and acquired. **Intrinsic chemoresistance** is displayed by tumor cells whose genetic and phenotypic characteristics make them ideally suited to withstand cytotoxic agents. **Acquired chemoresistance** can occur after prolonged exposure to chemotherapeutic agents, which disrupt only one of the many biochemical pathways involved in their pathogenesis. Unfortunately this approach often activates and strengthens the alternative pathways, resulting in chemo resistant mutations in the tumor cells and tumor relapse [18, 21, 22]. **Multidrug resistance, or MDR**, can also occur through a process of cross-resistance in which cancer cells mutate and acquire resistance to multiple structurally-related drugs and also to mechanistically different drugs, either via the over-expression of multidrug transporters or through altered apoptosis [21], resulting in decreased intracellular drug retention and altered tumor response [23].

2.4. The Patient — Compliance And Individuality

It may seem harsh to list the patient as an obstacle but, through no fault of their own, this is often the case. Genetic variation across individuals affects a drug's pharmacokinetics and pharmacodynamics [24], and a breakthrough with one patient cannot always be replicated in another. Also, each patient has different levels of tolerance to the discomfort and effects of chemotherapy, and in many cases a pre-existing condition or illness may complicate their cancer treatment or lead them to refuse it. Patients with comorbid illnesses and elderly patients are those most likely to forgo or discontinue chemotherapy [14].

3. CURRENT NANOTHERAPEUTICS: OVERCOMING THE OBSTACLES

3.1. More Accurate Detection And Diagnosis

Promising results have emerged from combining nanoparticle-based optical contrast agents with existing optical imaging technologies [9]. Their 'programmable' surface properties and potential for passive or active targeting make nanoparticles ideal for diagnostic imaging. The ability of nanoshells, constructed with a silica core and gold shell, to absorb specific wavelengths of light, has great potential for cancer imaging and therapeutic applications [4].

3.2. Quantum Dots

Semiconductor quantum dots are luminescent nanocrystals with great potential in both biological and biomedical applications [25]. Their photostability, fluorescence intensity, small size (2–10 nm) and tunable surfaces make them ideal for optical imaging and detecting hundreds of cancer biomarkers in blood assays or tissue biopsies at pg/mL concentrations [25]. The most commonly used agents in the quantum dots are selenides or sulfides of cadmium and zinc [12]. The wavelength of light emitted by the quantum dots depends on their size. The light emitted is much more intense and stable than their other fluorescent counterparts and hence very useful in optical imaging [12]. Cadmium selenide (CdSe), cadmium telluride (CdTe), indium phosphide (InP), and indium arsenide (InAs) are the most common quantum dot formulations used in biological applications [25]. The inorganic core is covered by an inorganic shell, which imparts greater photostability and increases the fluorescence properties of the core [26]. The surface of the shell is coated with another layer that enhances solubility and stability of quantum dots in the blood [26]. Often times, the surface coating is PEG as it has low toxicity and is biodegradable. A major limitation of quantum dots in imaging is a process called "Blinking". This is due to fluctuation of the quantum dots between the light emitting and non-emitting states. This limits the amount of signal obtained at a specific time [26].

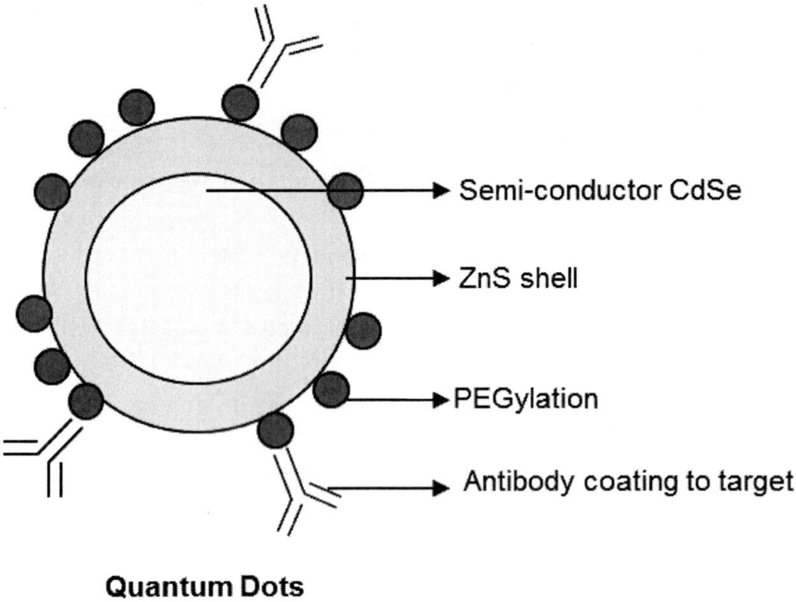

3.3. Magnetic Resonance Imaging

Recently, the development of nanoparticle systems to improve MRI for cancer imaging and diagnosis has made significant progress [8]. Magnetic nanoparticles usually consist of an inorganic nanoparticle core and a surface coating that provides stability in aqueous dispersions. This surface coating is manipulated to facilitate targeting, real-time monitoring or both [25]. Their success, particularly as contrast agents for MRI, is largely due to their enhanced proton relaxation and deep-tissue imaging capabilities, non-invasiveness and low toxicity [8, 25].

Supermagnetic iron oxide (SPIO) nanoparticles are now widely used as bowel contrast agents and have been used for some time in spleen/liver imaging. SPIO nanoparticles are readily taken up by macrophages present in the liver parenchyma (Kupffer cells) and, as liver tumors are usually devoid of macrophages, the macrophage-specific uptake of SPIOs increases the contrast between healthy and diseased tissue, allowing liver tumors or micro-metastases as small as 2–3 nm to be detected [25]. SPIO nanoparticles are biodegradable as the iron molecules released into the plasma upon degradation can bind hemoglobin. To avoid clearance of the SPIO nanoparticles, they are often coated with PEG, which enhances the circulation time during the imaging and treatment of prostate cancer. They are conjugated with an aptamer that binds with high specificity and affinity to a cell surface ligand on the prostate tumor cells. The aptamer binding to the cell surface antigen cause a localized increased accumulation of the SPIO that enables imaging. In addition, conjugation of doxorubicin to the SPIO nanoparticles allows the targeted delivery of the chemotherapeutic drug with minimal side effects [27].

3.4. Molecular Diagnostics

AuNPs (gold nanoparticles) have brought great benefits in this area, with increased sensitivity and specificity, multiplexing capability and short turnaround times. Aptamer-conjugated NPs can also be used for the collection and detection of multiple cancer cells [8, 28]. Gold nanoparticles scatter light intensely. Based on the size and shape of the gold nanoparticles, the scattering properties of the gold nanoparticles are also changed [29]. The light scattered by the gold nanoparticles have greater photostability than the other imaging agents commonly used [29]. Gold nanorods exhibit a phenomenon called the Surface Enhanced Raman Scattering (SERS), which is also used in cancer diagnosis. In addition, gold nanoshells and gold nanorods have been used to induce photothermal therapy [29]. This is an example for a "theragnostic" agent, as the gold nanorods not only assist in diagnosis of the cancer, but also help in ablation.

3.5. Improving Targeting, Transport And Delivery

Nanoparticles are increasingly utilized because of the multiple benefits that they offer [30]. Nanodelivery systems can make the use of chemotherapy drugs more safe and efficient by improving delivery, cell uptake and targeting, and have been shown to improve their pharmacokinetic profiles and enhance their targeting at the required site [21, 31]. This success relies on two main factors: 1] the EPR 2] The potential ability of nanodrug delivery systems to overcome the shortcomings of many anticancer drugs [20].

1. The EPR, or enhanced permeation retention effect, exists because of two properties of tumors. Firstly, tumor tissues have

increased vasculature which allows the entry of macromolecules and colloidal particles of diameter up to 600nm. Secondly, the lymphatic system is not effective in clearing the interstitial fluid from the tumor tissues [6]. Normal tissues other than the spleen, liver and kidney are impermeable to molecules that are larger than 2nm. Hence, nanoparticles can selectively target tumor tissues reducing toxic side effects [6]. Together, the enhanced permeation and retention properties of the tumor over the normal tissues cause the nanoparticle to have prolonged contact with the tumor cells. In addition, nanocarriers also release the drug slowly, ultimately resulting in reduced drug distribution and toxicity to normal tissues [6].

2. Once the nanoparticles reach the target tissue, cell surface receptors interact with ligand-coated nanoparticles leading to their uptake by endocytosis. Cellular uptake of uncoated nanoparticles is governed by their differences in size, shape and charge. It is suggested that positively charged nanoparticles are taken up more readily due to electrostatic attraction [32]. Interaction with specific serum proteins, results in the formation of a corona, promoting cell entry. Recent studies indicate that non-spherical molecules, such as rod-shaped structures, are internalized better than spherical structures [33]. Uptake of larger nanoparticles disrupts the membrane surface, thereby inducing cell death [34]. Non-specific uptake of the nanoparticles by the lung epithelial cells and red blood cells could cause toxic side effects.

3. Nanosized drug delivery systems can potentially overcome the shortcomings of many anticancer drugs, such as low aqueous solubility and stability and high nonspecific toxicity [20]. For example, paclitaxel nanoparticles stabilized with pluronic F68 are stable for years, while the same drug in dissolved form degrades completely in less than 48 hours [30, 35], and magnetic nanoparticles (MNPs) are increasingly used because their targeting ability reduces systemic distribution of cytotoxic compounds *in vivo* and enhances uptake at the target site, resulting in effective treatment at lower doses [8].

3.6. Nanodrug Delivery Systems

Nanodrug delivery can either use passive targeting mechanisms, such as the EPR effect, or active targeting mechanisms, using ligands directed against differentially overexpressed cell surface markers surface on tumor cells [20]. Drug encapsulation within nanoparticles can also enhance the bioavailability of drugs administered via routes other than intravenous; both insoluble and soluble drugs can be incorporated within nanoparticulate sols, extending their stability as they travel through the blood, which in turn improves their overall pharmacokinetic half-life [30].

By 'pre-programming' the degradation of nanoparticles in the body, prolonged drug release can be achieved, eliminating the need for repetitive dosages and enabling more sustained and consistent drug concentrations in the target area [30]. Brannon-Peppas and Blanchette have compared the uptake of nanoparticles with more hydrophobic surfaces with those of more hydrophilic surfaces. They concluded that a nanoparticle designed to be 100nm or less in diameter with a hydrophilic surface will have a longer circulation time and hence a greater ability to target the required site [17] due to reduced clearance by macrophages.

Nanodrug delivery systems can carry one or a combination of therapeutics, including cytotoxic agents, chemo sensitizers, small interference RNA (siRNA) and antiangiogenic agents [22]. The most commonly used platforms are described below.

Liposomes have been in use for the past several decades and are established as drug and imaging agent carriers with proven clinical efficacy [6]. They are artificial phospholipid vesicles 50 nm to ≥1 μm in size, either unilamellar or multilamellar (with one lipid layer or several, arranged in onion-like layers), with one or more aqueous compartments [6, 36]. The 'cargo' can be held in the aqueous compartment(s) or lipid layer [37]. Liposomal nanocarriers provide protection from degradation. Optimization of the pharmacokinetics of the encapsulated drug can improve drug accumulation in the tumor and reduce the adverse effects of bolus administration [37].

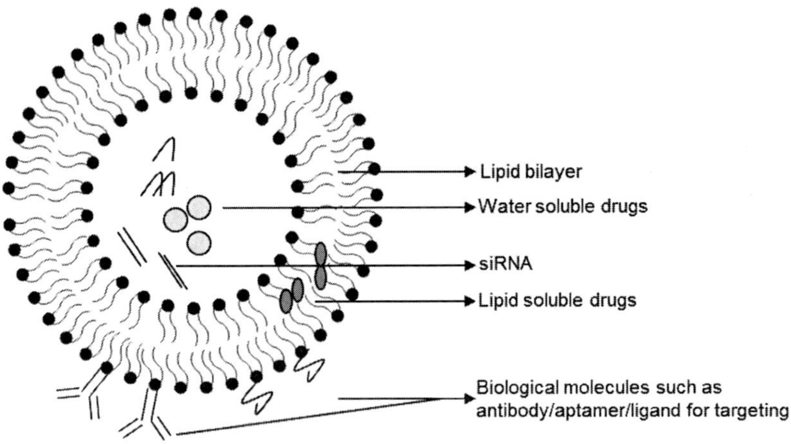

Liposome

Polymeric micelles consist of a hydrophobic core and a hydrophilic shell and are useful drug carriers, due to their tunable size and surface functions, high monodispersity and excellent stability. They have the ability to form hydrogels and are used for drug encapsulation or drug conjugation [38]. Under the right conditions, pluronics, the most well-known thermosensitive polymers, form a hydrogel at body temperature but are water soluble at 2-4°C. This allows them to be injected as a liquid but they form a hydrogel *in situ*, resulting in prolonged drug release of the encapsulated drug [36].

Dendrimers are globular macromolecular compounds consisting of an inner core, which can be manipulated to alter its shape and size, surrounded by a series of branches with surface functional groups. They can carry a multiple payload of active targeting molecule, diagnostic agent and therapeutic drug, and those with a hydrophobic core and hydrophilic surface groups can form micelles, which can then be designed for site-specific release of their payload, via pH and enzyme dependent mechanisms [39, 40].

Inorganic nanoparticles, such as gold nanoparticles, can be used as a cargo for drug delivery. Gold has a number of appealing surface properties, such as light scattering, which makes them attractive inorganic biomaterials for drug delivery when combined with nanoparticles. Due to their ease of synthesis, biocompatibility, and affluent functionalization, many drugs can be conjugated to the surface of gold through hydrophobic interactions. Gold–thiol conjugates are the most common due to their accurate and predictive functionalization. Various antibiotics, anticancer agents and oligonucleotides are also conjugated with gold nanoparticles to yield more viable drug delivery agents. Other inorganic nanoparticles that are frequently used in drug delivery and diagnostics include silica and iron oxide, which forms the core constituent of many inorganic nanoparticles [41].

Porous silica based nanoparticles are highly suitable for carrying hydrophobic drugs. These nanoparticles have a high surface-to-volume ratio and consists of large pores. The drug can be loaded on the nanoparticles by physical adsorption and covalent linkage [42]. Nanostructured mesoporous silicon (PSi), fabricated by electrochemical etching, have nanometer range pores that facilitate high drug loading capabilities, irrespective of different surface chemistries.

3.7. Nanoparticles As Therapeutic Agents

Nanoparticles can be used as a therapeutic agent themselves. Their ability to alter the substrate molecule, through a process called "intercrossing" upon excitation by light, is used to treat cancer cells in the photodynamic therapy. While in the photothermal therapy, the property of small inorganic molecules to generate heat upon excitation is taken advantage of in the inducing apoptosis or necrosis of cells.

3.7.1. Photothermal Therapy

Photothermal therapy (PTT) uses sensitizers that can absorb light in the near-infrared region and convert it to thermal energy, causing heat in the vicinity. The sensitizer used in PTT is usually inorganic molecules, such as gold or carbon nanoparticles. Thermal ablation therapy has been used in the treatment of cancer for many decades, but the damage to nearby tissues has limited the use of this technique in the treatment of cancer [43]. However, with the advent of photodynamic therapy (PDT), targeted destruction of the tumor cell has become possible. PEGylation and active targeting of Au nanotubes have been used in the treatment of many cancers [44].

3.7.2. Photodynamic Therapy

Photodynamic therapy (PDT) uses photosensitizers in the treatment of cancer or other disorders. Photosensitizers are molecules that can be excited by light, which then alters molecules in the vicinity, causing the release of singlet oxygen species (reactive oxygen species). ROS are capable of causing oxidative stress to the surrounding cells, causing apoptosis or necrosis [12]. Photosensitizers can be excited using lasers over a wide range of visible wavelengths. Because of the limited penetrability of visible light, photosensitizers can be used to treat only superficial tumors, such as skin, lung, esophagus, prostate, head and neck, colon and rectum to mention a few. Because the half-life of the reactive oxygen species is only a few milliseconds, this therapy can be used to cause targeted cell death in regions where the photosensitizer has accumulated. Photosensitizers can be coated with polyethylene glycol to prevent renal clearance and to enhance the circulation time in the blood. Further antibody conjugation to the surface can target the photosensitizer to the cancer cells that overexpress the antigen on the surface.

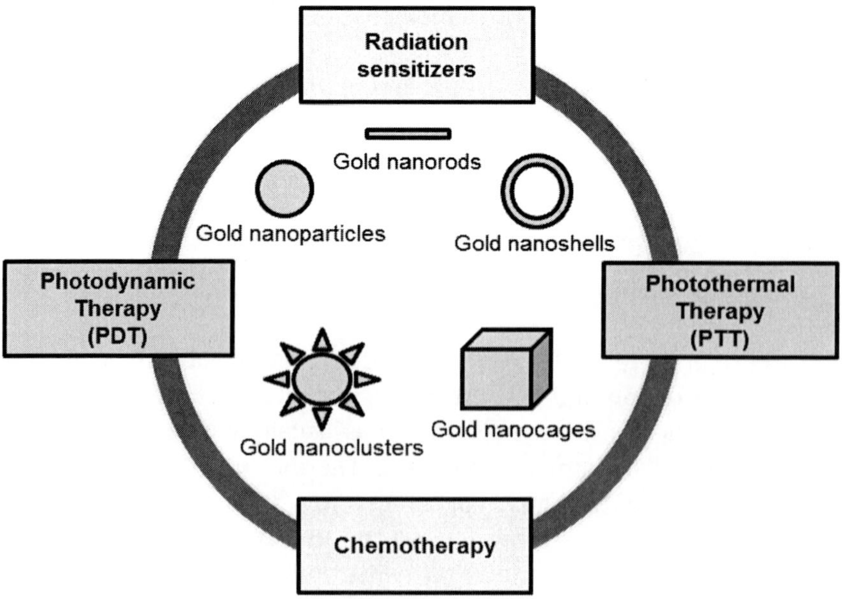

Combinational phototherapy

3.8. Overcoming Resistance

Nanovehicles carrying therapeutic drug combinations that not only target the tumor cells selectively, but also overcome the mechanisms of drug resistance are the focus of intensive research. This method has been proved especially effective in circumventing multidrug resistance (MDR) in multiple cancer models [21, 36]. MDR was reversed in *in vitro* and *in vivo* cancer models through the co-delivery of combinations of chemo sensitizing agents and chemotherapeutic agents [22].

3.9. Improving Therapy

Nanoshells are nanoparticle beads with a thin gold outer shell and a central silica core. By manipulating the thickness of the shell and core, the beads can be tuned to absorb and scatter specific wavelengths of light across the visible and near-infrared (NIR) spectrum, which is very useful in enhancing imaging properties [4].

Arguably, however, this ability to absorb light is most usefully exploited in thermal ablation therapy. For maximum efficacy, nanoshells with a silica core diameter of ~120 nm and a 10-nm gold shell are used in this therapy as they strongly absorb NIR light (~800 nm) and can then create intense heat that is fatal to cells [4]. As tissue chromophores do not absorb much energy in the NIR range, NIR light can penetrate several centimeters of human tissue without causing harm [4].

3.10. Improving Cancer Prevention

The complete prevention of cancer occurrence, claims Siddiqui et al, as an unachievable goal; cancer prevention describes 'slowing the process of carcinogenesis' and inhibiting its reoccurrence [45]. Inefficient systemic delivery and bioavailability of chemopreventive agents has so far limited their applicability to human medicine. However, Siddiqui et al have experimented with encapsulating a chemopreventive agent, epigallocatechin-3-gallate (EGCG), in polylactic acid [46] and polyethylene glycol (PEG) nanoparticles [45]. Nano-EGCG had a significantly longer half-life and had more than a 10-fold dose advantage over nonencapsulated EGCG in cell growth inhibition, proapoptotic, and angiogenic inhibitory effects. Curcumin derived from turmeric, when conjugated with polymeric amphiphile, mPEG-PA or PEG, has been shown to have more significant antiproliferative effects than the free curcumin [47, 48]. Another nanoparticle-based formulation, called solid lipid nanoparticles (SLN), is also being used as newer therapeutic modality to address the area of chemoprevention. The advantage is that they act like colloidal carriers which remain as solids at room and body temperature, and so can be efficiently used as alternatives to liposomes and other polymeric nanoparticles [36]. A multitude of approaches utilizing nanoparticles to combat these existing deficits in the chemopreventive strategies will re-captivate the 'silver bullet' for chemoprevention in the near future.

3.11. Improving Compliance

Nanotherapeutics can be less invasive than conventional diagnosis and treatment methods. This leads to shorter recovery times and a decreased risk of infection, and these advantages in turn should lead to a reduction in cost and improved life expectancy and quality [49].

4. THE FUTURE: POTENTIAL RISKS, REWARDS AND RESEARCH

4.1. New Risks: The Voice Of Caution

With its obvious potential for breakthroughs in so many fields, it is easy to view nanotechnology as an exclusively positive concept. However, it is not without risk and nanomaterials may present greater risks than their larger counterparts, as their greater relative surface and unique quantum effects mean they have a tendency to be more active and reactive [50]. Their potential to cause harm is harder to predict, as it is determined using factors such as surface area, rather than molecular structure, which is used to risk assess most other chemical hazards, and there are no proven toxicity screening methods to evaluate them. The scarcity of information about how nanomaterials may impact safety, health and the environment, along with the growing number and diversity of nanotechnologies and their associated engineered properties, has raised serious concerns. If nanomaterials escape the laboratory or manufacturing site, their degradation and interaction with substances in the environment would be unpredictable and potentially hazardous [30, 51].

When assessing the risk to patients, it is important to bear in mind that preclinical trials of nanodrugs may be less indicative of human risks than trials of standard medicines, and that nanomaterials can utilize unique mechanisms and routes of exposure, potentially bypassing the blood-brain barrier [25]. If inhaled, they may aggregate in the alveoli, where their increased surface area places a burden on mucociliary and macrophage clearance [52].

Like any other emerging area of interest in human health, nanotechnology also has its own demerits. A word of caution is that this research is still in its infancy to determine the unforeseen side effects pertaining to nanoparticle related therapies [53]. Although our understanding on the concepts regarding nanotherapeutics has come a long way, the exact nature of nanoparticulate drug interactions has not been tested vigorously. Studies in animals suggest alarming facts affecting the brain function [54-56]. With the limited current literature in humans, it is almost impossible to judge their safety over efficacy. Hence, until a stringent risk assessment strategy is employed, nanotherapeutics should not be viewed exclusively as a positive concept. It is important that, if nanotechnology is to move forward safely and sustainably, a thorough assessment of the biocompatibility and toxicity of nanoparticles is undertaken, with potential toxicities identified and their underlying mechanisms understood [57]. Research into the avoidance of health risks associated with nanotechnology may potentially be used to guide therapy, and vice versa [58].

5. NEW REWARDS: A BRIGHT FUTURE

5.1. Multifunction Nanovehicles

Advances in MRI contrasting agents promise a next generation of agents consisting of a core and coating conjugated to tumor-specific moieties for improved efficacy and tumor targeting [25]. Perche and Torchillin have suggested that a possible direction for research may be the coupling of ligands of different natures (antibodies, proteins, peptides and chemokines, hormone analogs) to target at least two tumor cell populations, providing more sensitive malignant lesion detection and reducing relapses [24, 37]

Shapira looks forward to the development of 'theragnostic' nanovehicles that carry four major components: a selective targeting moiety, a diagnostic imaging aid for localization of the malignant tumor and its metastases, a cytotoxic small molecule drug(s) or innovative therapeutic biological matter, and a chemosensitizing agent to neutralize drug resistance – the advent of "quadrugnostic" nanomedicine [59].

5.2. New Detection Methods And Diagnostic Devices

Nanoparticle probes, nanocantilever, nanowire and nanotube arrays are the subject of intensive research and are expected to solve the problem of early detection in the future [9]. Accurate localization of tumors and their metastases, *via* nanoparticles loaded with a diagnostic aid, could in future facilitate the harnessing of other therapies, such as radiotherapy, photodynamic therapy and surgery [59].

Heller group has described the goal of research as 'the development of a cancer therapy monitoring/diagnostic platform device'. This would provide real-time monitoring of patient blood for cancer cells, cell derived nanoparticulates (such as high molecular weight DNA fragments), and carry out cancer-related genotyping, gene expression and immunochemical analysis [60].

5.3. New Applications, New Targets

Superparamagnetic iron oxide nanoparticles (crystalline magnetite structures coated with dextran and dextran derivatives) are promising candidates for a number of applications, including magnetic resonance imaging and drug delivery [6]. Bharali and Mousa believe that a major potential application of these nanoparticles is the diagnosis and treatment of central nervous system (CNS) tumors, particularly if USPIOs (ultrasmall supermagnetic iron oxide particles) are used, as they can be utilized as intravascular contrast agents, as well as for cellular imaging [25] One USPIO already showing great promise is Combidex, which has been undergoing clinical trials for the detection of lymph node metastases [25].

Talekar et al predict that multifunctional superparamagnetic nanocarriers, with FR (folate receptor) targeting and pH mediated drug release, can be developed to achieve a decrease in tumor volume, as well as improved MRI sensitivity and decreased adverse effects [6]. Metal coordination complexes also offer a diversity of formulations and the prospect of mechanisms that differ from those of organic drugs, including ligand substitution and metal-and ligand-centered redox properties [31].

Therapeutic and imaging nanoparticles have normally used passive targeting to date, but active targeting needs to be used and further developed if drugs are to be delivered to specific classes of cells and specific intracellular sites in cancer cells [31].

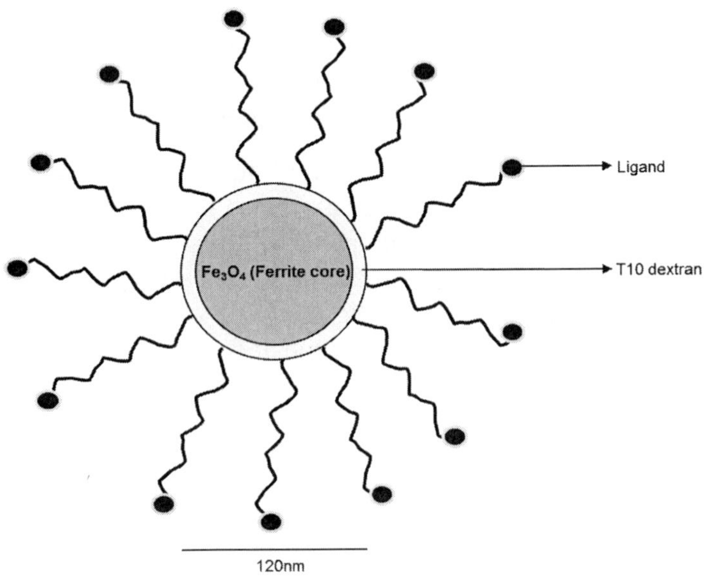

Superparamagnetic Iron oxide (Ferumoxtran-10)

5.4. Reducing The Side Effects

Nanoparticle encapsulation has already been shown to reduce unwanted accumulation of platinum in the kidneys from the platinum [59] prodrug mitaplatin, and reports show that metallodrugs loaded in nanoparticles cause less damage than the drugs on their own. So these formulations are predicted to be in line for further research and exploitation in the near future [31].

6. BENCH TO BEDSIDE: TRANSLATIONAL PERSPECTIVES

Nanotechnology has raised as many questions as it has answered, and spawned new and unpredicted fields [61]. With its vast array of potential applications in so many fields of science and industry, it is a prime candidate for multidisciplinary collaboration, and the urgent need to see laboratory breakthroughs translated to clinical successes is increasingly recognized. Biochemists are increasingly working with scientists from fields not usually associated with medicine, and the NIH's Nanomedicine Development Centers are staffed by multidisciplinary research teams, including biologists, physicians, mathematicians, engineers, and computer scientists, whose first task has been to research the chemical and physical properties of nanoscale biological structures [58]. Baseline work of this sort is vital if clinicians are to have the knowledge to develop new therapies.

Murday et al claim that translational research has been 'a powerful process that drives the clinical research engine', but feel that a stronger research infrastructure is needed in future to 'strengthen and accelerate this critical part of the clinical research enterprise [58]. Kawasaki and Player agree that scientists from all fields must make a strenuous effort to integrate and coordinate the research in an approach that might now be described as 'systems biology'. They hold up the 2004 article 'Electronic structure and bonding of Au on a SiO2 cluster: a nanobullet for tumors' [46], produced by physicists, as a prime example of how research in other fields can advance nanomedicine [46, 62].

7. CONCLUSIONS

Nanotherapeutics have already yielded significant breakthroughs in the detection, diagnosis and treatment of cancer, and appear to have the potential to yield many more, with extensive and focused routes of research planned for the future and the possibility of nanotechnology-based cancer prevention. But it is clear that nanotechnology must be thoroughly understood and its risks assessed if it is to be developed safely, and that the expertise of researchers in many fields needs to be brought together to move new discoveries out of the laboratory and into the clinical environment where patients can reap the benefits.

REFERENCES

1. Kostoff RN, Koytcheff, Raymond G. Lau, Clifford G.Y. Global Nanotechnology Research Literature Overview, Technological Forecasting and Social Change. 2007; 74(9): 1733-47.

2. Nazem A, Mansoori GA. Nanotechnology Solutions for Alzheimer's Disease: Advances in Research Tools, Diagnostic Methods and Therapeutic Agents. Journal of Alzheimer's Disease: JAD. 2008; 13(2): 199-223.

3. Piras AM, Dessy A, Chiellini F, Chiellini E, Farina C, Ramelli M, et al. Polymeric Nanoparticles for Hemoglobin-based Oxygen Carriers. Biochimica et biophysica acta. 2008; 1784(10): 1454-61.

4. Kim KY. Nanotechnology Platforms and Physiological Challenges for Cancer Therapeutics. Nanomedicine: Nanotechnology, Biology, and Medicine. 2007; 3(2): 103-10.

5. Ferrari M. Cancer Nanotechnology: Opportunities and Challenges. Nature Reviews Cancer. 2005; 5(3): 161-71.

6. Talekar M, Kendall J, Denny W, Garg S. Targeting of Nanoparticles in Cancer: Drug Delivery and Diagnostics. Anti-Cancer Drugs. 2011; 22(10): 949-62.

7. Venditto VJ, Szoka FC, Jr. Cancer Nanomedicines: So Many Papers and So Few Drugs! Advanced Drug Delivery Reviews. 2013; 65(1): 80-8.

8. Parveen S, Misra R, Sahoo SK. Nanoparticles: A Boon to Drug Delivery, Therapeutics, Diagnostics and Imaging. Nanomedicine: Nanotechnology, Biology, and Medicine. 2012; 8(2): 147-66.

9. Jabir NR, Tabrez S, Ashraf GM, Shakil S, Damanhouri GA, Kamal MA. Nanotechnology-based Approaches in Anticancer Research. International Journal of Nanomedicine. 2012; 7: 4391-408.

10. Siegel R, Naishadham D, Jemal A. Cancer Statistics, 2013. CA: A Cancer Journal for Clinicians. 2013; 63(1): 11-30.

11. Jain RK. Transport of Molecules in the Tumor Interstitium: A Review. Cancer Research. 1987; 47(12): 3039-51.

12. Thakor AS, Gambhir SS. Nanooncology: The Future of Cancer Diagnosis and Therapy. CA: A Cancer Journal for Clinicians. 2013.

13. Couvrer P R-TL, Poupon MF, Brasseur F, Puisieux F. Nanoparticles as Microcarriers for Anticancer Drugs 1990.

14. Kane B. Cancer Chemotherapy: Teaching Old Drugs New Tricks. Annals of Internal Medicine. 2001; 135(12): 1107-10.

15. Blanco E, Hsiao A, Mann AP, Landry MG, Meric-Bernstam F, Ferrari M. Nanomedicine in Cancer Therapy: Innovative Trends and Prospects. Cancer Science. 2011; 102(7): 1247-52.

16. Jain RK, Stylianopoulos T. Delivering Nanomedicine to Solid Tumors. Nature Reviews Clinical Oncology. 2010; 7(11): 653-64.

17. Brannon-Peppas L, Blanchette JO. Nanoparticle and Targeted Systems for Cancer Therapy. Advanced Drug Delivery Reviews. 2004; 56(11): 1649-59.

18. Cao Y, Wang B, Lou D, Wang Y, Hao S, Zhang L. Nanoscale Delivery Systems for Multiple Drug Combinations in Cancer. Future Oncology (London, England). 2011; 7(11): 1347-57.

19. Alabi C, Vegas A, Anderson D. Attacking the Genome: Emerging siRNA Nanocarriers from Concept to Clinic. Current Opinion in Pharmacology. 2012; 12(4): 427-33.

20. Vinogradov S, Wei X. Cancer Stem Cells and Drug Resistance: the Potential of Nanomedicine. Nanomedicine (London, England). 2012; 7(4): 597-615.

21. Ayers D, Nasti A. Utilisation of Nanoparticle Technology in Cancer Chemoresistance. Journal of Drug Delivery. 2012; 2012: 265691.

22. Hu CM, Zhang L. Nanoparticle-based Combination Therapy Toward Overcoming Drug Resistance in Cancer. Biochemical Pharmacology. 2012; 83(8): 1104-11.

23. Chen ZG. Small-molecule Delivery by Nanoparticles for Anticancer Therapy. Trends in Molecular Medicine. 2010; 16(12): 594-602.

24. Wheeler HE, Maitland ML, Dolan ME, Cox NJ, Ratain MJ. Cancer Pharmacogenomics: Strategies and Challenges. Nature Reviews Genetics. 2013; 14(1): 23-34.

25. Bharali DJ, Mousa SA. Emerging Nanomedicines for Early Cancer Detection and Improved Treatment: Current Perspective and Future Promise, Pharmacology & Therapeutics. 2010; 128(2): 324-35.

26. Madani SY, Shabani F, Dwek MV, Seifalian AM. Conjugation of Quantum Dots on Carbon Nanotubes for Medical Diagnosis and Treatment. International Journal of Nanomedicine. 2013; 8: 941-50.

27. Wang AZ, Bagalkot V, Vasilliou CC, Gu F, Alexis F, Zhang L, et al. Superparamagnetic Iron Oxide Nanoparticle-aptamer Bioconjugates for Combined Prostate Cancer Imaging and Therapy. ChemMedChem. 2008; 3(9): 1311-5.

28. Smith JE, Medley CD, Tang Z, Shangguan D, Lofton C, Tan W. Aptamer-Conjugated Nanoparticles for the Collection and Detection of Multiple Cancer Cells. Analytical Chemistry. 2007; 79(8): 3075-82.

29. Huang X, Jain PK, El-Sayed IH, El-Sayed MA. Gold Nanoparticles: Interesting Optical Properties and Recent Applications in Cancer Diagnostics and Therapy. Nanomedicine (London, England). 2007; 2(5): 681-93.

30. V U. Challenges for the Modern Science in its Descent Towards Nano Scale. Current Nanoscience. 2009; 5: 372-89.

31. Barry NP, Sadler PJ. Challenges for Metals in Medicine: How Nanotechnology May Help to Shape the Future. ACS nano. 2013; 7(7): 5654-9.

32. Thorek DL, Tsourkas A. Size, Charge and Concentration Dependent Uptake of Iron Oxide Particles by Non-phagocytic Cells. Biomaterials. 2008; 29(26): 3583-90.

33. Gratton SE, Ropp PA, Pohlhaus PD, Luft JC, Madden VJ, Napier ME, et al. The effect of Particle Design on Cellular Internalization Pathways. Proceedings of the National Academy of Sciences of the United States of America. 2008; 105(33): 11613-8.

34. Albanese A TP, Chan WC. The Effect of Nanoparticle Size, Shape, and Surface Chemistry on Biological Systems. Annu Rev Biomed Eng. 2012; 14: 1-16.

35. Oh KS SJ, Cho SH, Lee BS, Kim SY, Kim K, Jeon H, Kwon IC, Yuk SH. Paclitaxel-loaded Pluronic Nanoparticles Formed by a Temperature-induced Phase Transition for Cancer Therapy. J Control Release. 2010; 148(3): 344-50.

36. Mattheolabakis G, Rigas B, Constantinides PP. Nanodelivery Strategies in Cancer Chemotherapy: Biological Rationale and Pharmaceutical Perspectives. Nanomedicine (London, England). 2012; 7(10): 1577-90.

37. Perche F, Torchilin VP. Recent trends in Multifunctional Liposomal Nanocarriers for Enhanced Tumor Targeting. Journal of Drug Delivery. 2013; 2013: 705265.

38. Lim E-KJ, E.; Lee, K.; Haam, S.; Huh, Y.-M. Delivery of Cancer Therapeutics Using Nanotechnology. Pharmaceutics. 2013; 5: 294-317.

39. Alexis F, Rhee JW, Richie JP, Radovic-Moreno AF, Langer R, Farokhzad OC. New Frontiers in Nanotechnology for Cancer Treatment. Urologic Oncology. 2008; 26(1): 74-85.

40. Misra R, Acharya S, Sahoo SK. Cancer Nanotechnology: Application of Nanotechnology in Cancer Therapy. Drug Discovery Today. 2010; 15(19-20): 842-50.

41. Liong M, Lu J, Kovochich M, Xia T, Ruehm SG, Nel AE, et al. Multifunctional Inorganic Nanoparticles for Imaging, Targeting, and Drug Delivery. ACS nano. 2008;2(5):889-96.

42. Shahbazi MA HB, Santos HA. Nanostructured Porous Si-based Nanoparticles for Targeted Drug Delivery. Biomatter. 2012; 2(4): 296-312.

43. Huang X, Jain PK, El-Sayed IH, El-Sayed MA. Plasmonic Photothermal Therapy (PPTT) Using Gold Nanoparticles. Lasers in Medical Science. 2008; 23(3): 217-28.

44. Huang X, Jain PK, El-Sayed IH, El-Sayed MA. Determination of the Minimum Temperature Required for Selective Photothermal Destruction of Cancer Cells with the Use of Immunotargeted Gold Nanoparticles. Photochemistry and Photobiology. 2006; 82(2): 412-7.

45. Siddiqui IA, Adhami VM, Ahmad N, Mukhtar H. Nanochemoprevention: Sustained Release of Bioactive Food Components for Cancer Prevention. Nutrition and Cancer. 2010; 62(7): 883-90.

46. Kawasaki ES, Player A. Nanotechnology, Nanomedicine, and the Development of New, Effective Therapies for Cancer. Nanomedicine: Nanotechnology, Biology, and Medicine. 2005; 1(2): 101-9.

47. Li J, Wang Y, Yang C, Wang P, Oelschlager DK, Zheng Y, et al. Polyethylene Glycosylated Curcumin Conjugate Inhibits Pancreatic Cancer Cell Growth Through Inactivation of Jab1. Molecular Pharmacology. 2009; 76(1): 81-90.

48. Sahu A, Bora U, Kasoju N, Goswami P. Synthesis of Novel Biodegradable and Self-Assembling Methoxy Poly(ethylene glycol)-palmitate Nanocarrier for Curcumin Delivery to Cancer Cells. Acta Biomaterialia. 2008; 4(6): 1752-61.

49. Cheng Z AZA, Hui JZ, Muzykantov VR, Tsourkas A. Multifunctional Nanoparticles: Cost Versus Benefit of Adding Targeting and Imaging Capabilities. Science. 2012; 338(6109): 903-10.

50. Marchant GE, Lindor RA. Prudent Precaution in Clinical Trials of Nanomedicines. The Journal of Law, Medicine & Ethics: A Journal of the American Society of Law, Medicine & Ethics. 2012; 40(4): 831-40.

51. De Jong WH BP. Drug Delivery and Nanoparticles: Applications and Hazards. International Journal of Nanomedicine. 2008; 3(2): 133-49.

52. Shi H MR, Castranova V, Zhao J. Titanium Dioxide Nanoparticles: A Review of Current Toxicological Data. Part Fibre Toxicol. 2013.

53. Rose-James A, Sreelekha TT, George SK. Nanostrategies in the War against Multidrug Resistance in Leukemia. OncoDrugs. 2013;1 (1): p. 3e-9e.

54. Elder A, Gelein R, Silva V, Feikert T, Opanashuk L, Carter J, et al. Translocation of Inhaled Ultrafine Manganese Oxide Particles to the Central Nervous System. Environmental Health Perspectives. 2006; 114(8): 1172-8.

55. Ma L, Liu J, Li N, Wang J, Duan Y, Yan J, et al. Oxidative Stress in the Brain of Mice Caused by Translocated Nanoparticulate TiO2 Delivered to the Abdominal Cavity. Biomaterials. 2010; 31(1): 99-105.

56. Shimizu M, Tainaka H, Oba T, Mizuo K, Umezawa M, Takeda K. Maternal Exposure to Nanoparticulate Titanium Dioxide During the Prenatal Period Alters Gene Expression Related to Brain Development in the Mouse. Part Fibre Toxicol. 2009; 6:20.

57. Fadeel B, Garcia-Bennett AE. Better Safe Than Sorry: Understanding the Toxicological Properties of Inorganic Nanoparticles Manufactured or Biomedical Applications. Advanced Drug Delivery Reviews. 2010; 62(3): 362-74.

58. Murday JS, Siegel RW, Stein J, Wright JF. Translational Nanomedicine: Status Assessment and Opportunities. Nanomedicine: Nanotechnology, Biology, and Medicine. 2009; 5(3): 251-73.

59. Shapira A, Livney YD, Broxterman HJ, Assaraf YG. Nanomedicine for Targeted Cancer Therapy: Towards the Overcoming of Drug

Resistance. Drug Resistance Updates: Reviews and Commentaries in Antimicrobial and Anticancer Chemotherapy. 2011; 14(3): 150-63.

60. Michael Heller MJH. Nanotechnology for Cancer Diagnostics and Therapeutics. Nanomedicine: Nanotechnology, Biology and Medicine 2006; 2(4).

61. Sahoo SK, Labhasetwar V. Nanotech Approaches to Drug Delivery and Imaging. Drug Discovery Today. 2003; 8(24): 1112-20.

62. Sun Q, Wang Q, Rao BK, Jena P. Electronic Structure and Bonding of Au on a SiO2 Cluster: A Nanobullet for Tumors. Physical Review Letters. 2004; 93(18): 186803.

Chapter 3

Modeling of Nanotherapeutics Delivery Based on Tumor Perfusion

Anne L van de Ven[1,10,11], Behnaz Abdollahi[2,10], Carlos J Martinez[1,3], Lacey A Burey[4], Melissa D Landis[4], Jenny C Chang[4,5], Mauro Ferrari[5,6,7] and Hermann B Frieboes[2,8,9,11]

[1] *Department of Nanomedicine, The Methodist Hospital Research Institute, 6670 Bertner Avenue, Houston, TX 77030, USA*

[2] *Department of Electrical and Computer Engineering, University of Louisville, Louisville, KY, USA*

[3] *Department of Biology, Southwestern University, Georgetown, TX, USA*

[4] *The Methodist Hospital Cancer Center, The Methodist Hospital Research Institute, Houston, TX, USA*

[5] *Department of Medicine, Weill Cornell Medical College, New York, NY, USA*

[6] *The Methodist Hospital Research Institute, Houston, TX, USA*

[7] *Alliance for NanoHealth, Houston, TX, USA*

[8] *Department of Bioengineering, University of Louisville, 419 Lutz Hall, Louisville, KY 40208, USA*

[9] *James Graham Brown Cancer Center, University of Louisville, Louisville, KY, USA*

[10] *Shared first authorship.*

[11] *Authors to whom any correspondence should be addressed.*

ABSTRACT

Heterogeneities in the perfusion of solid tumors prevent optimal delivery of nanotherapeutics. Clinical imaging protocols for obtaining patient-specific data have proven difficult to implement. It is challenging to determine which perfusion features hold greater prognostic value and to relate measurements to vessel structure and function. With the advent of systemically administered nanotherapeutics whose delivery is dependent on overcoming diffusive and convective barriers to transport, such knowledge is increasingly important. We describe a framework for the automated evaluation of vascular perfusion curves measured at the single vessel level. Primary tumor fragments, collected from triple-negative breast cancer patients and grown as xenografts in mice, were injected with fluorescence contrast and monitored using intravital microscopy. The time to arterial peak and venous delay, two features whose probability distributions were measured directly from time-series curves, were analyzed using a fuzzy c-mean supervised classifier in order to rank individual tumors according to their perfusion characteristics. The resulting rankings correlated inversely with experimental nanoparticle accumulation measurements, enabling the modeling of nanotherapeutics delivery without requiring any underlying assumptions about tissue structure or function, or heterogeneities contained therein. With additional calibration, these methodologies may enable the investigation of nanotherapeutics delivery strategies in a variety of tumor models.

1. INTRODUCTION

Tumor vasculature is characterized by structural abnormalities that produce spatial and temporal heterogeneities in blood flow. The vasculature lacks a regular hierarchical network of large proximal vessels feeding into successively smaller vessels; instead, vessel interconnections are irregular in size and spacing [1, 2]. Endothelial cells lining these vessels have an altered morphology, pericytes (cells that support endothelial cells) are poorly attached or are absent, and the basement membrane is often abnormal. The resulting vessels are dilated, tortuous, saccular, and are vulnerable to collapse [1, 2]. The presence of fenestrations [3–5], combined with incomplete vascular walls [5], can yield localized regions of blood plasma leakage that alter macromolecule transport [6, 7] and increase interstitial pressure [8]. Collectively, these vascular abnormalities lead to regions of tumor tissue that are perfused poorly, intermittently or not at all [9, 10].

Non-uniformities in vascular perfusion hinder the transport of chemotherapeutics. The delivery of conventional chemotherapeutics relies on passive diffusion from the bloodstream into the tumor interstitium, and is therefore largely constrained by the drug circulation half-life, distance of travel and the pressure differential between the vasculature and tissue [11]. Nanotherapeutics, in which drugs are concentrated inside longer-circulating nanoscale delivery vehicles, have been developed to enhance drug accumulation within tumors. Early clinical successes, such as Doxil (liposome-encapsulated doxorubicin) and Abraxane (albumin-stabilized paclitaxel), rely on the enhanced permeation and retention (EPR) effect to passively accumulate in tumor fenestrations [12]. The overall efficacy of Doxil and other nanotherapeutics, however, remains variable due to patient-specific heterogeneities in tumor vascularization, interstitial pressure and drug retention [8]. Advances in multi-stage silicon nanovectors [13] promise to overcome many of these transport barriers, since the physical properties of these particles (size, shape, surface chemistry, etc) can be modulated to improve tumor-specific accumulation in an EPR-independent manner [14, 15]. The greatest challenge to the delivery of such nanotherapeutics lies in optimizing particles to leverage transport conditions that are not conducive to conventional chemotherapeutics delivery [16].

Tumor perfusion remains poorly understood, particularly with respect to what conditions lead to effective or poor treatment. Attempts to characterize tumor perfusion using static data, such as the measurement of microvessel density from patient biopsies, have shown mixed prognostic capacity [17, 18]. Clinical imaging modalities capable of monitoring perfusion dynamically, such as magnetic resonance imaging (MRI) [19], computed tomography (CT) [20], positron emission tomography (PET) [21] and Doppler sonography [22], have been used to produce time-series images that enable pixel-by-pixel analysis of contrast kinetics within tumors. Parameters measured from the resulting 'time–signal' curves are placed in pharmacokinetic (PK) models in order to extrapolate information regarding vascular anatomy and physiology. Principal features derived using PK models include the blood flow velocity, blood volume and mean transit time. Numerous methods have been proposed to extract these features in human tissues [23–31]. While the prognostic capacity of such an approach remains to be determined, MRI [32], CT [33] and PET [34] have demonstrated that tumor transport plays a role in treatment response, and that persistence of unfavorable perfusion characteristics (high blood volume fraction, rapid transit time, focal hyperpermeability and/or high fluorodeoxyglucose (FDG) metabolism) following chemotherapy correlates with a poor treatment response.

Due to the difficulties of relating clinical perfusion imaging with the underlying tumor structure and function, intravital microscopy (IVM) studies in live animals are becoming increasingly popular [35,36]. Using video-rate laser-scanning microscopy, blood flow velocity, flux and hematocrit can be measured by tracking trajectories of fluorescent red blood cells (RBCs) [37]. Concomitant injection of a fluorescent tracer allows measurement of shear rate [37], blood volume fraction [38] and tissue permeability [38–42]. These physiological parameters can be related to local variations in gene expression, enzyme activity, pH, metabolites and other parameters of interest (reviewed in [36]) by simultaneously imaging multiple fluorescent reporters. A major advantage of IVM is that tumor perfusion can be characterized on a vessel-by-vessel basis, potentially leading to insights into how local variations in perfusion can affect nanotherapeutics delivery and treatment response [43].

In this paper, we describe a theoretical framework for the automated evaluation of IVM perfusion curves in order to model the delivery of nanotherapeutics. Our hypothesis is that tumor-specific perfusion features may be used to model nanotherapeutics accumulation; thus, this framework aims to transcend the challenges posed by the typically abnormal tumor vasculature. Primary tumor fragments, collected from triple-negative breast cancer patients and grown as xenografts in mice, were injected with a bolus of a 40 kDa FITC–dextran tracer and monitored at 30 fps using IVM. The fluorescence intensity of each vessel was measured over time to yield a heterogeneous set of arterial and venous perfusion curves on a tumor-by-tumor basis. Two features were considered: the time to arterial peak and the venous delay, which acted as inputs for a fuzzy c-mean (FCM) supervised classifier. The data were classified into three defined groups (poorly vascularized, well vascularized and 'in between' vascularized), which were correlated to experimental nanoparticle accumulation measurements. We find that this approach enables an automated ranking of tumor vascular perfusion in order to model the delivery of nanotherapeutics. Using an independent validation set, we demonstrate that new samples can be mapped into the feature space to determine their perfusion ranking and hence estimate their nanoparticle retention. A major strength of this approach is that it enables the ranking of tumors and evaluation of their behavior in an automated manner without requiring PK models.

2. MATERIALS AND METHODS

2.1. Silicon particle fabrication

Plateloid nanoporous silicon particles of dimension 1000 × 400 nm were fabricated in the Microelectronics Research Center of The University of Texas at Austin [14]. Particles were fluorescently labeled for IVM as described in [14]. Particles were stored in IPA at 4 °C and then washed five times with phosphate-buffered saline immediately before use *in vivo*.

2.2. Animal models

BCM-2665, BCM-2147, BCM-4195 and BCM-3887 human cancer-in-mice xenografts were generated in SCID/beige mice (Harlan Laboratories, Wilmington, MA) by subcutaneous hetero-implantation of human tumor fragments in the mammary pad after gross removal of the epithelium [44]. These slow-growing tumor lines were selected for model calibration due to their highly reproducible vascularization from mouse to mouse. MDA-MB-231 triple-negative human breast cancer cells (ATCC) were grown orthotopically in nude mice as a validation set. Three days prior to imaging, mice received a one-time intravenous injection of DiD-labeled autologous RBCs (~3% hematocrit) [14] for visualization of blood flow dynamics. When tumors reached 3–5 mm in diameter, mice were anesthetized with isoflurane and prepared for IVM using an aseptic skin-flap procedure [14]. Tumors were cover slipped using a custom coverslip mount for the duration of the experiment. 1–4 h after particle injection, mice were sacrificed by gravity perfusion with saline followed by 10% neutral buffered formalin. All animal protocols were reviewed and approved by the Institutional Animal Care and Use Committee (IACUC) at The Methodist Hospital Research Institute.

2.3. Intravital microscopy image acquisition

Live animals were imaged on an upright Nikon A1R laser scanning confocal microscope customized for IVM [43]. First-pass perfusion was imaged using a 4 × magnification objective (3.2 × 3.2 mm) for 5 min at 30 frames per second (fps) immediately following an intravenous bolus of a 40 kDa FITC–dextran tracer (1 μM in 50 μl PBS; Invitrogen). High-resolution time-lapse images of particle accumulation were acquired across multiple fields-of-view (FOVs) for up to 4 h at 45–60 s intervals (7 fps) following a one-time intravenous injection of 5×10^8 particles. A minimum of 20 randomly selected, non-overlapping 1000 × 500 μm FOVs were acquired in parallel for each animal. All image acquisitions were performed by simultaneous excitation of tissue with 488, 541 and 640 nm lasers. Emissions were collected by photomultiplier tubes with band-pass filters of ~30–35 nm width centered at 525 nm (FITC–dextran tracer), 579 nm (silicon particles) and 670 nm (RBCs).

2.4. Quantification of particle accumulation

To determine particle accumulation as a function of time, the number of particles per FOV was quantified across each time-lapse video using image-processing techniques adapted from [14, 43]. The 12-bit images were split by color, the single pixel noise was removed using a minimum noise filter and individual particles were identified using a binary mask. Real-time particle accumulation curves (the number of particles mm^{-3}) were produced by automated counting of the appropriate particles in each FOV, summing particle counts across all FOVs at each time point and then dividing by the sampled volume [14]. All IVM quantifications were performed using Nikon NIS Elements v4.0 software.

2.5. Quantification of tracer perfusion

IVM first-pass perfusion videos acquired at 30 fps were processed as follows: stills were extracted at ten-frame intervals and aligned relative to each other, yielding 3 fps motion-stabilized videos. Circular regions-of-interest (ROIs) were randomly placed inside vessel segments between branching points, ensuring that there was at least 1 pixel of space between ROIs and vessel margins. Multiple arterioles, venules and capillaries (~10–200 μm diameter) representing the full spectrum of flow dynamics were selected for analysis, yielding approximately 30–60 ROIs per video. The mean fluorescence intensity of each ROI was measured and plotted as a function of time. Background fluorescence for intensity normalization was measured on a frame-by-frame basis using a non-perfused ROI. Measurement stability with regard to ROI placement was assessed by sampling sets of five identical ROIs within at least ten individual vessels per video. All IVM quantifications were performed using Nikon NIS Elements v4.0 software.

2.6. Perfusion classification

Tracer perfusion curves obtained for each tumor replicate were classified based on two features: the time to reach peak arterial perfusion and the delay between arterial and venous perfusion. Arterial and venous signals were distinguished on a video-by-video basis by plotting peak vessel intensity versus vessel diameter, which was found to yield two distinct vessel groupings. Randomly selected ROIs were monitored visually to confirm that the vessels were correctly grouped. The time to peak arterial perfusion was determined by normalizing each arterial curve to obtain a distribution density function. The highest peak was assigned the highest probability of the signal and the time to reach it was termed the *time to arterial peak*. Since the signals had different durations, the time to arterial peak was normalized by dividing by the signal duration. The perfusion signals were thus represented as random variables with a number of values, each with a different probability. The set of possible values associated with each random variable was mathematically treated as a distribution. The *venous delay*, defined as the lag time between tracer appearance in the arterial system and the venous system, was similarly assessed by obtaining distribution density functions and normalizing by the signal duration. Due to the complexity of the vascular network, no attempts were made to visually pair specific arteries with veins; instead, the vascular system was treated as a closed-loop system with a single input and output.

The time to arterial peak and venous delay were measured for each tumor replicate, with the final value representing the expectation (E) of all the probabilities for each set of veins and arteries:

$$E\,(\text{Feature 1}) = \sum_{i=1}^{n} P_{\text{vein}}(Y_i), \quad E\,(\text{Feature 2}) = \sum_{i=1}^{n} P_{\text{artery}}\,(X_i)\,.$$

where $P_{\text{vein}}(Y_i)$ is the probability of the venous delay and $P_{\text{artery}}(X_i)$ is the probability of the arterial peak.

2.7. Automated tumor ranking by fuzzy c-mean classification

Tumors were ranked according to degree of vascularization using an FCM classifier. Originally introduced by Bezdek [45], this technique ranks the data based on a membership grade assigned to each cluster. Two functions were utilized: a membership function (which establishes the degree of membership for points within a data cluster) and an objective function (which determines the position of the cluster center). Briefly, clustered data points were assigned an initial cluster center value. A membership function was then applied to determine the degree to which each given sample belongs to the cluster. The center of the clusters was changed iteratively to maximize the degree of belonging for all clustered data points. The unsupervised algorithm was stopped when the membership function became sufficiently small.

Tumors were ranked according to the time to arterial peak and venous delay by utilizing the objective function

$$\min\left\{J_m = \sum_{i=1}^{N}\sum_{j=1}^{c} u_{ij}^{m}\|x_i - c_j\|^2\right\}, \qquad 1 < m < \infty,$$

where *m* is the degree of fuzzification, $\|x_i - c_j\|^2$ is the distance (or norm) that specifies the similarity between the data and the center of the clusters, *cj* is a vector specifying the coordinates of the center of the clusters, *xi* is the vector of the input data and *uijm* is the membership degree of the *i*th input. Optimization of the objective function involved changing the exponential membership function in which

$$u_{ij} = \frac{1}{\sum_{k=1}^{c}\left(\frac{\|x_i - c_j\|}{\|x_i - c_k\|}\right)^{\frac{2}{m-1}}} \quad \text{and} \quad c_j = \frac{\sum_{i=1}^{N} u_{ij}^{m}.x_i}{\sum_{i=}^{N} u_{ij}^{m}}.$$

The condition $\|U^k - U^{k-1}\| < \varepsilon$ was implemented as the algorithm stop function. All FCM classifications were performed in an automated manner using Matlab 7.10.0 (R2010a).

2.8. Model validation

Model validation was performed in a blinded manner. Individual MDA-MB-231 tumors were classified based on arterial peak and venous delay measurements and then ranked by membership to the closest cluster center. Estimates of particle accumulation were generated by plotting tumor ranks on a curve calibrated with the training set (BCM-2665, BCM-2147, BCM-4195 and BCM-3887 tumors).

3. RESULTS

3.1. Nanotherapeutics delivery is heterogeneous from tumor to tumor

Real-time IVM of silicon particle accumulation in tumors revealed tumor-specific differences in particle accumulation. Particle accumulation was quantified across triple-negative breast tumor biopsies, which were collected from four different patients (BCM-2147, BCM-2665, BCM-3887 and BCM-4195) and grown as xenografts in immunocompromised SCID/Beige mice. Figure 1 shows sample images and kinetic data for the accumulation of 1000 × 400 nm particles in the vasculature of the 2147 and 4195 tumors. Mice treated with identical numbers of particles (5×10^8) showed distinct differences in the number of particles accumulated. Particle accumulation varied between tumors derived from different patients, as well as within tumor replicates. The 2147 mouse shown in figure 1, for example, accumulated particles at a density of ~27 900 particles mm^{-3}, whereas the 2147 replicates as a whole ($n = 3$) accumulated particles at a density of $27\,500 \pm 1450$ particles mm^{-3}. Similarly, the 4195 mouse shown in figure 1 accumulated particles at a density of ~2920 particles mm^{-3}, whereas 4195 replicates ($n = 4$) accumulated particles at a density of 3450 ± 400 particles mm^{-3}. The largest difference in particle accumulation was observed between tumors derived from different patients, leading us to speculate that tumor-specific differences in perfusion play an important role in nanoparticle delivery.

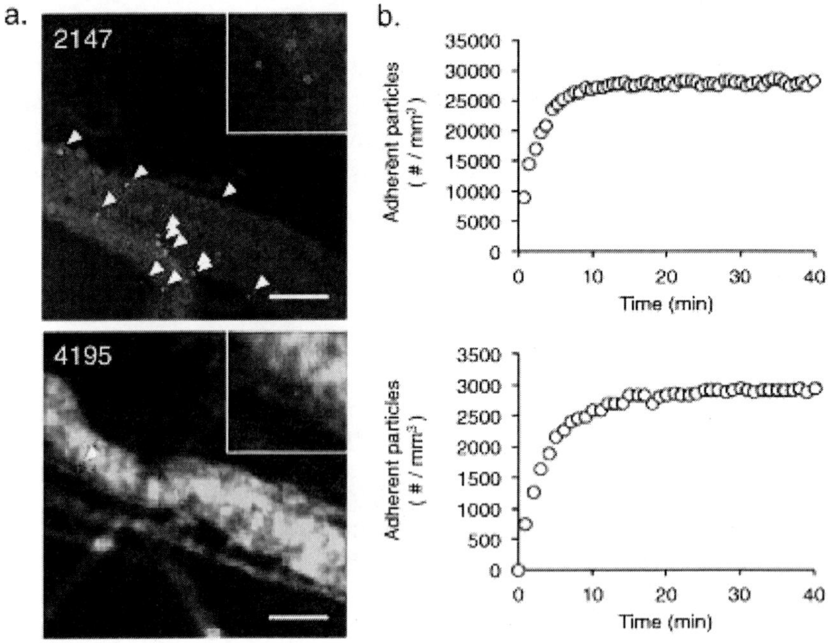

Figure 1. Accumulation of 1000 × 400 nm silicon particles in the vasculature of human breast cancer xenografts. (a) Representative IVM images of silicon particle (red) adhesion to the walls of perfused blood vessels, collected 1 h after particle injection. Vessel walls were delineated via a 40 kDa FITC–dextran tracer (green) and vessel perfusion was identified by the presence of moving RBCs (blue). Inset: a magnified view demonstrating that individual particles can be readily distinguished for quantification purposes. Scale bar = 50 μm. (b) Representative particle accumulation kinetics as measured by IVM, shown for individual 2147 and 4195 mice. Differential particle accumulation is observed, with the 2147 tumors showing more rapid particle accumulation and a higher quantity of adherent particles when compared to 4195 tumors.

3.2. Quantification of tracer first-pass perfusion

The first-pass perfusion of an intravenous bolus of a 40 kDa FITC–dextran tracer was recorded in real time (30 fps) using IVM. Representative IVM videos of the 2147 (video 1) and 4195 (video 2) tumors perfusion can be found in the online supplementary data (available fromstacks.iop.org/NJP/15/055004/mmedia). Frame-by-frame analysis of tracer intensity in selected ROIs yielded perfusion time curves for individual vessels. A representative video of the frame-by-frame analysis (video 3) can be found in the online supplementary data. Figure 2 highlights sample arterial and venous curves generated by the 2147 and 4195 tumors implanted into mice. Several key features can be observed: The arterial curves (red) are generally characterized by a rapid increase in fluorescence intensity which plateaus within the first minute, drops off and levels out. The venous curves (blue) demonstrate a more gradual increase in fluorescence intensity, resulting in a delayed plateau. A large number of such curves (~30–60) were generated for each implant, allowing characterization of intratumoral heterogeneity. Differences were observed in peak intensity, time to arterial peak and venous delay within each tumor, suggesting that vascularization can be heterogeneous within a given tumor. Independent stability analyses were performed for each video to confirm that ROI placement did not have a significant impact on the rate of tracer influx and that the variations in signal intensity at any given time point fell within the overall signal noise. Data were considered robust and included for classification when these conditions were met.

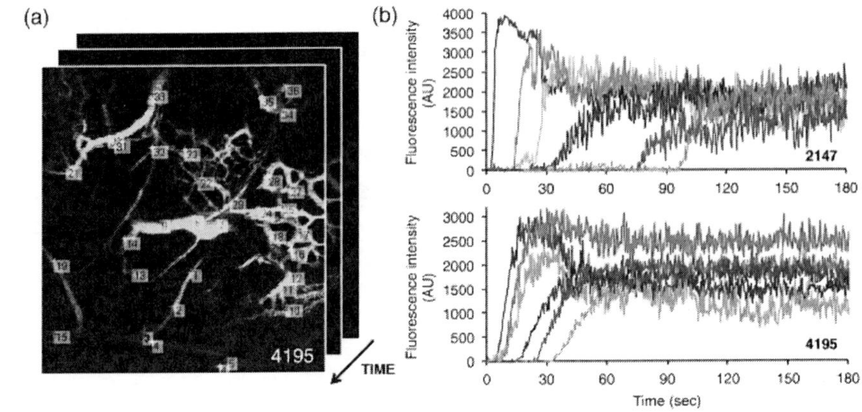

Figure 2. Quantification of tumor first-pass perfusion following injection of a 40 kDa FITC–dextran tracer. (a) Representative ROIs selected for time measurements of fluorescence intensity. Circular ROIs were randomly defined inside arterioles, venules and capillaries, between branching points, yielding approximately 30–60 ROIs per video. (b) Representative arterial (red) and venous (blue) perfusion-time curves of individual vessels, measured for single 2147 and 4195 tumors. Variations in the time to arterial peak and in venous delay are observed within each tumor. The videos from which the data have been derived can be found in the online supplementary data (available from stacks.iop.org/NJP/15/055004/mmedia).

3.3. Identification of tissue classifiers

Heterogeneities in intratumoral perfusion make it difficult to apply standard curve-fitting models for perfusion classification. The first-pass perfusion signal in tumor arteries, for example, does not necessarily rise very quickly to a maximum as would be expected in normal tissue. This was particularly evident for the 4195 and 3887 biopsy implants, in which a slow rise in arterial fluorescence was followed by little or no decrease, indicative that the tracer was already fully mixed in the blood by the time of arrival. In contrast, the 2147 and 2665 tumors behaved more like normal arteries in that their fluorescence intensity rapidly peaked and then declined immediately after the peak. These observations suggest that the time it takes for arterial flow to reach its peak is a critical feature of tumor perfusion. Accordingly, we generated a distribution density function in which the highest peak has the highest probability of signal, and the time to reach the peak following tracer entry was defined as the 'time to arterial peak'.

The perfusion of the tumor venous system showed distinct abnormalities as well. In normal tissue, the duration from the time blood enters an artery until it reaches the corresponding vein is a few seconds. In the tumors in this study, however, this process varied from a few seconds to over a minute. The 2147 tumor in figure 2, for example, showed a delay of ~30–90 s between when the tracer appeared in the arteries and when it appeared in the veins, whereas the 4195 tumor showed a venous delay of ~10–30 s. Thus, we postulated that venous delay is also an important feature of tumor perfusion. Accordingly, we applied statistical rules to measure the probability of this delay.

3.4. Classification of tumor vascularity

The time to arterial peak and venous delay was calculated for each biopsy implant and mapped to a single point within a two-dimensional feature space. The final value of a given feature is the expectation of all the probabilities of the vessels imaged over a 10 mm^2 FOV. Table 1 shows the results of the two features calculated for each implant. When plotted in a two-dimensional feature space, the complexity of the data becomes apparent (figure 3). The scattering of these points reflects both intra- and inter-tumoral heterogeneities. If no intra-tumoral heterogeneities were present, for example, we would expect to see four tight clusters of data, one for each set of tumor replicates. Since the data do not fall in a single line, a linear classification is not possible.

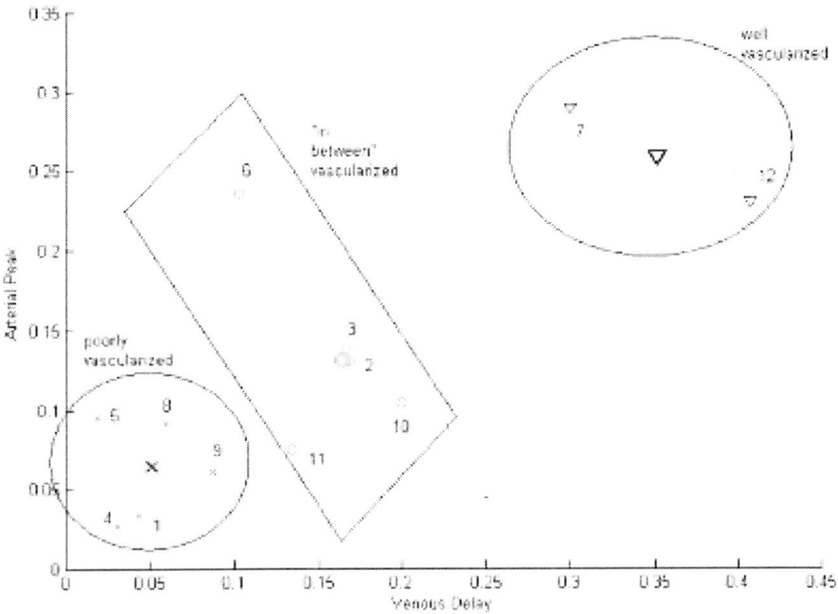

Figure 3. Application of the FCM classifier partitions the data set into three distinct categories. The numbers denote the individual tumor replicates as listed in table 1. Three classes are marked and the samples are shown with the same color as the center of the class. The red crosses represent poorly vascularized cases, the blue triangles belong to the well-vascularized class and the green circles denote the 'in between' cases.

The data were separated into three different classes based on the pattern of scatter: the first includes cases that are poorly vascularized (i.e. short time to peak and short venous delay), the second includes cases that are well vascularized (i.e. long time to peak and long venous delay) and the third class is neither poorly nor well vascularized ('in between' vascularized). These 'in between' cases can represent tumors of homogeneous vasculature with intermediate perfusion properties or tumors of heterogeneous vasculature with regions with differing perfusion properties. No restrictions were placed on the classification of very well or very poorly vascularized cases. Figure 3 shows the data set in the two-dimensional feature space after applying the FCM classifier.

Table 1. The calculated expectation of individual tumor features.

	Tumor type	Feature 1: venous delay	Feature 2: arterial peak
1	2147	0.0415	0.0342
2	2147	0.1608	0.1307
3	2147	0.1468	0.1381
4	2665	0.0300	0.0270
5	3887	0.0187	0.0952
6	3887	0.0961	0.2361
7	3887	0.2766	0.2896
8	3887	0.0540	0.0912
9	4195	0.0830	0.0609
10	4195	0.1822	0.1047
11	4195	0.1334	0.0751
12	4195	0.3526	0.2309

The data were ranked by taking into account both the distance of each data point to the center of its cluster and a weighted term for each of the measured features:

$$\text{rank}(p) = w1 \times \text{feature 1(venous delay)} + w2 \times \text{feature 2(arterial peak)},$$

where *p* is the tumor replicate in each class and *w*1 and *w*2 are the weighted terms for the venous delay and arterial peak, respectively. We note that there exist numerous optimization algorithms to determine such weighted terms [46, 47]. Here, the values for *w*1 and *w*2 were chosen by separately calculating the first moment of each feature in each class. Since each feature is described as a separate distribution function, *w*1 and *w*2 were selected so that *w*1 + *w*2 = 1. The other constraint, which is based on the observation that normal vasculature is usually associated with a higher probability of venous delay than rapidly perfused tumors, assigns a higher weight to *w*1. The ratio *r* of the mean of the two features in each class thus defines the second constraint as ($w1/w2 = r$). Using our experimental data, we calculate *w*1 = 0.6 and *w*2 = 0.4. Note that we do not choose the Euclidean distance from the samples to the center of the classes as the ranking criteria since the accuracy of such an approach is proportional to the sample number. Figure 4 shows the automated tumor ranking from poorly vascularized tumors (left) to well-vascularized tumors (right). Despite the small sample size, it can be observed that there is a large dynamic range (~9.5-fold) in the measured values. Interestingly, replicates from the same patient (No. 1–3 (2147), No. 5–8 (3887) and No. 9–12 (4195)) do not group together, which reflects intra-tumoral heterogeneities in growth and vascularization.

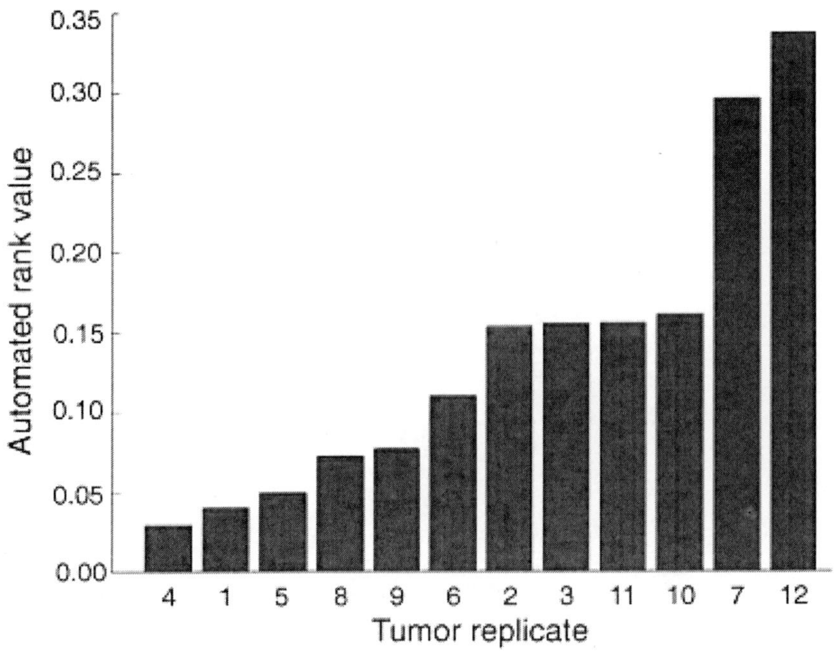

Figure 4. Automated ranking of the implants based on weighted feature probabilities.

Particle accumulation was measured for all tumor replicates evaluated here. Table 2 shows a comparison between tumor classification, automated ranking and particle accumulation on a tumor-by-tumor basis. Since the classification and ranking schemes do not show a consistent ranking, we cannot compare them directly with the experimental results. We therefore calculated the average value of these features for each patient. Comparison of the averaged patient ranking with the averaged experimental measurement suggests that tumors classified as 'poorly vascularized' would uptake the highest number of circulating particles, whereas tumors classified as 'well vascularized' would uptake the lowest number of particles. This trend is shown in figure 5, where the automated ranking appears inversely proportional to particle accumulation. Data were fit to a second-order polynomial based on the observation that 1000 × 400 nm plateloid particle accumulation is constrained by tumor-specific physiological transport phenomena [48]. The 2665 tumor, although a single replicate, had relatively little impact on the classification scheme and was therefore considered robust and included in the fit. Thus, the relationship between tumor rank and particle accumulation appears to be nonlinear, with small changes in the upper ranks yielding large changes in particle accumulation.

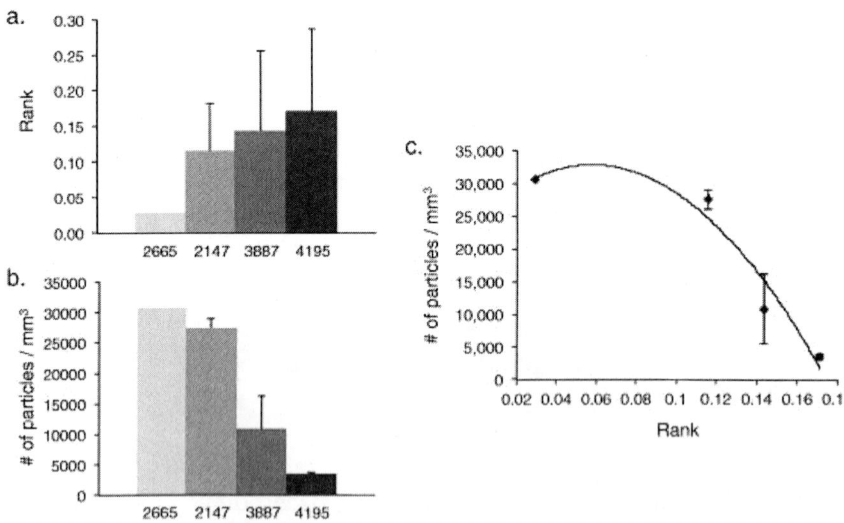

Figure 5. Comparison of tumor rank to experimentally observed particle accumulation. (a) Average tumor rank, grouped by patient number. Note that sample 2665 is a single replicate. (b) Average particle accumulation, grouped by patient. Particle accumulation is observed to be inversely proportional to tumor rank. (c) Plot of the nonlinear relationship between the average particle accumulation and the average tumor rank.

Table 2. Comparison between classification, automated ranking and experimentally derived nanoparticle accumulation measurements. Mean values for each tumor type are given, followed by the individual measurements. Mean values are presented as ±1 standard deviation. Tumor vascularity is indicated by − (poorly vascularized), ± (in between) or + (well vascularized).

	Patient	Vascularity classification	Automated rank value		Particle accumulation (number of particles mm^{-3})	
1	2147	−	0.1160 ± 0.0661	(0.0397)	27 500 ± 1450	(28 690)
2	2147	±		(0.1534)		(25 880)
3	2147	±		(0.1550)		(27 930)
4	2665	−	0.0293	(0.0293)	30 620	(30 620)
5	3887	−	0.1434 ± 0.1116	(0.0493)	10 810 ± 5400	(8080)
6	3887	±		(0.1560)		(18 800)
7	3887	+		(0.2959)		(9410)
8	3887	−		(0.0722)		(6960)
9	4195	−	0.1714 ± 0.1157	(0.0768)	3450 ± 400	(3410)
10	4195	±		(0.1617)		(3620)
11	4195	−		(0.1103)		(2920)
12	4195	+		(0.3369)		(3850)

Triple-negative MDA-MB-231 xenografts were generated for model validation. Grown simultaneously in littermates for 30 days under identical conditions, these tumors nevertheless demonstrated significant differences in tumor vascularization, particle accumulation and ranking. Figure 6(a) highlights the morphological differences observed under brightfield illumination and following FITC–dextran injection. Cumulative particle accumulation, as measured by IVM, was found to vary by as much as ~30-fold across the five tumors studied (figure 6(b)). These tumors were individually classified and ranked in a blinded manner (table 3).

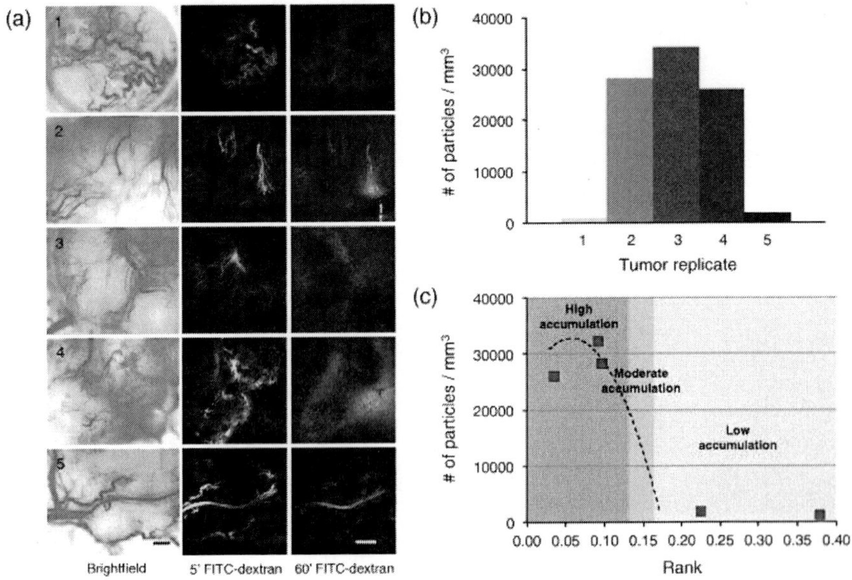

Figure 6. Vascularization, particle accumulation and ranking of MDA-MB-231 xenografts. (a) Brightfield and fluorescence microscopy images of five individual tumors grown under identical conditions (top to bottom: rows 1–5). Significant differences in vascular morphology were observed, as well as local differences in vessel permeability resulting in tracer extravasation. Scale bar = 200 μm. (b) Cumulative particle accumulation, as measured by IVM, ranged widely from ~1000 to 34 000 particles mm^{-3}. (c) Predicted (dashed line) and measured (blue solid square) particle accumulation values, plotted by tumor rank. The degree of particle accumulation was categorized by position along the predicted accumulation curve (from figure 5(c)). High accumulation: >20 000 particles mm^{-3}; moderate accumulation: 5000–20 000; low accumulation: <5000 particles mm^{-3}.

The calculated tumor ranks were found to range from 0.035 (tumor 4, poorly vascularized) to 0.378 (tumor 1, well vascularized). Figure 6(c) shows the predicted and measured particle accumulation values, plotted by tumor rank. The three tumors predicted to show high particle accumulation (>20 000 particles mm^{-3}) correlated in a statistically significant manner (two-tailed test with $\alpha = 0.05$) with the model prediction ($R = 0.99$ as measured by Pearson product moment correlation), while those with relatively high ranks (>0.18) showed low particle accumulation as expected.

Table 3. Automated classification and ranking of MDA-MB-231 tumors. Tumor vascularity is indicated by – (poorly vascularized), ± (in between) or + (well vascularized).

	Vascularity classification	Automated rank value	Particle accumulation (number of particles mm^{-3})	
			Predicted	Measured
1	+	0.3779	0	1070
2	–	0.0977	28 940	28 310
3	–	0.0920	29 960	34 300
4	–	0.0352	31 610	26 070
5	±	0.2245	0	1900

4. DISCUSSION

The collection and interpretation of perfusion data present significant challenges at both the clinical and the preclinical level. In a clinical setting, it is difficult to acquire morphological and perfusion information simultaneously following a single dose of contrast agent; thus most researchers have to choose between studying dynamic or architectural features [19]. While early evidence suggests that a careful combination of both data sets may ultimately improve the accuracy of breast cancer imaging [49, 50], researchers are yet to identify perfusion features that may have diagnostic or prognostic value. For this reason, we utilized IVM, a preclinical imaging modality with high spatial (≤2 μm) and high temporal (≤30 fps) resolution that is uniquely suited for studying tumor pathophysiology in animal models [36]. Collection of data at these scales allows us to detect heterogeneities in tumor vascular structure and function, but at the same time introduces new complexities into the data analysis.

Here we utilized IVM to simultaneously collect both perfusion and particle accumulation kinetics in patient-derived xenografts. Vessel perfusion was measured on a vessel-by-vessel basis, in order to yield a large set of arterial and venous perfusion curves whose variability reflects local differences in vessel structure and function. Features of interest were directly extracted from the measured data sets by using an FCM supervised classifier. Since our goal was to model nanoparticle accumulation based on tumor perfusion characteristics that vary with location and time, we chose not to extrapolate global tumor parameters such as the mean transit time or blood volume (see the appendix). While such measurements might serve as acceptable classifiers, interpolation of each data set into a single-intensity curve would effectively discard all measurements of intratumoral heterogeneity.

To analyze our complex sets of perfusion measurements, we developed a framework to automatically perform tumor classification and ranking without relying on PK models. Traditional dynamic imaging techniques require PK models to analyze the time dependence of contrast signals in order to extrapolate features such as the tumor blood volume, blood flow, permeability and the size of the extravascular space. The accuracy of such models is ultimately limited by the underlying complexity of the tumor pathophysiology and our ability to model these complexities [51]. For this reason, we chose to rank tumors based on direct measurements of the raw data, without using PK models as an intermediary. Although our data sets failed to yield a simple relationship between the shape of the perfusion curves and tumors from specific patients, we were able to extract the time to arterial peak and venous delay as discriminating features for tumor classification and ranking. By measuring these two features from experimental IVM data sets, we showed that individual tumors could be automatically ranked according to tumor perfusion. Calibration of the model with IVM measurements of particle accumulation allowed estimation of tumor behavior without requiring any underlying assumptions about tissue structure or function, or heterogeneities contained therein.

The calculated ranks are a direct reflection of tumor heterogeneity, since the classified features incorporate the probabilities collected over a large number of vessels. If no intratumoral heterogeneities were present, for example, we would expect replicates derived from the same patient to yield identical results. Instead, differences in both tumor perfusion and particle accumulation are observed from patient to patient, as well as within tumor replicates. When tumor ranks are averaged by patient, it appears that particle accumulation is preferentially associated with poorly vascularized tumors (e.g. short venous delay and short time to arterial peak). This relationship, plotted in figure 5(c), is dependent on tumor heterogeneity. As tumor perfusion becomes more heterogeneous (with respect to the venous delay or time to peak), the tumor rank will shift along the accumulation curve. Thus, we expect changes in tumor perfusion to yield differences in nanotherapeutics delivery.

The xenograft tumor sets studied here highlight the importance of selecting appropriate animal models for the study of biophysical transport phenomena. Xenografts grown from human cell lines are generally fast growing and show large variations in vascularization from mouse to mouse. As a result, the statistical power animal studies is largely dependent on the scope, quality and amount of samples analyzed. Our findings suggest that tumors implanted as tissue fragments, while generally slower growing (~2–4 months), show a higher degree of reproducibility when evaluated in terms of tissue perfusion and particle accumulation. This allowed us to calibrate the model with a small set of tumors. In contrast, tumors derived from MDA-MB-231 cells varied much more widely than the tumor lines, translating into a ~10-fold range in ranking. Predictions of particle accumulation in individual tumors matched well with experimentally measured values, supporting our hypothesis that tumor-specific perfusion features may be used to model nanotherapeutics accumulation.

This observation has interesting implications for patient therapy. Successful nanotherapy relies largely on the number of nanoparticles that are retained by tumor tissue [43]. Patients treated with anti-angiogenic agents, for example, may accumulate different numbers of nanotherapeutics and thus respond very differently after vascular remodeling. Vascular normalization via VEGF targeting has been reported to elevate blood perfusion [52] and modulate nanotherapeutics size selectivity [53]. It is not yet known, however, how decreases in vessel leakiness may compromise the advantages gained from increased convection. Based on our model, we would expect vascular normalization to improve particle delivery by simultaneously increasing perfusion and decreasing intratumoral heterogeneity. Such a hypothesis could be readily tested in animals using the methodologies outlined here.

From a clinical perspective, there is great interest in identifying tumor-specific perfusion parameters that govern nanotherapeutics delivery. Patient eligibility for nanotherapeutics is generally indicated after failure of prior chemotherapy. The IVM data presented here suggest that select groups of patients may highly benefit from nanotherapy while others may not. Based on our initial findings, we propose three ranges of particle accumulation: high (>20 000 particles mm^{-3}), moderate (5000–20 000) and low (<5000 particles mm^{-3}). We previously calculated that therapeutic silicon particles retained at a density of >15 000 particles mm^{-3} are likely to deliver sufficient drug for achieving therapeutic benefit at subclinical doses [43]. Thus, tumors whose rankings yield moderate to high accumulation are expected to benefit the most from the use of nanotherapeutics over conventional chemotherapy. The approach described here, which combines the high spatial and temporal resolution of IVM with mathematical modeling, is a powerful tool for studying this issue in pre-clinical models. Both perfusion and particle accumulation, for example, can be studied in the same animal on a vessel-by-vessel basis in order to identify the mechanisms driving particle delivery and accumulation. Since we expect nanoparticle delivery to vary based on physical properties such as particle size, shape and surface chemistry [14], a large variety of different nanoparticles may be imaged via IVM and utilized to create a library of perfusion model calibrations. While IVM itself is not suitable for use in patients, the ultimate goal of such studies would be to identify specific parameters that can be measured using existing clinical instruments for personalized selection of appropriate nanotherapeutics.

Although these analyses were performed with only a small set of tumors, they serve to highlight the importance of tumor ranking. The methodology we describe here allows an unbiased, automated comparison between different tumors. New samples can be mapped directly into the feature space in order to determine their perfusion ranking. The number of classes and their center positions are readily adapted using this learning methodology so that the model becomes further refined as it receives more inputs. Each input results in a discrete rank value that can be used to quantitatively compare the pathophysiology of one tumor against other measured tumors. Such rankings can be correlated with a variety of quantifiable physiological parameters in order to evaluate the behavior of a given tumor. The same methodology could be applied to a variety of different cancer types to generate tumor-specific information. We expect this to be particularly useful for glioblastoma, where perfusion parameters are thought to correlate with tumor grade, aggressiveness and prognosis [54–57]. Furthermore, estimates of particle accumulation based on perfusion characteristics could be coupled with advances in multiscale models of tumor vasculature and blood flow [58] in order to predict response to treatment. In our recent works, we have simulated the effect of tumor vascularization and blood flow on particle transport and accumulation within solid tumors [43, 59]. Theoretical calculations of arterial peak and venous delay, generated via such models, could be automatically evaluated using the framework proposed herein, allowing improved estimation of particle accumulation in combination with patient-specific measurable characteristics such as vascular density and tumor size [59].

We note that additional features can be extracted from the perfusion curves beyond the two described here, such as single-vessel flow rate and tracer/particle throughput, in order to improve model sensitivity and specificity. In this pilot study, we describe the simplest automated method for estimating particle delivery based on readily identifiable tumor perfusion characteristics. Clustering of our data sets shows that the relationship between tumor rank and particle accumulation is nonlinear and that tumor rank is not always reproducible across tumor replicates. A single, general deterministic definition for particle accumulation is unlikely to found, and as such, makes it difficult to assign a sensitivity and specificity as is common with clustering techniques. Nevertheless, our initial implementation enabled us to determine that there is an inverse relationship between particle accumulation number and vascularization rank, and that this holds true for the test data set. While it is still unclear at this time how many features are needed for model improvement, increasing the sample size and feature number is expected to greatly improve the statistical significance of such studies.

In summary, here we present an automated technique for the theoretical modeling of nanotherapeutics delivery based on heterogeneous sets of whole arterial and venous perfusion curves collected at the single vessel level. Unlike conventional perfusion studies, in which tumor tissue and its vasculature are treated as individual homogeneous compartments for the extrapolation of PK parameters, tumors were classified and ranked without requiring any underlying assumptions about tissue structure or function, or heterogeneities contained within. The time to arterial peak and venous delay, measured directly from the experimental data, proved sufficient for discriminating between individual tumors. The resulting tumor rankings correlated inversely with experimental nanoparticle accumulation measurements, allowing the estimation of nanotherapeutics delivery. With proper calibration, these methodologies may enable the study of a variety of nanoparticles in different tumor models.

ACKNOWLEDGMENTS

This work was supported by an NIH/NCI Physical Sciences—Oncology Center (PS-OC) Young Investigator Trans-Network Award to AV and HF as a part of the Methodist (U54CA143837) and USC (U54CA143907) PS-OC Centers. LB, ML and JC acknowledge funding from the NIH (R01CA138197 and U54CA149196-01) and the Breast Cancer Research Foundation. MF acknowledges funding from NIH/NCI PS-OC grant number U54CA143837 and additional research support from DoD/BCRP (W81XWH-09-1-0212), NIH/NCI (U54CA151668) and Ernest Cockrell Jr Distinguished Endowed Chair.

REFERENCES

1. Jain R K 1988 Determinants of tumor blood flow: a review Cancer Res. **48** 2641–58

2. Vakoc B J et al 2009 Three-dimensional microscopy of the tumor microenvironment in vivo using optical frequency domain imaging Nature Med. **15** 1219–23

3. Jain R K 1987 Transport of molecules across tumor vasculature Cancer Metastasis Rev. **6** 559–93

4. Roberts W G and Palade G E 1997 Neovasculature induced by vascular endothelial growth factor is fenestrated Cancer Res. **57** 765–72

5. Hashizume H, Baluk P, Morikawa S, McLean J W, Thurston G, Roberge S, Jain R K and McDonald D M 2000 Openings between defective endothelial cells explain tumor vessel leakiness Am. J. Pathol. **156**1363–80

6. Matsumura Y and Maeda H 1986 A new concept for macromolecular therapeutics in cancer chemotherapy: mechanism of tumoritropic accumulation of proteins and the antitumor agent smancsCancer Res. **46** 6387–9

7. Maeda H, Wu J, Sawa T, Matsumura Y and Hori K 2000 Tumor vascular permeability and the EPR effect in macromolecular therapeutics: a review J. Control. Release **65** 271–84

8. Fang J, Nakamura H and Maeda H 2011 The EPR effect: unique features of tumor blood vessels for drug delivery, factors involved and limitations and augmentation of the effect Adv. Drug Deliv. Rev. **63**136–51

9. Jain R K and Stylianopoulos T 2010 Delivering nanomedicine to solid tumors Nature Rev. Clin. Oncol.**7** 653–64

10. Pozrikidis C and Farrow D A 2003 A model of fluid flow in solid tumors Ann. Biomed. Eng. **31** 181–94

11. Hobbs S K, Monsky W L, Yuan F, Roberts W G, Griffith L, Torchilin V P and Jain R K 1998 Regulation of transport pathways in tumor vessels: role of tumor type and microenvironment Proc. Natl Acad. Sci. USA **95** 4607–12

12. Duggan S T and Keating G M 2011 Pegylated liposomal doxorubicin: a review of its use in metastatic breast cancer, ovarian cancer, multiple myeloma and AIDS-related Kaposi's sarcoma Drugs **71** 2531–58

13. Godin B, Tasciotti E, Liu X, Serda R E and Ferrari M 2011 Multistage nanovectors: from concept to novel imaging contrast agents and therapeutics Acc. Chem. Res. **44** 979–89

14. van de Ven A et al 2012 Rapid tumoritropic accumulation of systemically injected plateloid particles and their biodistribution J. Control. Release **158** 148–55

15. Parodi A et al 2013 Biomimetic camouflage imparts cell-like activity to synthetic particles Nature Nanotechnol. **8** 61–8

16. Michor F, Liphardt J, Ferrari M and Widom J 2011 What does physics have to do with cancer? Nature Rev. **11** 657–70

17. Uzzan B, Nicolas P, Cucherat M and Perret G R-Y 2004 Microvessel density as a prognostic factor in women with breast cancer Cancer Res. **64** 2941–55

18. Hlatky L, Hahnfeldt P and Folkman J 2002 Clinical application of antiangiogenic therapy: microvessel density, what it does and doesn't tell us J. Natl Cancer Inst. **94** 883–93

19. Sinha S and Sinha U 2009 Recent advances in breast MRI and MRS NMR Biomed. **22** 3–16

20. Jain R 2011 Perfusion CT imaging of brain tumors: an overview Am. J. Neuroradiol. **32** 1570–7

21. Laking G and Price P 2010 Radionuclide imaging of perfusion and hypoxia Eur. J. Nucl. Med. Mol. Imaging **37** S20–29

22. Cosgrove D and Lassau N 2010 Imaging of perfusion using ultrasound Eur. J. Nucl. Med. Mol. Imaging**37** S65–85

23. Fieselmann A, Kowarschik M, Ganguly A, Hornegger J and Fahrig R 2011 Deconvolution-based CT and MR brain perfusion measurement: theoretical model revisited and practical implementation detailsInt. J. Biomed. Imaging **2011** 467563

24. Klotz E and Konig M 1999 Perfusion measurements of the brain: using dynamic CT for the quantitative assessment of cerebral ischemia in acute stroke Eur. J. Radiol. **30** 170–84

25. Tuominen T 2004 Perfusion Deconvolution via EM Algorithm (Aalto: Department of Engineering Physics and Mathematics, Helsiniki University of Technology)

26. Brix G, Griebel J, Kiessling F and Wenz F 2010 Tracer kinetic modelling of tumour angiogenesis based on dynamic contrast-enhanced CT and MRI measurements Eur. J. Nucl. Med. Mol. Imaging **37** S30–51

27. Miles K A and Griffiths M R 2003 Perfusion CT: a worthwhile enhancement? Br. J. Radiol. **76** 220–31

28. Konstas A A, Goldmakher G V, Lee T Y and Lev M H 2009 Theoretic basis and technical implementations of CT perfusion in acute ischemic stroke: part 2. Technical implementations Am. J. Neuroradiol. **30** 885–92

29. Kudo K, Sasaki M, Yamada K, Momoshima S, Utsunomiya H, Shirato H and Ogasawara K 2010 Differences in CT perfusion maps generated by different commercial software: quantitative analysis by using identical source data of acute stroke patients Radiology **254** 200–9

30. Hermoye L, Annet L, Lemmerling P, Peeters F, Jamar F, Gianello P, Van Huffel S and Van Beers B E 2004 Calculation of the renal perfusion and glomerular filtration rate from the renal impulse response obtained with MRI Magn. Reson. Med. **51** 1017–25

31. Kind T, Houtzager I, Faes T J and Hofman M B 2010 Evaluation of model-independent deconvolution techniques to estimate blood perfusion Conf. Proc. IEEE Eng. Med. Biol. Soc. **2010** 2602–7

32. Reddick W E, Taylor J S and Fletcher B D 1999 Dynamic MR imaging (DEMRI) of microcirculation in bone sarcoma J. Magn. Reson. Imaging **10** 277–85

33. Sahani D V, Kalva S P, Hamberg L M, Hahn P F, Willett C G, Saini S, Mueller P R and Lee T-Y 2005 Assessing tumor perfusion and treatment response in rectal cancer with multisection CT: initial observations Radiology **234** 785–92

34. Dunnwald L K et al 2008 Tumor metabolism and blood flow changes by positron emission tomography: relation to survival in patients treated with neoadjuvant chemotherapy for locally advanced breast cancer J. Clin. Oncol. **26** 4449–57

35. Tozer G M, Ameer-Beg S M, Baker J, Barber P R, Hill S A, Hodgkiss R J, Locke R, Prise V E, Wilson I and Vojnovic B 2005 Intravital imaging of tumour vascular networks using multi-photon fluorescence microscopy Adv. Drug Deliv. Rev. **57** 135–52

36. Jain R K, Munn L L and Fukumura D 2002 Dissecting tumour pathophysiology using intravital microscopy Nature Rev. **2** 266–76

37. Kamoun W S, Chae S S, Lacorre D A, Tyrrell J A, Mitre M, Gillissen M A, Fukumura D, Jain R K and Munn L L 2010 Simultaneous measurement of RBC velocity, flux, hematocrit and shear rate in vascular networks Nature Methods **7** 655–60

38. Brown E B, Campbell R B, Tsuzuki Y, Xu L, Carmeliet P, Fukumura D and Jain R K 2001 In vivomeasurement of gene expression, angiogenesis and physiological function in tumors using multiphoton laser scanning microscopy Nature Med. **7** 864–8

39. Yuan F, Dellian M, Fukumura D, Leunig M, Berk D A, Torchilin V P and Jain R K 1995 Vascular permeability in a human tumor xenograft: molecular size dependence and cutoff size Cancer Res. **55**3752–6

40. Lichtenbeld H C, Yuan F, Michel C C and Jain R K 1996 Perfusion of single tumor microvessels: application to vascular permeability measurement Microcirculation **3** 349–57

41. Gerlowski L E and Jain R K 1986 Microvascular permeability of normal and neoplastic tissuesMicrovasc. Res. **31** 288–305

42. Yuan F, Leunig M, Berk D A and Jain R K 1993 Microvascular permeability of albumin, vascular surface area and vascular volume measured in human adenocarcinoma LS174T using dorsal chamber in SCID mice Microvasc. Res. **45** 269–89

43. van de Ven A L, Wu M, Lowengrub J, McDougall S, Chaplain M A, Cristini V, Ferrari M and Frieboes H 2012 Integrated intravital microscopy and mathematical modeling to optimize nanotherapeutics delivery to tumors AIP Adv. **2** 011208

44. Zhang X et al 2011 A renewable tissue resource of phenotypically stable human breast cancer xenografts for preclinical studies Cancer Res. **71** P5-21–01

45. Bezdek J C, Ehrlich R and Full W 1984 FCM: the fuzzy c-means clustering algorithm Comput. Geosci.**10** 191–203

46. Goldberg D E 1989 Genetic Algorithms in Search, Optimization and Machine Learning (Reading, MA: Addison-Wesley Professional)

47. Sra S, Nowozin S and Wright S J 2011 Optimization for Machine Learning (Cambridge, MA: MIT Press)

48. van de Ven A L et al 2013 submitted

49. Schnall M D et al 2006 Diagnostic architectural and dynamic features at breast MR imaging: multicenter study Radiology **238** 42–53

50. Huang W, Fisher P R, Dulaimy K, Tudorica L A, O'Hea B and Button T M 2004 Detection of breast malignancy: diagnostic MR protocol for improved specificity Radiology **232** 585–91

51. Tofts P S et al 1999 Estimating kinetic parameters from dynamic contrast-enhanced T(1)-weighted MRI of a diffusable tracer: standardized quantities and symbols J. Magn. Reson. Imaging **10** 223–32

52. Sorensen A G et al 2012 Increased survival of glioblastoma patients who respond to antiangiogenic therapy with elevated blood perfusion Cancer Res. **72** 402–7

53. Chauhan V P, Stylianopoulos T, Martin J D, Popovic Z, Chen O, Kamoun W S, Bawendi M G, Fukumura D and Jain R K 2012 Normalization of tumour blood vessels improves the delivery of nanomedicines in a size-dependent manner Nature Nanotechnol. **7** 383–8

54. Law M, Young R J, Babb J S, Peccerelli N, Chheang S, Gruber M L, Miller D C, Golfinos J G, Zagzag D and Johnson G 2008 Gliomas: predicting time to progression or survival with cerebral blood volume measurements at dynamic susceptibility-weighted contrast-enhanced perfusion MR imagingRadiology **247** 490–8

55. Law M, Yang S, Babb J S, Knopp E A, Golfinos J G, Zagzag D and Johnson G 2004 Comparison of cerebral blood volume and vascular permeability from dynamic susceptibility contrast-enhanced perfusion MR imaging with glioma grade Am. J. Neuroradiol. **25** 746–55

56. Jain R, Ellika S K, Scarpace L, Schultz L R, Rock J P, Gutierrez J, Patel S C, Ewing J and Mikkelsen T 2008 Quantitative estimation of permeability surface-area product in astroglial brain tumors using perfusion CT and correlation with histopathologic grade Am. J. Neuroradiol. **29** 694–700

57. Law M, Oh S, Johnson G, Babb J S, Zagzag D, Golfinos J and Kelly P J 2006 Perfusion magnetic resonance imaging predicts patient outcome as an adjunct to histopathology: a second reference standard in the surgical and nonsurgical treatment of low-grade gliomas Neurosurgery **58** 1099–1107

58. Wu M, Frieboes H B, McDougall S, Chaplain M A, Cristini V and Lowengrub J 2013 The effect of interstitial pressure on tumor growth: coupling with the blood and lymphatic vascular systems J. Theor. Biol. **320** 131–51

59. Frieboes H B, Wu M, Lowengrub J, Decuzzi P and Cristini V 2013 A computational model for predicting nanoparticle accumulation in tumor vasculature PLoS ONE **8** e56876

60. Abels B, Klotz E, Tomandl B F, Kloska S P and Lell M M 2010 Perfusion CT in acute ischemic stroke: a qualitative and quantitative comparison of deconvolution and maximum slope approach Am. J. Neuroradiol. **31** 1690–8

61. Chan A A and Nelson S J 2004 Simplified gamma-variate fitting of perfusion curves IEEE Int. Symp. on Biomedical Imaging: Nano to Macro **2** 1067–70

62. Madsen M T 1992 A simplified formulation of the gamma variate function Phys. Med. Biol. **37** 1597

Chapter 4

Delivery of Nanoparticles to Brain Metastases of Breast Cancer using a Cellular Trojan Horse

Mi-Ran Choi & Rizia Bardhan & Katie J. Stanton-Maxey & Sunil Badve & Harikrishna Nakshatri & Keith M. Stantz & Ning Cao & Naomi J. Halas & Susan E. Clare

Department of Surgery, Indiana University School of Medicine, Indianapolis, IN 46202, USA

ABSTRACT

As systemic cancer therapies improve and are able to control metastatic disease outside the central nervous system, the brain is increasingly the first site of relapse. The blood–brain barrier (BBB) represents a major challenge to the delivery of therapeutics to the brain. Macrophages originating from circulating monocytes are able to infiltrate brain metastases while the BBB is intact. Here, we show that this ability can be exploited to deliver both diagnostic and therapeutic nanoparticles specifically to experimental brain metastases of breast cancer.

Keywords: Breast cancer Brain metastasis Gold-silica nanoshell Nanoparticle Blood–brain barrier

1 INTRODUCTION

Brain metastases are a significant clinical challenge. They are diagnosed in 100,000–170,000 patients/year in the United States (Posner 1992; Weil et al. 2005) and outnumber primary brain tumors by a ratio of 10 to 1 (Cairncross and Posner 1983; Walker et al. 1985; Posner 1992). They are estimated to occur in 20–40 % of all cancer patients (Cairncross and Posner 1983; Posner 1995). The incidence rate of brain metastasis is thought to be increasing as a function of the aging population, better treatment of non-central nervous system (CNS) disease and improved imaging techniques. The most common primary tumor sites are lung (40–50 %), breast (13–17 %), melanoma (11–17 %), renal (6–16 %), and GI tract (4–6 %) (Barnholtz-Sloan et al. 2004; Klos and O'Neill 2004). At least 10 % of patients with primary small cell lung cancer (SCLC) have brain metastasis at diagnosis (Hochstenbag et al. 2000; Grossi et al. 2001), however a more recent prospective study of 432 patients in the Netherlands found the rate to be 18 % (Seute et al. 2004). Patients with locally advanced non-small cell lung cancer are at the highest risk for brain metastasis, with some studies reporting greater than 50 % of patients developing brain metastasis over the course of the disease (Stuschke et al. 1999).

Breast cancer metastatic to the brain is most prevalent in the triple negative (Lin et al. 2008) and HER2+ subpopulations (Bendell et al. 2003; Clayton et al. 2004; Lin and Winer 2007; Stemmler et al. 2006; Yau et al.2006), where the median survival time ranges from 2 to 16 months and the mean 1-year survival is ~20 % (Mahmoud-Ahmed AS 2002). Since targeted therapies against HER2+ disease are able to successfully control non-CNS disease, the brain is increasingly being seen as the first site of relapse (Burstein et al. 2005). Currently, the mainstays of treatment for metastatic brain tumors are whole brain radiation therapy (WBRT), surgery, stereotactic radiosurgery or a combination of these modalities. However, significant neurotoxicity has been reported with the use of WBRT, resulting in endocrine dysfunction, significant memory loss and dementia (Sneed et al. 1999; Patchell and Regine 2003; Lo et al. 2005).

Drug uptake into the brain is limited by numerous factors, including physical barriers such as the blood–brain barrier (BBB) and the blood–cerebrospinal fluid (blood–CSF) barrier, and a substrate's affinity for specific transport systems located at both of these interfaces (Graff and

Pollack 2004; Pardridge 2005). Despite recent indications that chemical modulation of the BBB may be feasible (Carman et al. 2011), under physiological conditions, drugs and other substances can enter the brain only by passive transcellular diffusion, receptor-mediated transcytosis, or through the action of specific carrier systems. While in general, the more lipid-soluble a molecule is, the more readily it will penetrate the BBB and blood–CSF barrier to reach targets in the CNS, many lipid-soluble therapeutics have much lower brain permeability than would be predicted on the basis of their solubility (Begley 2004; Muldoon et al. 2007). In an experimental model of brain metastases of breast cancer, cytotoxic concentrations of paclitaxel were reached only in a subset (<10 %) of the "leakiest" metastases (Lockman et al. 2010), and this therapy was unable to reduce the metastatic burden in the brain over the period of the study. All of these factors render the brain a "sanctuary" site for metastases.

More than two decades ago, Fidler and colleagues provided evidence that macrophages of blood monocyte origin can infiltrate experimental brain metastases while the blood–brain barrier is intact (Schackert et al. 1988). Even earlier, Morantz and colleagues had quantified the content of macrophages in clinical specimens (Morantz et al.1979). They examined 12 metastases to the brain from a variety of primary tumors. The mean content of macrophages was 24 % with a range of 4 to 70 %. The specific means by which macrophages are recruited to the metastasis is largely unknown. Primary brain tumors such as gliomas produce MCP1 and HGF/SF1, which attract monocytes (Strik et al. 2004). Whether there are similar immunomodulatory cytokines and chemokines elaborated by intracranial metastases has been "poorly investigated to date" (Strik et al. 2004).

The use of monocyte/macrophages as delivery vehicles to the CNS has been investigated in situations other than malignancy. Afergan et al. demonstrated the delivery of serotonin to the brain by monocytes, which had phagocytosed nano-liposomes containing this otherwise brain impermeant drug (Afergan et al. 2008). Dou and colleagues utilized bone marrow derived macrophages as carriers of and depots for antiretroviral drugs to treat and attenuate the symptoms of HIV-associated neurocognitive disorder (Dou et al. 2009). Therefore, we hypothesized that nanoparticle-laden monocytes/macrophages would home in to intracranial metastatic deposits by crossing the blood–brain barrier following injection into the systemic circulation. If successful, this would open the door to the use of monocytes/macrophages for the delivery of therapeutic nanovectors as well as nanoformulated therapeutics to malignant intracranial lesions.

2 MATERIALS AND METHODS

2.1 Fabrication of gold (Au) nanoshells

Au nanoshells (NS) $[r_1, r_2] = [66, 80]$ nm were fabricated by seed mediated electroless plating of Au onto silica spheres as previously reported (Oldenburg et al. 1998; Brinson et al. 2008). Briefly, monodisperse silica nanospheres of 66 ± 2 nm radii were synthesized by the hydrolysis of tetraethylorthosilicate (TEOS) in basic solution via the Stoeber method (Stoeber et al. 1968). The silica particles are redispersed in ethanol and functionalized with (3-aminopropyl) triethoxysilane (APTES, Sigma) overnight. These amine-terminated silica nanospheres were washed twice to remove excess amines and redispersed in ethanol. The precursor nanoparticles were prepared by decorating the silica particles with small gold colloid (2–3 nm) fabricated by the method reported by Duff et al. (1993). The precursor particles were left unperturbed for 24 h at room temperature, following which they were washed and redispersed in H_2O (10 mL). A plating solution was prepared in an amber bottle by mixing potassium carbonate (anhydrous, Fisher, Fairlawn, NJ) with 1 % $HAuCl_4$ solution in H_2O (200 mL). The plating solution was aged for 48 h before using it to fabricate the nanoshells. A continuous gold shell was grown around the silica nanospheres by mixing the plating solution with different aliquots of the precursor particles and bubbling $CO_{(g)}$ for 10 s (Brinson et al. 2008). The reaction was scaled up to obtain the appropriate volume of nanoshells; the nanoshells were washed twice and finally redispersed in H_2O.

2.2 Isolation of Monocytes from Buffy Coat

Human whole blood was obtained from the Indiana Blood Center (Indianapolis, IN) for the isolation of monocytes. Lymphocytes, monocytes, and platelets, i.e., the buffy coat, were isolated using Ficoll (GE Healthcare Biosciences, Piscataway, NJ) density gradient centrifugation. Monocytes were separated from the other components of the buffy coat using MicroBeads conjugated to monoclonal mouse anti-human CD14 antibodies and MACS® cell separation system (Miltenyi Biotec, Auburn, CA).

2.3 Imaging of gold-silica nanoshells loaded in monocytes/macrophages

Five thousand monocytes/macrophages were incubated in 200 µl RPMI media supplemented with M-CSF with 8.3×10^8 nanoshells for 3 days at 37 °C, 5 % CO_2. The visualization was performed using a Bio-Rad Radiance 2100 MP Rainbow Confocal/Multiphoton System. The images were acquired using the ×10 objective.

2.4 Imaging of red fluorescence microspheres loaded in monocytes/macrophages

Specimens for confocal fluorescence microscopy were prepared by pipetting 50 µL of the red fluorescently labeled microsphere suspension (FluoSpheres® NeutrAvidin® labeled microspheres; 0.04 µm; red fluorescent, excitation 580 nm, emission 605 nm; Molecular Probes, Invitrogen, Carlsbad, CA) onto the glass bottom of 35 mm glass bottom dishes (MatTek Corporation, Ashland, MA). The dishes were left at room temperature for 30 min to allow time for the particles to settle. Three thousand macrophages suspended in 100 µL of RPMI media were added to the glass bottom and the dishes were incubated at 37 °C for 1 h to allow the cells to attach. Three milliliters of RPMI supplemented with M-CSF was added to the cells and they were incubated for 3 days at 37 °C, 5 % CO_2.

2.5 Imaging of gold nanospheres and red fluorescence microspheres loaded in monocytes/macrophages

Electron microscopy specimens were prepared by adding 50 µL of the red fluorescently labeled microsphere suspension to a Thermanox coverslip [cut in half], which was placed in a 35 mm tissue culture dish. 50 µL of gold streptavidin conjugate, 20 nm were added to the same coverslip followed by 300,000 macrophages in 100 µL of media. Dishes were incubated at 37 °C for 1 h in order for the cells to attach. Three milliliters of RPMI supplemented with M-CSF was added to the dish and the dishes were incubated for 3 days at 37 °C, 5 % CO_2. Cells were then fixed in 2 % paraformaldehyde, 2 % glutaraldehyde in 0.1 M PO_4 buffer.

2.6 Establishment of the brain metastatic tumor xenografts

The human MDA-MB-231 BR "brain-seeking" (231-BR) cell line expressing enhanced green fluorescent protein (eGFP) was produced and kindly provided by Dr. Patricia S Steeg (National Cancer Institute, Bethesda, MD). The cells were maintained in RPMI1640 (Cellgro, Mediatech, Inc., Manassas, VA) supplemented with 10 % fetal bovine serum (Gibco, Invitrogen, Grand Island, NY) and 1 % antibiotic–antimycotic (Invitrogen, Carlsbad, CA). Cells were kept in a humidified atmosphere with 5 % CO_2 at 37 °C. eGFP expression in the cells was confirmed by fluorescent microscopy. Prior to beginning, the study protocol was approved by the Institutional Animal Care and Use Committee of the Indiana University School of Medicine. All experiments were conducted in accordance with the NIH guidelines for the care and use of laboratory animals. Six- to eight-week-old athymic *nu/nu* female mice (Harlan Sprague–Dawley Inc., Indianapolis, IN) were used to establish human breast metastatic tumor xenografts in the brain. A cell suspension of eGFP expressing 231-BR cell line (231-BR-eGFP) in the exponential growth phase was prepared in a concentration of 250,000 cells in 100 µl HBSS. Under isoflurane anesthesia, the cells were inoculated into the left cardiac ventricle of three mice. After 4 weeks, the mice evidenced symptoms of brain metastasis, e.g., hind limb paralysis. Mice were sacrificed; brains were removed and fixed in 10 % buffered formalin (Protocol™, Fisher Scientific, Kalamazoo, MI). Following paraffin-embedding, 5-µm sections were cut and the sections viewed using an Olympus BX41 fluorescence microscope fitted with a ×40 FITC filter.

A second group of 12 mice underwent intracardiac injection with the 231-BR-eGFP cells as above. Upon evidence of cerebral metastasis, monocytes were isolated and loaded with red fluorescent microspheres as follows: 20.8×10^7 monocytes in 25 mL of RPMI media (Cellgro, Mediatech, Inc., Manassas, VA) supplemented with 10 % fetal bovine serum (Gibco, Invitrogen, Grand Island, NY) and 1 % antibiotic–

antimycotic (Invitrogen, Carlsbad, CA) were incubated with 50 μl of red fluorescent FluoSpheres® NeutrAvidin®-labeled microspheres (0.04 μm; excitation 580 nm, emission 605 nm; Molecular Probes, Invitrogen, Carlsbad, CA) in a VueLife® FEP cell culture bag (American Fluoroseal Corporation, Gaithersburg, MD) overnight at 37 °C, 5 % CO_2. To remove any unphagocytosed red fluorescent microspheres, cells were washed with PBS twice followed by centrifugation. A total of 4.1×10^7 cells were collected. The presence of the red fluorescent microspheres in the cells was confirmed by fluorescence microscopy. The cell concentration was adjusted to 10^7/100 μl by adding 410 μl PBS to the cell pellet. One hundred microliters of the cell suspension was injected into the systemic circulation via the tail vein; 24 h after injection of the monocytes/macrophages, the mice were euthanized.

2.7 Biodistribution analysis of mouse organs following injection of monocytes/macrophages loaded with red fluorescent microspheres

Following the systemic injection of monocytes/macrophages containing the fluorescently labeled microspheres, mice were sacrificed and the brain, lung, liver, and the heart were dissected. The presence and location of metastatic tumor foci (green fluorescence) and monocytes/macrophages loaded with the red fluorescent microspheres in these organs was determined using an optical imaging system, Berthold NightOwl Optical Imager (Berthold Technologies, Oak Ridge, TN) loaded with Berthold Winlight 32 software (Berthold Technologies). The images of green fluorescence and red fluorescence were taken after exposure times of 100 and 500 ms, respectively. The intensity of the fluorescence in different area of the organs was measured using the signal intensity bar.

2.8 Immunofluorescence analysis of monocytes/macrophages in the green fluorescent brain metastatic tumor cells

After imaging, brains were bisected along the sagittal plane, and fixed by perfusion in 4 % paraformaldehyde overnight at 4 °C. For further fixation the brain hemispheres were transferred to 20 % sucrose solution and fixed overnight at 4 °C. The fixed brain was frozen in

Tissue-Tek O.C.T. compound (Sakura Finetec, Torrance, CA). Brains were sectioned serially in 5-µm increments, processed for immunofluorescent staining and imaging. eGFP expressing tumor cells in brain metastases and red fluorescent microspheres were detected by confocal microscopy using Olympus FV1000 MPE (Olympus, Center Valley, PA). In order to determine if the red fluorescent microspheres were contained within human monocytes/macrophages, brain sections were stained with anti-human CD68 antibodies (clone C-18; Santa Cruz Biotechnology, Santa Cruz, CA) labeled with APEX Pacific Blue fluorochrome. The labeling of the antibodies was performed using APEX Pacific Blue™ Antibody labeling Kit (Molecular Probes, Invitrogen, Carlsbad, CA) according to the manufacturer's instruction.

3 RESULTS AND DISCUSSION

This study was designed as a pilot to test whether loaded monocytes/macrophages are able to maneuver around the BBB and actively deliver nanoparticles to intracranial metastasis with the potential, to be realized, to deliver effective therapy. In a previous publication, the efficient phagocytosis of gold nanoshells by monocytes/macrophages was demonstrated (Choi et al. 2007). Phagocytosis of nanoshells is so avid, in fact, that the monocytes/macrophages are rendered black in optical imaging (Fig. 1). This appears to occur without exception in every monocyte/macrophage in culture.

To detect the presence of the nanoparticle-laden macrophages in the brain, fluorescently labeled microspheres were used to track macrophage location. Although fluorescent nanoshells have been demonstrated that combine both diagnostic and therapeutic functions in the same nanoparticle,(Bardhan et al. 2008, 2009a, 2009b; Tam et al.2007) here we chose to investigate delivery by a "cocktail" of two different types of nanoparticles, one therapeutic and one contrast agent. Prior to commencing the in vivo experiment, it was determined if monocytes would phagocytose the fluorescently labeled microspheres as avidly as gold nanoshells. Avid uptake of the fluorescently labeled microspheres was observed, as shown in Fig. 2. Although it appears

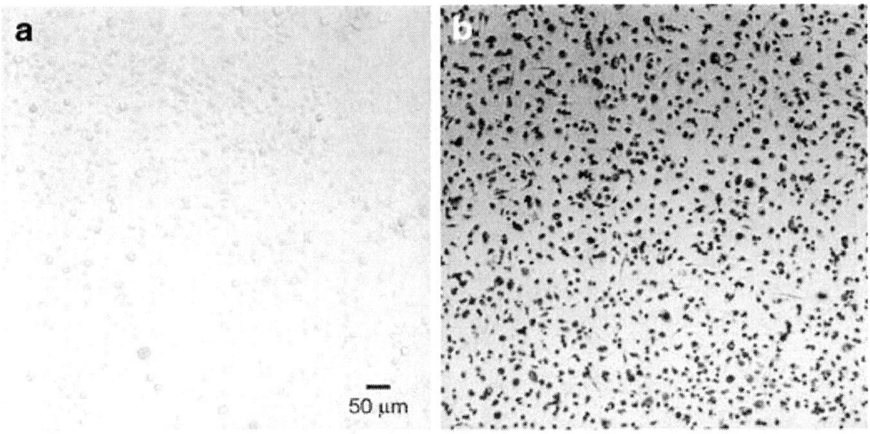

Figure 1. Phagocytosis of gold-silica nanoshells by macrophages. Photomicrographs of transmitted light images of macrophages (control) (**a**) and following 3 days incubation with nanoshells (**b**). The visualization was performed using a Bio-Rad Radiance 2100 MP Rainbow Confocal/Multiphoton System. The images were acquired using the ×10 objective

from this two-dimensional photomicrograph that the uptake is within the nucleus, with three-dimensional imaging it can be observed that the microspheres are perinuclear, which is confirmed by transmission electron microscopy (TEM) imaging. The TEM image also shows a much larger number of microspheres phagocytosed in relation to the numbers of gold conjugate. As with the phagocytosis of the nanoshells, the phagocytosis of the microspheres and gold conjugates appears to be robust in every monocyte/macrophage exposed to the nanoparticles.

To test the hypothesis that systemically injected, nanoparticle-laden monocytes/macrophages would home in to intracranial metastatic deposits by crossing the blood–brain barrier a mouse model of breast cancer metastatic to the brain, the human MDA-MB-231 BR "brain-seeking" (231-BR) cell lines expressing enhanced green fluorescent protein (eGFP), was utilized (Yoneda et al. 2001; Palmieri et al. 2007). Twelve mice underwent intracardiac injection of the 231-BR cells of

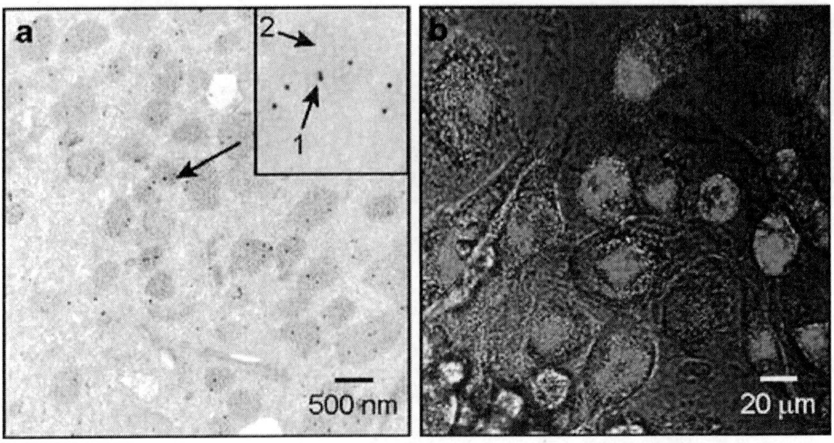

Figure 2. Cellular uptake of gold-silica nanoshells and red fluorescent microspheres by monocytes/macrophages. **a**Transmission electron micrograph of monocytes/macrophages incubated with nanoparticles reveals intracellular localization of gold conjugates (*arrow 1 in inset*) as well as the ingested red fluorescent microspheres located in the vacuoles in the cytoplasm (*arrow 2 in inset*). **b** Fluorescence microscopy imaging shows significant intensity of red fluorescence (580/605 nm) indicating the presence of intracellular red fluorescent microspheres

which three died following injection. The remaining nine mice underwent tail vein injection of the nano-laden macrophages; at necropsy it was determined that six of these nine mice had actually developed brain metastasis, three had not. Imaging of the freshly dissected brains of mice injected 24 h earlier with the loaded macrophages reveals that the green [metastasis] and red [microspheres] fluorescence overlap each other with maximal intensity in a posterior direction (Fig. 3). This suggests that the microspheres have been successfully delivered to the metastases.

Confocal microscopy of the brain sections reveals eGFP expressing tumor cells forming brain metastases (Fig. 4a). Red fluorescence from the microspheres was observed within the metastases of two of the six mice with brain metastases. To determine if the red fluorescent microspheres were contained within human macrophages, brain sections were stained with anti-human CD68 antibodies labeled with APEX Pacific Blue fluorochrome. As observable in Fig. 4b, the

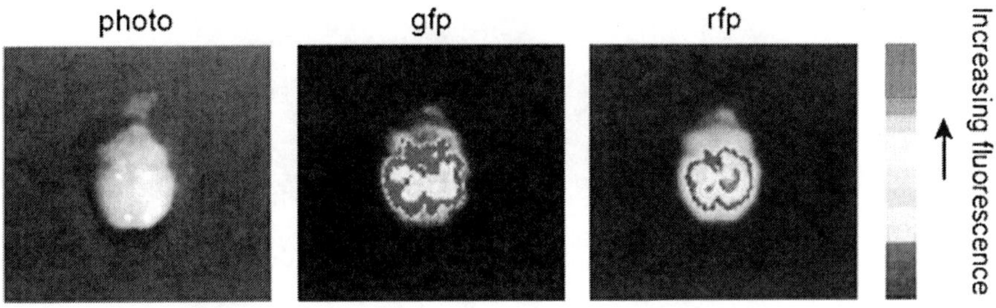

Figure 3. Ex vivo images of whole brain of mice injected with monocytes/macrophages loaded with red fluorescent microspheres. The presence and location of metastatic brain tumor foci (green fluorescence) and macrophages loaded with the red fluorescent microspheres was determined after resection using an optical imaging system. The images of green fluorescence (green fluorescent protein, *gfp*) and red fluorescence (red fluorescent particles, *rfp*) were taken after exposure times of 100 and 500 ms, respectively. The intensity of the fluorescence in different area of the brain is measured using the signal intensity bar. Values are normalized relative to the exposure times

microspheres are contained with the macrophages, which are intercalated within the metastases. Tail vein injection in athymic *nu/nu* mice is technically challenging given the small size of this vessel. In the four mice for which no delivery of nanoparticles is observed, the hypothesis is that the needle transversed the vein and the macrophage suspension infiltrated the subcutaneous tissue surrounding the tail vein rather than entering it and the systemic circulation.

Whole-body fluorescence imaging of mice following the systemic injection of macrophages containing the fluorescently labeled microspheres shows an initial [within minutes] and temporary residence in the lungs followed by residence in the liver and spleen which occurs over hours to days (Fig. 5 and data not shown).

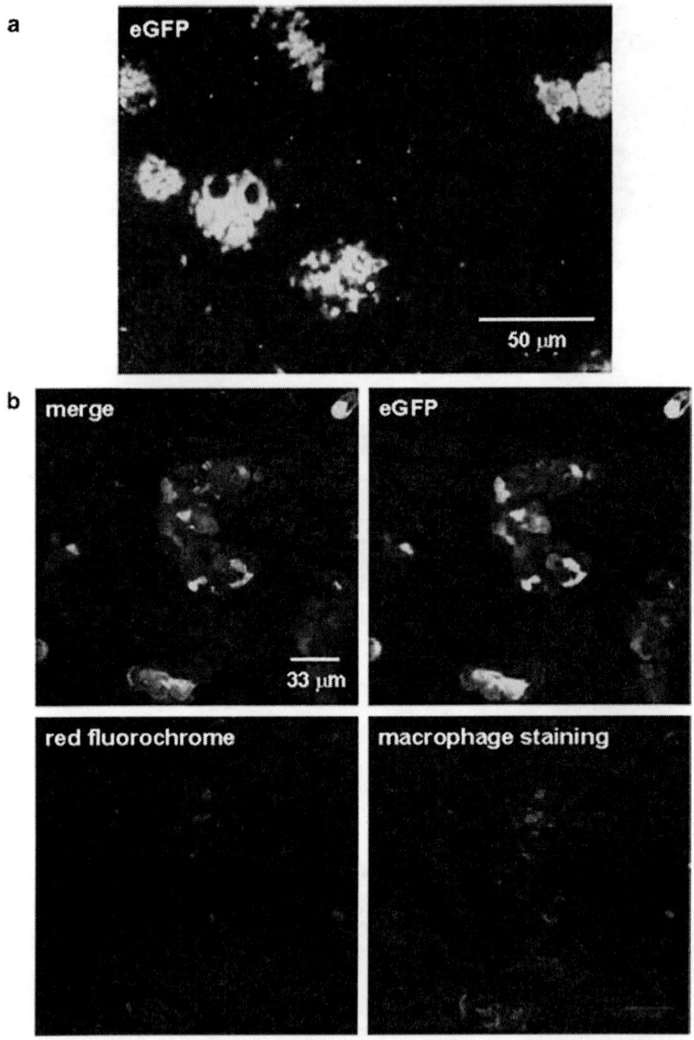

Figure 4. Histologic images of brain metastatic tumor cells. **a** Paraffin-embedded section of the brain of a control mouse showing the formation of metastatic brain lesions derived from eGFP expressing breast cancer cells. **b** Macrophages loaded with red fluorescent nanospheres infiltrating the brain metastases detected by immunofluorescent staining using anti-human CD68 antibodies labeled with APEX Pacific Blue fluorochrome. *Green fluorescence* is emitted by the brain metastatic tumor cells. *Red fluorescence* and *blue fluorescence* result from the red fluorescent nanospheres included within the macrophages and the macrophage staining, respectively

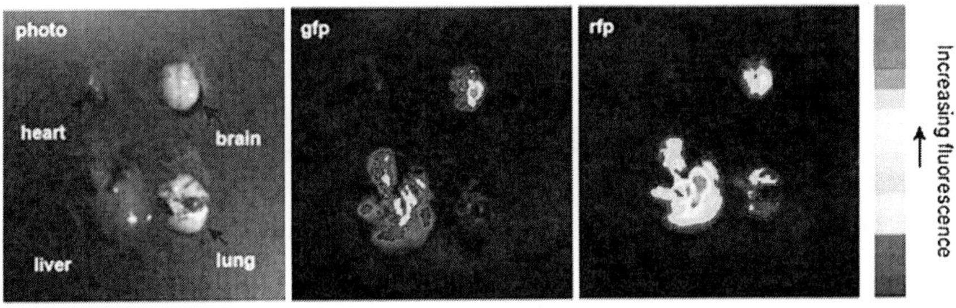

Figure 5. Biodistribution images of mouse organs following injection of monocytes/macrophages loaded with red fluorescent nanospheres. The distribution of metastatic tumor foci (*green fluorescence*) and macrophages loaded with the red fluorescent nanospheres in the brain, lung, liver, and the heart was determined after resection using an optical imaging system. The images of *green fluorescence* (green fluorescent protein, *gfp*) and red fluorescence (red fluorescent particles, *rfp*) were taken after exposure time of 600 ms. The intensity of the fluorescence in different area of the organs is measured using the signal intensity bar. There is abundant uptake of microsphere-laden macrophages in the liver. Brain metastases are located in the left hemisphere of the brain. The distribution of the *red fluorescence* within the brain overlaps that of the green fluorescence suggesting that the microsphere-laden macrophages are co-located with the cerebral metastases

Our work is focused on the treatment of metastases from breast cancer. This is a critical unmet clinical need. The purpose our study was to test the hypothesis that nanoparticle-laden monocytes/macrophages would home in to intracranial metastatic deposits by crossing the blood–brain barrier following injection into the systemic circulation. The activated macrophages not only cross the BBB but as shown in Fig. 3, they envelop the metastatic cells delivering the loaded nanoparticle to less than a cell width away from the nearest metastatic cell. This "Trojan Horse" delivery method has been designed to address the challenges to successful cancer nanotherapeutics posed by the tumor microenvironment. It takes advantage of the recruitment of macrophages to the metastatic lesions; this is active transport of the nanovectors likely the result of the productions of chemoattractant(s) by the metastasis, which does not require the Enhanced Permeability and Retention effect or diffusion of the nanovector.

Injection of monocytes/macrophages into the systemic circulation resulted in residence in the liver and lungs as well as transport to the brain metastasis. This result was predictable. Previous studies have demonstrated that when marrow derived mononuclear cells or peritoneal macrophages are injected into the systemic circulation they home to the same tissues and have a distribution similar to endogenous macrophages (Kennedy and Abkowitz 1998; Freeman et al. 1999). This distribution is to treatment advantage. Monocyte/macrophages as delivery vehicles can be envisioned as a pan-metastatic treatment because, in addition to the brain, the lungs and liver are frequent sites of metastatic disease. What is unknown and to be determined in follow-on studies is the exact percentage of the administered dose that actually crosses the BBB. Also to be determined is the rate at which the macrophage will discharge its cargo and whether or not it will be necessary to destroy the macrophage for this to happen.

4 CONCLUSIONS

To our knowledge, we report the first successful demonstration of the active delivery, using macrophages, of nanoparticles to brain metastases and it paves the way for testing this method to deliver other nanovectors including nanorods, hollow nanospheres in the sub-100- and sub-50 nm range as well as nanoformulated therapeutics.

ACKNOWLEDGMENTS

This work was funded by The Breast Cancer Research Foundation (S.E.C., M.C.); Susan G. Komen for the Cure®, grant number SAC 110004 (S.B.) and grant number SAC110025 (H.N.); the Robert A. Welch Foundation (N.J.H.; C-1220), and The Division of General Surgery, Indiana University School of Medicine (S.E.C.).

OPEN ACCESS

REFERENCES

1. Afergan E, Epstein H, Dahan R, Koroukhov N, Rohekar K, Danenberg HD, Golomb G (2008) Delivery of serotonin to the brain by monocytes following phagocytosis of liposomes. J Contr Release 132(2):84–90

2. Bardhan R, Grady NK, Halas NJ (2008) Nanoscale control of near-infrared fluorescence enhancement using Au nanoshells. Small 4:1716–1722.

3. Bardhan R, Chen WX, Perez-Torres C, Bartels M, Huschka RM, Zhao LL, Morosan E, Pautler RG, Joshi A, Halas NJ (2009a) Nanoshells with targeted simultaneous enhancement of magnetic and optical imaging and photothermal therapeutic response. Adv Funct Mater 19(24):3901–3909.

4. Bardhan R, Grady NK, Cole JR, Joshi A, Halas NJ (2009b) Fluorescence Enhancement by Au Nanostructures: Nanoshells and Nanorods. ACS Nano.

5. Barnholtz-Sloan JS, Sloan AE, Davis FG, Vigneau FD, Lai P, Sawaya RE (2004) Incidence proportions of brain metastases in patients diagnosed (1973 to 2001) in the Metropolitan Detroit Cancer Surveillance System. J Clin Oncol 22(14):2865–2872.

6. Begley DJ (2004) ABC transporters and the blood–brain barrier. Curr Pharm Des 10(12):1295–1312

7. Bendell JC, Domchek SM, Burstein HJ, Harris L, Younger J, Kuter I, Bunnell C, Rue M, Gelman R, Winer E (2003) Central nervous system metastases in women who receive trastuzumab-based therapy for metastatic breast carcinoma. Cancer 97(12):2972–2977.

8. Brinson BE, Lassiter JB, Levin CS, Bardhan R, Mirin N, Halas NJ (2008) Nanoshells made easy: improving Au layer growth on nanoparticle surfaces. Langmuir 24(24):14166–14171.

9. Burstein HJ, Lieberman G, Slamon DJ, Winer EP, Klein P (2005) Isolated central nervous system metastases in patients with HER2-overexpressing advanced breast cancer treated with first-line trastuzumab-based therapy. Ann Oncol 16(11):1772–1777

10. Cairncross JG, Posner JB (1983) The management of brain metastases. Oncology of the nervous system. Nijhoff, Boston

11. Carman AJ, Mills JH, Krenz A, Kim D-G, Bynoe MS (2011) Adenosine receptor signaling modulates permeability of the blood–brain barrier. J Neurosci 31:13272–13280

12. Choi MR, Stanton-Maxey KJ, Stanley JK, Levin CS, Bardhan R, Akin D, Badve S, Sturgis J, Robinson JP, Bashir R, Halas NJ, Clare SE (2007) A cellular Trojan Horse for delivery of therapeutic nanoparticles into tumors. Nano Lett 7(12):3759–3765.

13. Clayton AJ, Danson S, Jolly S, Ryder WD, Burt PA, Stewart AL, Wilkinson PM, Welch RS, Magee B, Wilson G, Howell A, Wardley AM (2004) Incidence of cerebral metastases in patients treated with trastuzumab for metastatic breast cancer. Br J Cancer 91(4):639–643.

14. Dou H, Grotepas CB, McMillan JM, Destache CJ, Chaubal M, Werling J, Kipp J, Rabinow B, Gendelman HE (2009) Macrophage delivery of nanoformulated antiretroviral drug to the brain in a murine model of neuroAIDS. J Immunol 183(1):661–669

15. Duff DG, Baiker PP, Edwards A (1993) A new hydrosol of gold clusters. 1. Formation and particle size variation. Langmuir 9:2301–2309

16. Freeman BJ, Roberts MS, Vogler CA, Nicholes A, Hofling AA, Sands MS (1999) Behavior and therapeutic efficacy of beta-glucuronidase-positive mononuclear phagocytes in a murine model of mucopolysaccharidosis type VII. Blood 94(6):2142–2150

17. Graff CL, Pollack GM (2004) Drug transport at the blood–brain barrier and the choroid plexus. Curr Drug Metabol 5(1):95–108

18. Grossi F, Scolaro T, Tixi L, Loprevite M, Ardizzoni A (2001) The role of systemic chemotherapy in the treatment of brain

metastases from small-cell lung cancer. Crit Rev Oncol Hematol 37(1):61–67

19. Hochstenbag MM, Twijnstra A, Wilmink JT, Wouters EF, ten Velde GP (2000) Asymptomatic brain metastases (BM) in small cell lung cancer (SCLC): MR-imaging is useful at initial diagnosis. J Neurooncol 48(3):243–248

20. Kennedy DW, Abkowitz JL (1998) Mature monocytic cells enter tissues and engraft. Proc Natl Acad Sci U S A 95(25):14944–14949

21. Klos KJ, O'Neill BP (2004) Brain metastases. Neurologist 10(1):31–46.

22. Lin NU, Winer EP (2007) Brain metastases: the HER2 paradigm. Clin Cancer Res 13(6):1648–1655

23. Lin NU, Claus E, Sohl J, Razzak AR, Arnaout A, Winer EP (2008) Sites of distant recurrence and clinical outcomes in patients with metastatic triple-negative breast cancer: high incidence of central nervous system metastases. Cancer 113(10):2638–2645.

24. Lo SS, Chang EL, Suh JH (2005) Stereotactic radiosurgery with and without whole-brain radiotherapy for newly diagnosed brain metastases. Expert Rev Neurother 5(4):487–495.

25. Lockman PR, Mittapalli RK, Taskar KS, Rudraraju V, Gril B, Bohn KA, Adkins CE, Roberts A, Thorsheim HR, Gaasch JA, Huang S, Palmieri D, Steeg PS, Smith QR (2010) Heterogeneous blood-tumor barrier permeability determines drug efficacy in experimental brain metastases of breast cancer. Clin Cancer Res 16(23):5664–5678.

26. Mahmoud-Ahmed ASS, Lee SY et al (2002) Results of whole brain radiotherapy in patients with brain metastases from breast cancer: a retrospective study. Int J Radiat Oncol Biol Phys 54:810–817

27. Morantz RA, Wood GW, Foster M, Clark M, Gollahon K (1979) Macrophages in experimental and human brain tumors. Part 2: studies of the macrophage content of human brain tumors. J Neurosurg 50(3):305–311.

28. Muldoon LL, Soussain C, Jahnke K, Johanson C, Siegal T, Smith QR, Hall WA, Hynynen K, Senter PD, Peereboom DM, Neuwelt EA (2007) Chemotherapy delivery issues in central nervous system malignancy: a reality check. J Clin Oncol 25(16):2295–2305

29. Oldenburg SJ, Averitt RD, Westcott SL, Halas NJ (1998) Nanoengineering of optical resonances. Chem Phys Lett 288:243–247

30. Palmieri D, Bronder JL, Herring JM, Yoneda T, Weil RJ, Stark AM, Kurek R, Vega-Valle E, Feigenbaum L, Halverson D, Vortmeyer AO, Steinberg SM, Aldape K, Steeg PS (2007) Her-2 overexpression increases the metastatic outgrowth of breast cancer cells in the brain. Cancer Res 67(9):4190–4198

31. Pardridge WM (2005) The blood–brain barrier: bottleneck in brain drug development. NeuroRx 2(1):3–14

32. Patchell RA, Regine WF (2003) The rationale for adjuvant whole brain radiation therapy with radiosurgery in the treatment of single brain metastases. Tech Canc Res Treat 2(2):111–115

33. Posner JB (1992) Management of brain metastases. Rev Neurol (Paris) 148(6–7):477–487

34. Posner JB (1995) Neurologic complications of cancer. Davis, Philadelphia

35. Schackert G, Simmons RD, Buzbee TM, Hume DA, Fidler IJ (1988) Macrophage infiltration into experimental brain metastases: occurrence through an intact blood–brain barrier. J Natl Canc Inst 80(13):1027–1034

36. Seute T, Leffers P, ten Velde GP, Twijnstra A (2004) Neurologic disorders in 432 consecutive patients with small cell lung carcinoma. Cancer 100(4):801–806.

37. Sneed PK, Lamborn KR, Forstner JM, McDermott MW, Chang S, Park E, Gutin PH, Phillips TL, Wara WM, Larson DA (1999) Radiosurgery for brain metastases: is whole brain radiotherapy necessary? Int J Radiat Oncol Biol Phys 43(3):549–558

38. Stemmler HJ, Kahlert S, Siekiera W, Untch M, Heinrich B, Heinemann V (2006) Characteristics of patients with brain metastases receiving trastuzumab for HER2 overexpressing metastatic breast cancer. Breast 15(2):219–225

39. Stoeber W, Fink A, Bihb EJ (1968) Controlled growth of monodisperse silica spheres in the micron size range. J Colloid Interface Sci 26:62–69

40. Strik HM, Stoll M, Meyermann R (2004) Immune cell infiltration of intrinsic and metastatic intracranial tumours. Anticancer Res 24(1):37–42

41. Stuschke M, Eberhardt W, Pottgen C, Stamatis G, Wilke H, Stuben G et al (1999) Prophylactic cranial irradiation in locally advanced non-small cell lung cancer after multimodality treatment: long-term follow-up and investigations of late neuropsychologic effects. J Clin Oncol 17:2700–2709

42. Tam F, Goodrich GP, Johnson BR, Halas NJ (2007) Plasmonic enhancement of molecular fluorescence. Nano Lett 7:496–501.

43. Walker AE, Robins M, Weinfeld FD (1985) Epidemiology of brain tumors: the national survey of intracranial neoplasms. Neurology 35(2):219–226

44. Weil RJ, Palmieri DC, Bronder JL, Stark AM, Steeg PS (2005) Breast cancer metastasis to the central nervous system. Am J Pathol 167(4):913–920

45. Yau T, Swanton C, Chua S, Sue A, Walsh G, Rostom A, Johnston SR, O'Brien ME, Smith IE (2006) Incidence, pattern and timing of brain metastases among patients with advanced breast cancer treated with trastuzumab. Acta Oncol 45(2):196–201

46. Yoneda T, Williams PJ, Hiraga T, Niewolna M, Nishimura R (2001) A bone-seeking clone exhibits different biological properties from the MDA-MB-231 parental human breast cancer cells and a brain-seeking clone in vivo and in vitro. J Bone Miner Res 16(8):1486–1495

Chapter 5

Nanocarriers for Diagnosis and Targeting of Breast Cancer

Arun Sharma, Nitin Jain, and Rashmi Sareen

Department of Pharmaceutics, School of Pharmaceutical Sciences, Shoolini University, Bajhol, Solan, Himachal Pradesh 173229, India

ABSTRACT

Breast cancer nanotherapeutics is consistently progressing and being used to remove the various limitations of conventional method available for the diagnosis and treatment of breast cancer. Nanoparticles provide an interdisciplinary area for research in imaging, diagnosis, and targeting of breast cancer. With advanced physicochemical properties and better bioavailability, they show prolonged blood circulation with efficient tumor targeting. Passive targeting mechanisms by using leaky vasculature, tumor microenvironment, or direct local application and active targeting approaches using receptor antibody, amplification in the ability of nanoparticles to target specific tumor can be achieved. Nanoparticles are able to reduce cytotoxic effect of the active anticancer drugs by increasing cancer cell targeting in comparison to conventional formulations. Various nanoparticles-based formulations are in the preclinical and clinical stages of development; among them, polymeric drug micelles, liposomes, dendrimer, carbon nanotubes, and nanorods are the most common. In this review, we have discussed the role of nanoparticles with respect to oncology, by particularly focusing on the breast cancer and various nanodelivery systems used for targeting action.

1. INTRODUCTION

The development and inventions of various nanoscale technologies have provided new field of research among chemistry, biology, toxicology, medicine, material science, engineering, and mathematics. Nanotechnology is the manipulation of cellular and molecular components of matter. Nanotechnology yields the incredibly small particles of size ranging between tens to hundred nanometers. These small particles are known as nanoparticles, which are considered as the engineered materials mainly cluster of molecules, atoms, and molecular fragments. These innovations are referred to as nanomedicines by the National Institute of Health and have the potential of carrying chemotherapeutic agents to the targeted site. Being a nanotechnologically engineered material, nanocarriers must have four characteristics of its own such as size of the material should be in nanometer, properties of the material should be in nanoscopic dimensions, behavior of the material should be displayable with suitable mathematical expression, material should be man-made [1]. Rationale behind the development on nanocarriers is that polymeric particles, metal, and semiconductors have unique structural, magnetic, optical, and electronic properties which make them a suitable drug delivery carrier for targeting [2].

Nanoscale devices form the concept of biodegradable, self-assembled nanoparticles which can be targeted to the cancer-affected area and can be used as contrast imaging agents [3]. Breast cancer is a major ongoing public health problem, and at present, there are less curative options for the patients suffering from breast cancer, while emerging nanotechnologies give a promising new approach for the early detection and treatment of breast cancer. Nanoparticles provide an interdisciplinary area for research in imaging, diagnosis and targeting of breast cancer (Figure 1).

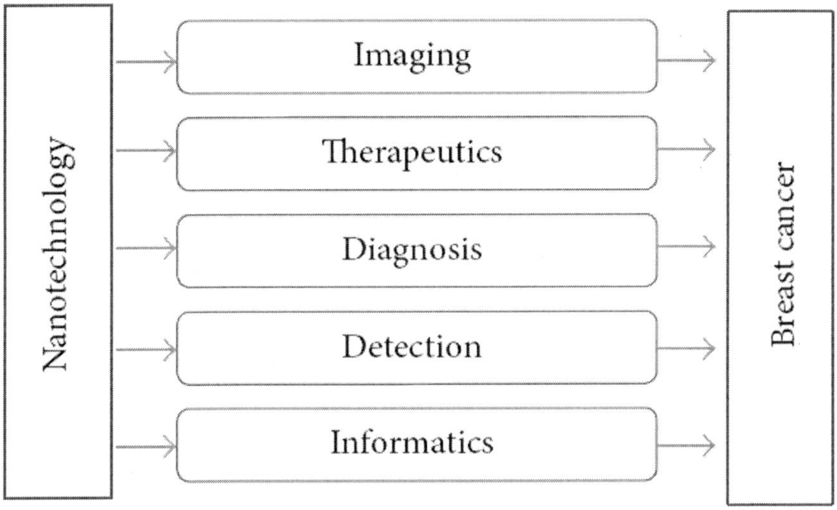

Figure 1: Area of nanotechnology in breast cancer.

2. HUMAN BREAST CANCER

It is also called prostate cancer which originates from breast tissue. Breast cancer is most frequently diagnosed in women; approximately up to 7% of breast cancers are being diagnosed in women having their age below 40 years and less than 4% in women below the age of 35 years [4]. In young women, the breast cancer is uncommon [5]. Breast cancer is a heterogeneous disease and has different subtypes, which are based on the expression level of progesterone receptor, estrogen receptor, and HER-2/neu receptor (human epidermal growth factor receptor 2) [6]. Breast cancer stem cells play a major role in growth and formation of metastastic breast cancer. Breast cancer stem cells have a potential for undergoing self-renewal and side by side give rise to daughter cells which results in the formation of tumor cells in bulk having self-replicating potential. Breast cancer stem cells make small-small part of most tumors, whereas in others like in melanoma it comprises 25% of total mass [7]. Based on the TNM (tumor nodes metastasized) system, breast cancer can be divided into four stages: based on the size of tumor (T), whether the tumor has spread to the lymph nodes (N) in the armpits or not, and whether the tumor has metastasized (M).

Types of stages in breast cancer are as follows.(1)Stage 0: it consists of three types of breast carcinoma.(a)Ductal carcinoma in situ (DCIS): this condition is noninvasive and the abnormal cells are found in lining of the breast duct, but the spreading of the abnormal cells is not outside the tissues of breast.(b)Lobular carcinoma in situ (LCIS): in this condition, the abnormal cells are present in the lobules of the breast. This rarely occurs as invasive cancer. Presence of abnormal cells in lobules increases the risk of breast cancer.(c)Paget disease of the nipple: in this condition, abnormal cells are found in nipple only.(2)Stage I: it is divided into two stages Ia and Ib.(a)Stage Ia: tumor is 2 cm or small and not found outside the breast.(b)Stage Ib: small clusters are found in the lymph nodes and either tumor is 2 centimeters or not found in breast.(3)Stage II: it is divided into Stage IIa and Stage IIb.(a)Stage IIa: tumor is found to be larger than 2 cm but not larger than 5 cm. Cancer has not spread to the lymph nodes.(b)Stage IIb: tumor is larger than 2 cm but not greater than 5 cm. Cancer spreads to 1 to 3 axillary lymph nodes or to the lymph node near the breastbone.(4)Stage III: it is divided into IIIa and IIIb.(a)Stage IIIa: the tumor is larger than 5 cm and cancer spreads to 1 to 3 axillary lymph nodes.(b)Stage IIIb: the tumor spreads to 9 axillary lymph nodes.(c)Stage IIIc: tumor may be of any size causing swelling or ulcer and has spread to chest wall. Cancer has spread to 10 or more axillary lymph nodes.

In treatment point of view, Stage IIIc is divided into operable and inoperable.

(5) Stage IV: cancer has spread to other parts of the body, mostly to lungs, bone, or liver.

Now nanotechnology comes up with a bright way to overcome the problem related to breast cancer. Many researchers focus on different types of nanotechnology-based drug delivery system and their mechanism of action in such type of carcinoma. Various types of nanoparticles are used for the detection of breast carcinoma; among these, carbon nanorods (gold nanorods [8]), nanowires (Au nanowires [9]), and nanobarcodes are the most common. Semiconductor quantum dots (QDs) are a new advancement in nanotechnology; these are small nanoscale light-emitting particles and are better in comparison to fluorescent protein and organic dyes. Unique electronic and optical properties of semiconductor quantum dots make them suitable agents for cellular and in vivo biomolecular imaging [10]. Yu et al. had synthesized cadmium oxide-selenium powdered QD of 2-nanometer diameter approximately that produces a blue emission and a 7-nanometer diameter quantum dots showing red light emission [11]. Superimposed optical images and X-ray have shown high resolution and high sensitivity for the location of not only bigger breast cancer but also for small abnormal tumor daughter cells. Chemotherapy in the form of nanoparticles can be delivered by active and passive pathway. Nanotechnology is used in molecular cancer diagnosis by employing biomarker and nanoparticles probes. Multiple ligands can be conjugated on tiny single nanoparticles and provide a multivalent effect for increased specificity and binding affinity, hence used as suitable diagnostic agent.

3. CHEMOTHERAPEUTIC NANOPARTICLES

Chemotherapeutic drugs are "cytotoxic" in nature, which means cell-killing drugs. They play a vital role in the management and treatment of both initial-stage breast cancer and advanced breast cancer. Cytotoxic chemotherapy is essential for palliation of women with hormone-insensitive or hormone-refractory breast cancer and is administered into human body by taking therapeutic goals into consideration such as relief from pain, disease progression, relief from symptoms, prolonged life of patient, and improvement in mood disturbances of suffering women [12]. It is administered orally or by intravenous injection. It works systemically by killing cancer cells throughout the body along with normal cells, which leads to various short-term and long-term side effects. Mostly chemotherapy is used in advanced breast cancer, but may also be used to treat early-stage breast cancer. By using nanoparticles as carrier, cytotoxic side effects may be reduced and targeting may be achieved.

Even the most advanced chemotherapeutic agents do not differentiate between normal cells and cancerous cells efficiently, which leads to nonspecific distribution of drug in the body and causes systemic toxicity and adverse effects [13]. The maximum allowable dose of the drug gets limited; in order to achieve the desired therapeutic effect in the tumor tissue, large quantity of drug has to be administered in order to achieve anticancer effect, but this is not economical and undesirable toxicity may also appear [13, 14]. Nanoparticles are the promising carrier system for the targeted delivery of chemotherapeutic agents by using both active and passive targetings, and systemic toxicity or normal cell toxicity can be avoided [14].

4. ACTIVE AND PASSIVE DRUG DELIVERY

Mostly the nanoparticles accumulate in tumor cells as expected because of pathophysiological characteristics of tumor blood supplying vessels. There is an increased demand of oxygen and nutrients to the tumor cells or tissue as it is increasing in size as well as in its shape. In order to supply nutrients and oxygen, new blood capillary system is being developed which is not developed properly and hence becomes permeable to some particles of specific size [15]. Types of targeting are shown in Figure 2.

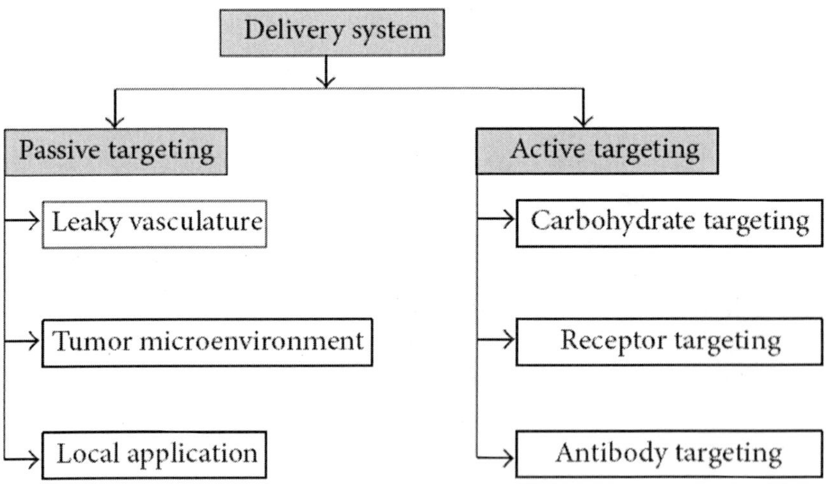

Figure 2: Types of targeting by nanodelivery system.

4.1. Passive Targeting by Nanoparticles

Passive targeting can differentiate between normal and tumor tissues and has the advantage of direct permeation to tumor tissue (Figure 3).

Drug administered passively in the form of prodrug or inactive form, when exposed to tumor tissue, becomes highly active. Nanoparticles that are expected to show localization on specific tissues or at specific sites of disease follow the biological mechanisms such as ERS (enhanced retention system) or EPS (enhanced permeation system) effect. To prolong the circulation and to achieve increased targeting efficiency, the size should be below 100 nanometers in diameter and the surface of the nanoparticles should be hydrophilic in nature in order to circumvent clearance by macrophages. The hydrophilic surface of the nanoparticles provides protection against plasma protein adsorption to the surface, and this can be made possible by using hydrophilic polymer coating, like polyethylene glycol (PEG), polysaccharides, poloxamines, or poloxamers or by using block or branched amphiphilic copolymer [16, 17]. Passive targeting system is further classified into (a) leaky vasculature, (b) tumor microenvironment, and (c) local drug application.

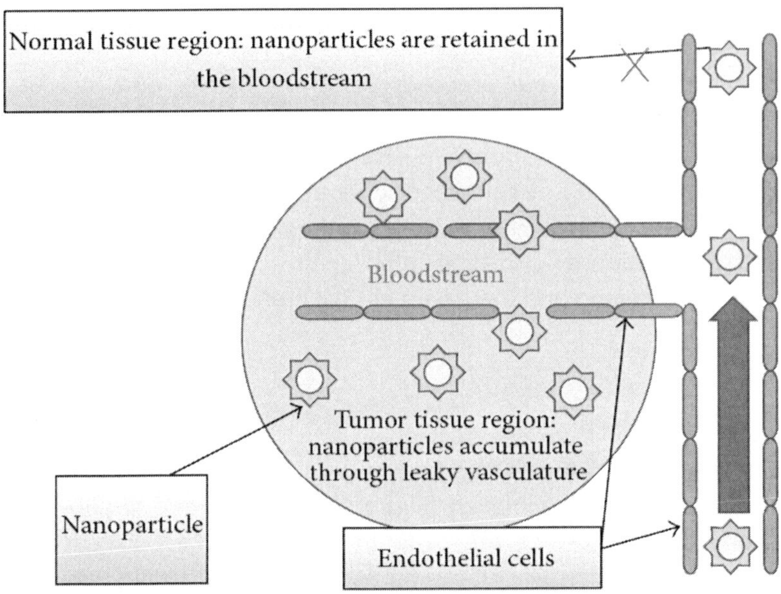

Figure 3: Passive targeting.

(1) Leaky Vasculature. Maeda and Matsumura had first displayed the enhanced permeation and retention effect by using polymer to form

nanoparticles. Concept of enhanced permeability and retention is based on two factors [18]. (a) The capillary endothelium system in malignant tissue shows more permeation to macromolecules in comparison to normal tissue endothelium; this makes circulating polymeric nanoparticles permeable into the tumor. (b) Tumor lacks lymphatic drainage; hence, more drug gets accumulated in side tumor tissue. By using a suitable biodegradable polymer, the concentration of drug gets 10 to 100 times higher than that of free circulating drug.

(2) Tumor Microenvironment. Tumor microenvironment provides the advantage of the passive drug targeting. Active state of chemotherapeutic agent is conjugated with tumor-specific material and administered into the body. When this drug-polymer conjugate reaches its desired destination, tumor environment converts into more active form. This phenomenon is called tumor activated prodrug therapy. Mansour et al. had developed an albumin-bound form of doxorubicin and showed in an in vitro study, that doxorubicin was efficiently cleaved by matrix metalloproteniase-2 [19].

(3) Local Drug Application. Direct application of the chemotherapeutic agent locally to tumor site prevents systemic toxicity and increased concentration of drug at the tumor site. Nomura et al. had synthesized intratumoral injection of mitomycin c-dextran conjugate; this results in increased concentration of anticancer drug at tumor site and decreased systemic toxicity [20]. Prabha and Labhasetwar had worked on nanoparticles-mediated wild-type p53 gene for breast cancer and observed the sustained and increased antiproliferative effect [21].

4.2. Active Targeting

By conjugating the nanoparticles with a drug to desired target site, an active targeting may be achieved (Figure4). Active targeting allows the increased accumulation of the drug in cancer tissue. Directing the nanoparticles to the cancer cell can be done by the following ways. This approach is basically based on the specific interactions, like lectin carbohydrate, ligand receptor, and antibody-antigen [22].

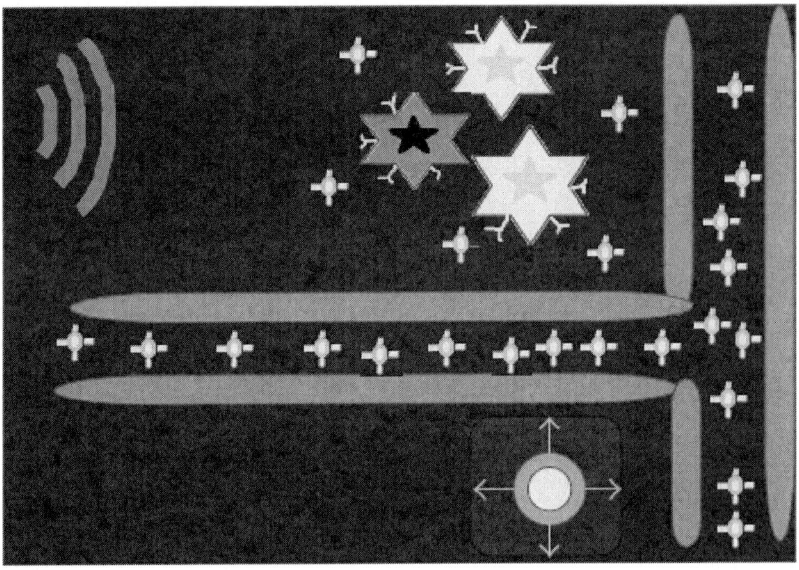

Figure 4: Active targeting.

(1) Carbohydrate-Directed Targeting. An excellent example of active drug targeting is lectin carbohydrate. Carbohydrates present on the surface of tumor cell are different than those in the normal cell. Lectin is a nonimmunological protein, which is capable of binding and recognizing the glycoproteins which are present on the surface of the cell. Certain carbohydrates interact with lectins to form the cell-specific binding moieties. These carbohydrates moieties can be used for target drug delivery system for lectins (lectin direct targeting); similarly, lectins can also be used for the targeting of the surface carbohydrates (reverse lectin targeting). Specific carbohydrate present on tumor can be targeted and anticancer effect may be achieved.

(2) Receptor Targeting. Endocytosis plays a major role in this type of active targeting. Ideally drug is being conjugated to polymer carrier; this carrier gets incorporated into the cell and localized at the cell surface. Once the drug-polymer conjugate reaches the tumor intracellular environment, dissociation of drug takes place and anticancer effect is being achieved.

Three essential molecules can be delivered by this targeting system:(a)antigen or receptors,(b)drug-polymer conjugates, and(c)ligands or antibodies.

(3) Antibody Targeting. Kirpotin et al. had described the evidence of monoclonal antibody mechanism for targeting nanoparticles to solid tumor tissue in vivo. Prepared formulation was targeted towards the HER-2 (human epidermal growth factor receptor 2) cancer and was prepared by conjugating the anti-HER-2 monoclonal antibody fragments with liposomal-grafted polyethylene glycol chain. Increased cellular uptake of the drug was observed; hence, antibody targeting provides the new opportunities for drug delivery system in breast cancer [22].

5. TYPES OF NANODELIVERY SYSTEM

Different types of nanodelivery system having different physicochemical properties with different materials have been formulated so far in order to cure diseases. Most commonly studied among these are polymeric micelles, dendrimers, liposomes, carbon nanotubes, and nanorods (Table 1).

Table 1: Types of nanocarriers for drug delivery.

Sr. no.	System	Structure	Characteristics	Example of compounds	References
1	Polymeric micelles	Hydrophobic core and hydrophilic shell are formed by assembling amphiphilic block copolymer	(a) Efficient carrier system for hydrophilic drug (b) Biodegradable, self-assembling, and biocompatible (c) Potential targeting (d) Functional modification	PEG-b-p(LA-CO-MCG) PEG-B-PCL Curcumin micelles	[1–3]
2	Dendrimers	Synthetic polymer forming nanosized branched structure with repeated units and regular pattern	(a) Uniformity in size, shape, and branch length (b) Tuned pharmacokinetics and biodistribution (c) Increased surface area, increased loading (d) Targeting is achieved	G4 PAMAM-D DOX-PPI-FA	[3, 4]
3	Liposomes	Lipid bilayer memberane forming self assembled closed colloidal structures	(a) Biocompatible (b) Longer duration of circulation (c) Amphiphilic	DOX-p18-4 Pegylated liposomal of doxorubicin	[1, 4]
4	Carbon nanotubes	Benzene ring forming carbon cylindrical structure	(a) Multiple function (b) Chemical modification (c) Water soluble and biocompatible	SWNTs-PTX SWNTs-siRNA	
5	Nanorods	Metals or semiconducting materials forming rod shape structure.	(a) Efficient loading (b) Increased surface area (c) Biocompatible (d) Specific tumor targeting	HER-PEG-GNRs ZnO-NRs-DNR PPDME-ZnO-NRs	[1, 4, 5]

PEG-b-p(LA-CO-MCG)-CISPLATIN, PEG-B-PCL (polyethylene glycol-paclitaxel), G4 PAMAM-D (G4 polyamidoamine dendrimer), DOX-PPI-FA (doxorubicin-polypropylene imine-folic acid), DOX-p18-4 (doxorubicin-peptide ligands), SWNTs-PTX (single-walled carbon nanotubes-paclitaxel), SWNTs-siRNA (single-walled carbon nanotubes-small interfering RNA), HER-PEG-GNRs (herceptin-polyethylene gold nanorods), ZnO-NRs-DNR (zinc oxide-nanorods daunorubicin), PPDME-ZnO-NRs (protoporphyrin dimethyl ester-zinc oxide-nanorods).

5.1. Polymeric-Based Drug Carrier

The drug is either covalently bound or physically entrapped in polymer matrix, depending on the method of preparation [23]. Polymers can be divided into two groups: natural and synthetic polymers. Polymers like chitosan, albumin, and heparin occur naturally and have been a choice of material for the delivery of DNA, protein, and oligonucleotides as well as drug. Gradishar et al. had formulated conjugate of paclitaxel with serum albumin to form nanoparticles formulation. This drug-polymer conjugate has been applied for the treatment of metastatic breast [24].

Among synthetic polymers, N-(2-hydroxypropyl)-methacrylamide copolymer (HPMA), poly-1-glutamic acid (PGA), polystyrene maleic anhydride copolymer, and polyethylene glycol (PEG) are common. Polycaprolactone and polyalkyl cyanoacrylates are widely used polymers in nanodelivery. PGA is the first biodegradable polymer to be used for conjugate synthesis [25]. HPMC and PEG are nonbiodegradable synthetic polymers which are most widely used [26].

5.1.1. Polymeric Micelles

Micelles are generally colloidal particles having a size range usually in between 5 and 100 nanometers in diameter. Micelles mainly consist of surface active agents (surfactant) or amphiphiles, which are made up of two different regions, hydrophobic tail and mostly hydrophilic head. Amphiphiles exist as monomers in aqueous medium at low concentration as a true solution. By increasing the concentration of amphiphiles, self-assembled aggregations are being formed called micelles within the narrow concentration window [27]. The concentration above which the micelles formation takes place is called CMC (critical micelles concentration). Above the CMC, the micelles are being formed by the dehydration of the hydrophobic tails with favorable entropy. Van der Waals bonds are responsible for the formation of micelle core by combining hydrophobic polymers in symmetrical way. Conventional oral administration of anticancer drugs showed reduced absorption and reduced bioavailability [27].

Polymeric micelles provide an excellent advantage of smaller size in comparison to liposomes. Polymer selection plays an important role in the formation of micelles, and the selection for the micelles formation is based on the characteristics of both hydrophobic and hydrophilic block polymers. Hydrophilic outer shell of the micelles gives steric stability and prevents rapid uptake of formulation by reticulo endothelial system and provides longer duration of circulation time inside the body [28]. Hydrophobic and hydrophilic polymers are the block polymers for the formation of the micelles which assemble themselves in an aqueous environment to form hydrophobic core which is being stabilized by hydrophilic shell. By arranging these block polymers, different patterns of micelles are being formed; hence, these polymers are called diblock copolymer (A-B type copolymers), triblock copolymer (A-B-C type copolymer), and grafted polymers [29].

Xue et al. had developed biodegradable diblock amphiphilic copolymer (mPEG-b-p(LA-CO-MCG) having carboxylate group for platinum chelation. The cytotoxicity of the drug-polymer conjugate towards breast cancer was lower than of cisplatin but comparable to that of oxaliplatin. This polymer conjugate showed the potential use as a targeted carrier vehicle due to its reduced side effect [30]. Zhang et al. had developed a combination of salinomycin and octreotide-modified paclitaxel-loaded PEG-B-PCL polymer micelles. This combination therapy showed improved treatment of breast cancer. Combination was designed in order to eradicate both breast cancer stem cells and breast cancer cells which cannot be eradicated by conventional chemotherapy. Elimination of cancer cell is based on the mechanism of receptor-mediated endocytosis [31]. Octreotide-modified paclitaxel follows the active targeting mechanism, whereas salinomycin follows the passive targeting mechanism. Liu et al. had formulated curcumin-loaded biodegradable self-assembled polymeric micelles called as curcumin polymeric micelles which showed good water solubility and had met the intravenous administration requirements. Sustained release and lower cytotoxicity of curcumin polymer micelles may serve as candidate for antimetastasis agent for breast cancer [32].

Polymer-based imaging with near-infrared (NIR) fluorophores provides efficient advantages for tumor imaging, such as improved plasma half-lives, large surface area, less toxicity, stability, and improved targeting. For in vivo imaging of tumor, NIR fluorophores are increasing its hold [33]. Along this, NIR fluorophores do not require expensive instruments, a local cyclotron, or incontinent radionuclide-labeling step [34]. Kim et al. have developed NIR Cy5.5-labeled hydrophobically modified glycol chitosan nanoparticles (HGC-Cy5.5) with molecular weight ranging from

20 to 250 kDa. In vivo biodistribution study revealed that low-molecular-weight HGC-Cy5.5 showed faster clearance from the body in comparison to high-molecular-weight HGC-Cy5.5, whereas high-molecular-weight HGC-Cy5.5 had high tumor targeting capacity than low-molecular-weight HGC-Cy5.5. These probes provide promising imaging agents, which are used to detect solid tumor [35]. Kim et al. have developed NIR fluorescent-activatable polymeric nanoparticles (Cy5.5) linked effector caspase-specific peptide having efficient biocompatibility and cell permeability. These nanoparticles were specifically apoptosis sensitive nanoparticles (80–100 nm). This probe could be used as an imaging agent for apoptosis in single cells [36].

5.1.2. Dendrimer

Nanosized branched structures are called dendrimer. The name comes from the Greek word "dendron" which means tree-like structures. With various architectural variations, uniformity in size, branching length, shape and increased surface area can be achieved. Dendrimers show higher biocompatibility and certain changes in the structure of dendrimers; pharmacokinetic parameters can also be predictable. Hence, dendrimers can be optimal and unique carrier system for anticancer drug [37, 38]. Dendrimer can be grown towards outward direction from the central core; this process is known as divergent method designed by Newkome and Tomalia [39–41], or it may be formulated by the Frechet's method, in which the dendrimers are made toward inside direction, that is, from the periphery to inner core [42]. Dendrimers are also described on the basis of the branching unit they consist of, like dendrimer with central branch core molecule is considered as generation 0 (G0) and with each successive addition of increased branching point they may be considered as G1, G2 and so forth. Dendrimers may be categorized by terminal generation, like G6 consists of polymer with five generations of branching points. Dendrimers form the globular shape and attain higher diameter with increasing branching generation [43]. Dendrimers and dendrons are monodispersed and usually highly symmetric, spherical compounds. Dendrimer can be used as carrier system for the treatment of diseases like AIDS, cancer, malaria, and so forth.

Wang et al. had synthesized G4 polyamidoamine dendrimer (G4 PAMAM-D) conjugate with antisense oligodeoxynucleotides (ASODN). The conjugate showed more stability less toxicity, and increased bioavailability. In vivo studies on xenograft mice model showed that the conjugate has more accumulating efficiency to inhibit tumor vascularisation of breast tumor than naked ASODN [44]. Gupta et al. had conjugated doxorubicin (DOX) to polypropylene imine (PPI) as well as folic acid to fifth-generation polypropylene imine. The conjugated ligands DOX-PPI-FA and PPI-FA have less haemolytic activity, thus more stable and less toxic [45]. Fluorescence studies showed higher cellular uptake by tumor cell of the formulated conjugate ligand. Results of the study revealed that folic-acid-conjugated PPI dendrimers may be a better choice for anticancer drug targeting in the future.

Samuelson et al. have developed translocator protein (TSPO) dendrimer imaging agent with significantly increased targeting and imaging characteristics. The reported study revealed that TSPO can be used as an imaging agent in brain, breast, and ovarian cancer as well as in prostate carcinoma. The main synthesizing material used to produce TSPO dendrimer was 1-(2-chlorophenyl) isoquinoline-3-carboxylic acid (ClPhIQ acid). Hence, TSPO targeted dendrimer is a real-time imaging agent for breast cancer [46].

5.1.3. Liposomes

Liposomes drug delivery system can change the biodistribution and pharmacokinetics of the drug in such a way that it shows overall improvement in the pharmacological properties of chemotherapeutic agents [47–49]. Due to the success achieved by the liposomal-based chemotherapeutic agents in clinical trials, liposomal formulations are currently used for the treatment of the breast cancer like Doxil liposomal preparation [50]. Liposomes consist of lipid bilayer membrane which surrounds the aqueous core. Depending on the solubility of active pharmaceutical ingredient, either it is loaded to lipid membrane or to the hydrophobic core. On the basis of lamellarity and size, liposomes are classified into three: small unilamellar vesicles, large unilamellar vesicles, and multilamellar vesicles [51]. At present, various kinds of cancer drugs have been loaded to this lipid-based system by using different preparation methods. Liposomes are the potential carrier system for anticancer drugs due to the following three pharmacological parameters.

(a) Liposomes provide slow and sustained release. (b) Liposomes are able to reduce cytotoxicity of chemotherapeutic agents by altering the biodistribution of entrapped drug. (c) Liposomes enhance the drug accumulation.

Doxil, a liposomal-based formulation which consists of cholesterol and high phase-transition temperature phospholipid hydrogenated soy phosphatidylcholine (HSPC) gives a stable drug delivery system with enhanced biocompatibility, efficacy and reduced cytotoxic effects [52]. Anthracycline doxorubicin, an active cytotoxic agent, when encapsulated inside the aqueous core of the liposome, significantly shows decrease in the cardiotoxicity [53]. Hence, higher dose of the chemotherapeutic agents can be given to the patient as in the form of liposomal drug delivery system, which can transfer significant amount of the anticancer drug to the desired targeted site.

Shahun et al. had formulated liposomes of doxorubicin (DOX) which is actively targeted to breast cancer by using engineered peptide ligands, P18-4. The effect of the peptide ligand on breast cancer with respect to accumulation cytotoxicity and growth inhibition was studied by varying the molar ratio of P18-4. It was found that the engineered P18-4 peptide can improve the antitumor efficacy by using optimum density [54]. Urbinati et al. had incorporated histone deacetylase inhibitors (HADCi) which belong to class 1 trichostatin and PXD 101 into liposome in large amounts. Phosphatidylcholine, cholesterol, and distearoyl phosphoethanolamine-polyethylene glycol were used to make liposomes and were used in a ratio of 64 : 30 : 6. Liposomes were checked for their toxicity and were measured in MCF-7, T47-D, SKbr 3, and MDA-MB-231 breast cancer cell lines. Formulation made by Urbinati et al. showed improvement in drug accumulation not only in breast cancer but other cancers also get eradicated [55]. Park had prepared pegylated liposome as a suitable drug carrier for doxorubicin. The study revealed the substantial efficacy towards the breast cancer and reduced toxicity of anticancer drug. Pegylated liposomal doxorubicin can be used either in combination with other chemotherapeutics or as monotherapy for breast cancer. Pegylated liposomal formulation can further be used for molecular targeting [56].

Dagar et al. had developed vasoactive intestinal peptide receptors (VIP-R) as a breast cancer targeted imaging with increased pharmacokinetics, biodistribution and with a better imaging ability. VIP-R, a 28-amino-acid mammalian neuropeptide, was attached covalently to the surface of the sterically stabilized liposomes (SSL) which was further encapsulated to a radionuclide (Tc99 m-HMPAO). Presented study revealed that VIP-R is 5 times more expressive in human breast cancer in comparison to other imaging probes. SSL without VIP showed significantly less accumulation than Tc99 m-HMPAO-encapsulated SSL with VIP [57].

5.1.4. Carbon Nanotubes

The allotropes of carbon with a cylindrical nanoshape structure are called carbon nanotubes. Carbon nanotubes belong to the fullerene structure. Representation of the carbon nanotubes is similar to the rolled sheets of graphene rings. A carbon nanotube provides the variety of promising biomedical applications in comparison to other nonmaterials. Carbon nanotubes are more dynamic and are used potentially not only in cancer cell imaging but are also used for drug delivery system. The unique biological and chemical properties, hollow monolithic structure, nanoneedle shape, and the ability of carbon nanotubes to incorporate any functional group make them a suitable carrier system for chemotherapeutic agents. This allows a passive diffusion of carbon nanotubes across the lipid bilayer, or it may attach to the surface of the cell and subsequent endocytosis (engulfing by cells) takes place [58, 59].

Carbon nanotubes can be categorized into two as follows.(1)Single-walled carbon nanotubes (SWCNTs).(2)Multiwalled carbon nanotubes (MWCNTs).

SWCNTs consist of one layer of graphene sheet with diameter of 1-2 nm and length varies from 50 to several hundred nanometers. On the other hand, MWCNTs are multiple layers of SWCNTs which are coaxially arranged with diameter variation of 5 to 100 nm. SWCNTs and MWCNTs have different mechanisms of cell penetration. By using confocal microscopy imaging, it has been observed that SWCNTs have the ability to incorporate inside the cells, whereas MWCNTs are not incorporated into the cells. Size of the carbon nanotube also affects the cellular uptake; due to this, SWCNTs show localized effect in cell and prolonged distribution [60]. Drug can either be loaded into the carbon nanotubes or be attached to the surface of the carbon nanotube. Attachment of anticancer drug can be done by either noncovalent bonding or covalent bonding, which includes electrostatic interactions π-π stacking and hydrophobic interactions [61]. Research has been done by Wu et al. to deliver an anticancer drug, 10-hydroxyl camptothecin (HCPT), by covalent attachment on the outer surface of the MWCNT. Similarly, succinic anhydride was reacted with HCPT to obtain carboxylic groups on its surface; amino acids were then incorporated to the MWCNTs. Carbon nanotubes coated with HCPT and amino group were functionalized by carboxylic group. This enhances the cell uptake of MWCNTs-HCPT and increased blood circulation with high drug accumulation to the tumor [62]. Liu et al. had conjugated paclitaxel (PTV) to branched polyethylene glycol chain on SWNTs. SWNTs-PTX conjugate exhibited higher drug accumulation, higher bioavailability, and little toxicity. Murine 4T1 breast cancer model shows suppression in tumor growth, enhanced permeation and retention. SWNTs-PTX delivery is the promising treatment for cancer therapy in the future, with higher efficacy and minimum cytotoxic effect [63]. Chen et al. had developed nanocarbon tube by chemical functionalization of SWNTs (f-SWCNTs) with DSPE-PEG-amine. The conjugate bounded to small interfering RNA (SiRNA) was targeting towards breast cancer. Disulfide bond was used for siRNA-mediated gene targeting. Resulting study shows that there is increase in the uptake of SWNTs-SiRNA by 83.55% into the breast carcinoma B-cap-37. Proliferation inhibition was found to be 44.53% for 72 hours in B-cap-37 cells. This novel strategy of chemical functionalization is effective carrier system and is a very advanced or significant therapy for breast cancer in the future [64].

Avti and Sitharaman have developed europium-catalyzed single-walled carbon nanotubes (Eu-SWCNTs) as cellular imaging probe for breast cancer cells. These probes, when excitated at 365 nm and 458 nm wavelengths, showed bright red luminescence. Mechanism of uptake of Eu-SWCNTs is endocytosis, and it was demonstrated in the study that Eu-SWCNTs showed 95%–100% labeling efficiency. The study revealed that Eu-SWCNT is an excellent cellular imaging probe for breast cancer, having excitation value with invisible range [65].

5.1.5. Nanorods

Morphologically the nanorods are nanoscale materials in nanotechnology. Their dimension varies from 1–100 nm and they can be synthesized chemically. Nanorods have a high surface area and are biocompatible, hence, a promising approach for breast cancer. For gold nanorods, because of their special physicochemical properties, they are widely used for imaging, biosensing, photothermal therapy, and for drug delivery system. Inert and nontoxic nature of gold nanorods makes them a suitable nanomedicines carrier system applicable in biomedical field [66, 67]. Different cellular uptake patterns are being followed by the single gold nanoparticle and aggregated gold nanoparticles, and during their uptake these particles interact with the compartments of cellular membrane [68, 69]. Eghtedari et al. had functionalized gold nanorods (GNRs) for in vivo targeting to breast cancer which was grown on athymic nude mouse. Herceptin (HER), a monoclonal antibody, was used to functionalize the gold nanorods by molecular recognition of tumor cells of breast along with PEG (polyethylene glycol). Eghtedari et al. revealed the in vitro stability study of fabricated herceptin-PEG-gold nanorods in blood and in vivo study for breast cancer in nude mice model for breast carcinoma. To achieve a successful targeting to in vivo cancer cell, extra engineering efforts are required to make them stable inside the microenvironment of the cancer cells, biocompatible, have prolonged circulation in the blood to reach targeted site, and able to search cancer cells and bind to them. To prolong the circulation time, gold nanoparticles must be protected from reticuloendothelial system, and for this polyethylene glycol (PEG) has shown a promising effect [70].

Connor et al. had studied the cytotoxic effect of gold nanoparticles as noncytotoxic under suitable experiment condition. Small size of nanorods makes them potentially useful for drug delivery and gene therapy, hence, provides drug delivery system with lower cytotoxicity towards normal cell and increased chemotherapeutic efficiency towards abnormal cancer cell [71]. Xiao et al. had developed multifunctional water-soluble gold nanorods (GNRs) as a nanocarrier for tumor targeting. pH-sensitive behaviour of GNRs causes the release of drug, by minimizing the cytotoxic nonspecific systemic distribution of anticancer drug, during circulation inside the human body side by side increasing the efficiency of anticancer drug to targeting tumor [72].

Likewise, zinc oxide nanorods (ZnO) also provide a promising approach in cancer for imaging and drug delivery system for cancer therapy. ZnO nanorods are self-organizing nanomaterials which can be grown on any substance with high quality of crystalline and amorphous properties. This provides ZnO nanorods with large surface area to volume ratio and higher efficiency for photoimaging. Generally, white light is being observed in photonic device and potentially used in photodynamic therapy. Photosensitizers are being taken by cancer cell in photodynamic therapy for cancer followed by exposure to white light [73]. Zhang et al. had fabricated zinc oxide (ZnO) nanorods as a drug carrier for the anticancer drug daunorubicin (DNR) in photodynamic therapy, by using simple one-step solid-state reaction at a normal room temperature in the air. The investigation revealed that the combination of ZnO-nanorods-DNR has induced remarkable decrease in cytotoxicity of anticancer drug and considerable increase in the cancer cell targeting mediated by reactive oxygen species (ROS) in human hepatocarcinoma cells (SMMC-7721 cells) [74]. Kishwar et al. had conjugated developed ZnO nanorods (ZnO-NRs) with protoporphyrin dimethyl ester (PPDME) and used it in the treatment of breast cancer. ZnO nanorods were developed on borosilicate glass capillaries tip by using aqueous chemical growth technique. Developed PPDME-conjugated ZnO-NRs have induced cell localized toxicity indicating potential application in necrosis of breast carcinoma.

Wang et al. have developed multifunctional nanoparticles of gold and pearls consisting of single amine-modified gold nanorod, and Fe_3O_4 "pearls" were used to give final touch with the help of carboxyl group. Reported study demonstrated the effectiveness of the gold nanorod in breast cancer photothermal ablation and dual-mode imaging of breast cancer [75].

6. CONCLUSION

Human breast cancer is still an extremely complex and dangerous disease with multiple questions. Nanotechnology is a fast emerging area of science with potential for imaging, monitoring, diagnosing, and delivery of drug to specific targeted tumor cells. Nanoparticles offer the advanced methods of tumor targeting with improved efficacy and decreased toxicity. Many nanoparticle formulations are already in clinical practices. Ongoing efforts by researchers, scientists, and other medical personnel in the field of nanotechnology will consistently produce the new platform for nanoparticles. In the near future, nanotechnology will not only show a greater application in oncology, but the discipline of medicines will also be benefitted.

CONFLICT OF INTERESTS

The authors report no conflict of interests.

ACKNOWLEDGMENT

The authors would like to offer highest regard and gratitude to the reverend Professor P. K. Khosla (Vice Chancellor, Shoolini University) for this perennial guidance, inspiration, and encouragement to complete this paper.

REFERENCES

1. T. Tanaka, P. Decuuzzi, M. Ferrai, et al., "Nanotechnology for breast cancer therapy," Biomed Micro Devices, vol. 11, no. 1, pp. 49–63, 2009.

2. S. Nie, Y. Xing, G. J. Kim, et al., "Nanotechnology application in cancer," Annual Review of Biomedical Engineering, vol. 9, pp. 257–288, 2007.

3. R. Sinha, G. J. Kim, S. Nie, and D. M. Shin, "Nanotechnology in cancer therapeutics: bioconjugated nanoparticles for drug delivery," Molecular Cancer Therapeutics, vol. 5, no. 8, pp. 1909–1917, 2006.

4. L. A. Brinton, M. E. Sherman, J. D. Carreon, and W. F. Anderson, "Recent trends in breast cancer among younger women in the United States," Journal of the National Cancer Institute, vol. 100, no. 22, pp. 1643–1648, 2008.

5. O. Leary, Sheaffer, Phillips, et al., Cancer Epidemiology in Older Adolescents and Young Adults 15 to 29 Years of Age, Including SEER Incidence and Survival: 1975–2000, National Cancer Institute (NIH), 2006, Pub. No. 06–5767.

6. B. G. Haffty, Q. Yang, M. Reiss et al., "Locoregional relapse and distant metastasis in conservatively managed triple negative early-stage breast cancer," Journal of Clinical Oncology, vol. 24, no. 36, pp. 5652–5657, 2006.

7. M. Shackleton, E. Quintana, E. R. Fearon, and S. J. Morrison, "Heterogeneity in cancer: cancer stem cells versus clonal evolution," Cell, vol. 138, no. 5, pp. 822–829, 2009.

8. X. Huang, I. H. El-Sayed, W. Qian, and M. A. El-Sayed, "Cancer cell imaging and photothermal therapy in the near-infrared region by using gold nanorods," Journal of the American Chemical Society, vol. 128, no. 6, pp. 2115–2120, 2006.

9. S. J. Patil, A. Zajac, T. Zhukov, and S. Bhansali, "Ultrasensitive electrochemical detection of cytokeratin-7, using Au nanowires based biosensor," Sensors and Actuators B, vol. 129, no. 2, pp. 859–865, 2008.

10. S. Nie, Y. Xing, G. J. Kim, et al., "Nanotechnology application in cancer," Annual Review of Biomedical Engineering, vol. 9, pp. 257–288, 2007.

11. W. W. Yu, L. H. Qu, W. Z. Guo, and X. G. Peng, "Experimental determination of the extinction coefficient of CdTe, CdSe, and CdS nanocrystals," Chemistry of Materials, vol. 15, no. 14, pp. 2854–2860, 2003.

12. K. Cho, X. Wang, S. Nie, Z. Chen, and D. M. Shin, "Therapeutic nanoparticles for drug delivery in cancer," Clinical Cancer Research, vol. 14, no. 5, pp. 1310–1316, 2008.

13. R. Sinha, G. J. Kim, S. Nie, and D. M. Shin, "Nanotechnology in cancer therapeutics: bioconjugated nanoparticles for drug delivery," Molecular Cancer Therapeutics, vol. 5, no. 8, pp. 1909–1917, 2006.

14. P. Geels, E. Eisenhauer, A. Bezjak, B. Zee, and A. Day, "Palliative effect of chemotherapy: objective tumor response is associated with symptom improvement in patients with metastatic breast cancer," Journal of Clinical Oncology, vol. 18, no. 12, pp. 2395–2405, 2000.

15. Jones and A. L. Harris, "New developments in angiogenesis: a major mechanism for tumor growth and target for therapy," Cancer Journal from Scientific American, vol. 4, no. 4, pp. 209–217, 1998.

16. S. M. Moghimi and A. C. Hunter, "Poloxamers and poloxamines in nanoparticle engineering and experimental medicine," Trends in Biotechnology, vol. 18, no. 10, pp. 412–420, 2000.

17. E. K. Park, S. B. Lee, and Y. M. Lee, "Preparation and characterization of methoxy poly(ethylene glycol)/poly(ε-caprolactone) amphiphilic block copolymeric nanospheres for tumor-specific folate-mediated targeting of anticancer drugs," Biomaterials, vol. 26, no. 9, pp. 1053–1061, 2005.

18. H. Maeda and Y. Matsumura, "Tumoritropic and lymphotropic principles of macromolecular drugs,"Critical Reviews in Therapeutic Drug Carrier Systems, vol. 6, no. 3, pp. 193–210, 1989.

19. M. Mansour, J. Drevs, N. Esser et al., "A new approach for the treatment of malignant melanoma: enhanced antitumor efficacy of an albumin-binding doxorubicin prodrug that is cleaved by matrix metalloproteinase 2," Cancer Research, vol. 63, no. 14, pp. 4062–4066, 2003.

20. T. Nomura, A. Saikawa, S. Morita et al., "Pharmacokinetic characteristics and therapeutic effects of mitomycin C-dextran conjugates after intratumoural injection," Journal of Controlled Release, vol. 52, no. 3, pp. 239–252, 1998.

21. S. Prabha and V. Labhasetwar, "Nanoparticle-mediated wild-type p53 gene delivery results in sustained antiproliferative activity in breast cancer cells," Molecular Pharmacology, vol. 1, no. 3, pp. 211–219, 2004.

22. D. B. Kirpotin, D. C. Drummond, Y. Shao et al., "Antibody targeting of long-circulating lipidic nanoparticles does not increase tumor localization but does increase internalization in animal models,"Cancer Research, vol. 66, no. 13, pp. 6732–6740, 2006.

23. M. Rawat, D. Singh, S. Saraf, and S. Saraf, "Nanocarriers: promising vehicle for bioactive drugs,"Biological and Pharmaceutical Bulletin, vol. 29, no. 9, pp. 1790–1798, 2006.

24. W. J. Gradishar, S. Tjulandin, N. Davidson et al., "Phase III trial of nanoparticle albumin-bound paclitaxel compared with polyethylated castor oil-based paclitaxel in women with breast cancer," Journal of Clinical Oncology, vol. 23, no. 31, pp. 7794–7803, 2005.

25. C. Li, "Poly(L-glutamic acid)-anticancer drug conjugates," Advanced Drug Delivery Reviews, vol. 54, no. 5, pp. 695–713, 2002.

26. R. Duncan, "The dawning era of polymer therapeutics," Nature Reviews Drug Discovery, vol. 2, no. 5, pp. 347–360, 2003.

27. V. P. Torchilin, "Micellar nanocarriers: pharmaceutical perspectives," Pharmaceutical Research, vol. 24, no. 1, pp. 1–16, 2007.

28. M. L. Adams, A. Lavasanifar, and G. S. Kwon, "Amphiphilic block copolymers for drug delivery," Journal of Pharmaceutical Sciences, vol. 92, no. 7, pp. 1343–1355, 2003.

29. M.-C. Jones and J.-C. Leroux, "Polymeric micelles—a new generation of colloidal drug carriers,"European Journal of Pharmaceutics and Biopharmaceutics, vol. 48, no. 2, pp. 101–111, 1999.

30. Y. Xue, X. Tang, J. Huang et al., "Anti-tumor efficacy of polymer-platinum(II) complex micelles fabricated from folate conjugated PEG-graft-α,β-poly [(N-amino acidyl)-aspartamide] and cis-dichlorodiammine platinum(II) in tumor-bearing mice," Colloids and Surfaces B, vol. 85, no. 2, pp. 280–288, 2011.

31. Y. Zhang, H. Zhang, X. Wang, J. Wang, X. Zhang, and Q. Zhang, "The eradication of breast cancer and cancer stem cells using octreotide modified paclitaxel active targeting micelles and salinomycin passive targeting micelles," Biomaterials, vol. 33, no. 2, pp. 679–691, 2012.

32. L. Liu, L. Sun, W. Qijie, et al., "Curcumin loaded polymeric micelles inhibit breast tumor growth and spontaneous pulmonary metastasis," International Journal of Pharmaceutics, vol. 44, no. 1-2, pp. 175–182, 2013.

33. R. Weissleder, C.-H. Tung, U. Mahmood, and A. Bogdanov Jr., "In vivo imaging of tumors with protease-activated near-infrared fluorescent probes," Nature Biotechnology, vol. 17, no. 4, pp. 375–378, 1999.

34. X. Chen, P. S. Conti, and R. A. Moats, "In vivo near-infrared fluorescence imaging of integrin α vβ3 in brain tumor xenografts," Cancer Research, vol. 64, no. 21, pp. 8009–8014, 2004.

35. S. E. Kim, I. C. Kwon, H. R. Song, and K. Park, "Insight of key factors influencing tumor targeting characteristics of Glycol Chitosan-based nanoparticles and in vivo applications," Macromolecular Research, vol. 20, no. 11, pp. 1109–1117, 2012.

36. K. Kim, M. Lee, H. Park et al., "Cell-permeable and biocompatible polymeric nanoparticles for apoptosis imaging," Journal of the American Chemical Society, vol. 128, no. 11, pp. 3490–3491, 2006.

37. C. C. Lee, J. A. MacKay, J. M. J. Fréchet, and F. C. Szoka, "Designing dendrimers for biological applications," Nature Biotechnology, vol. 23, no. 12, pp. 1517–1526, 2005.

38. S. Svenson and D. A. Tomalia, "Dendrimers in biomedical applications—reflections on the field,"Advanced Drug Delivery Reviews, vol. 57, no. 15, pp. 2106–2129, 2005.

39. D. A. Tomalia, H. Baker, J. Dewald et al., "Dendritic macromolecules: synthesis of starburst dendrimers,"Macromolecules, vol. 19, no. 9, pp. 2466–2468, 1986.

40. D. A. Tomalia, H. Baker, J. Dewald et al., "A new class of polymers: starburst dendritic macromolecules,"Polymer Journal, vol. 17, no. 1, pp. 117–132, 1984.

41. G. R. Newkome, Z.-Q. Yao, G. R. Baker, and V. K. Gupta, "Cascade molecules: a new approach to micelles. A [27]-arborol," Journal of Organic Chemistry, vol. 50, no. 11, pp. 2003–2004, 1985.

42. C. J. Hawker and J. M. J. Fréchet, "Preparation of polymers with controlled molecular architecture. A new convergent approach to dendritic macromolecules," Journal of the American Chemical Society, vol. 112, no. 21, pp. 7638–7647, 1990.

43. S. Svenson and D. A. Tomalia, "Dendrimers in biomedical applications—reflections on the field,"Advanced Drug Delivery Reviews, vol. 57, no. 15, pp. 2106–2129, 2005.

44. P. Wang, X.-H. Zhao, Z.-Y. Wang, M. Meng, X. Li, and Q. Ning, "Generation 4 polyamidoamine dendrimers is a novel candidate of nano-carrier for gene delivery agents in breast cancer treatment,"Cancer Letters, vol. 298, no. 1, pp. 34–49, 2010.

45. U. Gupta, S. K. D. Dwivedi, H. K. Bid, R. Konwar, and N. K. Jain, "Ligand anchored dendrimers based nanoconstructs for effective targeting to cancer cells," International Journal of Pharmaceutics, vol. 393, no. 1-2, pp. 186–197, 2010.

46. L. E. Samuelson, M. J. Dukes, C. R. Hunt, J. D. Casey, and D. J. Bornhop, "TSPO targeted dendrimer imaging agent: synthesis, characterization, and cellular internalization," Bioconjugate Chemistry, vol. 20, no. 11, pp. 2082–2089, 2009.

47. D. R. Khan, E. M. Rezler, J. Lauer-Fields, and G. B. Fields, "Effects of drug hydrophobicity on liposomal stability," Chemical Biology and Drug Design, vol. 71, no. 1, pp. 3–7, 2008.

48. R. R. C. New, Liposomes: A Practical Approach, Oxford University Press, Oxford, UK, 1st edition, 1990.

49. E. M. Rezler, D. R. Khan, J. Lauer-Fields, M. Cudic, D. Baronas-Lowell, and G. B. Fields, "Targeted drug delivery utilizing

protein-like molecular architecture," Journal of the American Chemical Society, vol. 129, no. 16, pp. 4961–4972, 2007.

50. D. R. Khan, "The use of nanocarriers for drug delivery in cancer therapy," Journal of Cancer Science and Therapy, vol. 2, no. 3, pp. 58–62, 2010.

51. R.-D. Hofheinz, S. U. Gnad-Vogt, U. Beyer, and A. Hochhaus, "Liposomal encapsulated anti-cancer drugs," Anti-Cancer Drugs, vol. 16, no. 7, pp. 691–707, 2005.

52. T. A. Elbayoumi and V. P. Torchilin, "Tumor-specific antibody-mediated targeted delivery of Doxil reduces the manifestation of auricular erythema side effect in mice," International Journal of Pharmaceutics, vol. 357, no. 1-2, pp. 272–279, 2008.

53. Gabizon, "Pegylated liposomal doxorubicin: metamorphosis of an old drug into a new form of chemotherapy," Cancer Investigation, vol. 19, no. 4, pp. 424–436, 2001.

54. M. Shahun, R. Soudy, H. M. Aliabadi, et al., "Engineered breast tumor targeting peptide ligand modified liposomal doxorubicin and the effect of peptide density on anticancer activity," Biomaterials, vol. 34, no. 16, pp. 4089–4097, 2013.

55. G. Urbinati, V. Marsaud, V. Plassat, E. Fattal, S. Lesieur, and J. M. Renoir, "Liposomes loaded with histane deacetylase inhibitors for breast cancer therapy," International Journal of Pharmaceutics, vol. 379, no. 1, pp. 184–193, 2010.

56. J. W. Park, "Liposome-based drug delivery in breast cancer treatment," Breast Cancer Research, vol. 4, no. 3, pp. 95–99, 2002.

57. S. Dagar, A. Krishnadas, I. Rubinstein, M. J. Blend, and H. Önyüksel, "VIP grafted sterically stabilized liposomes for targeted imaging of breast cancer: in vivo studies," Journal of Controlled Release, vol. 91, no. 1-2, pp. 123–133, 2003.

58. N. G. Sahoo, H. Bao, Y. Pan et al., "Functionalized carbon nanomaterials as nanocarriers for loading and delivery of a poorly water-soluble anticancer drug: a comparative study,"

Chemical Communications, vol. 47, no. 18, pp. 5235–5237, 2011.

59. C. Lamprecht, I. Liashkovich, V. Neves et al., "AFM imaging of functionalized carbon nanotubes on biological membranes," Nanotechnology, vol. 20, no. 43, Article ID 434001, 2009.

60. B. Kang, S. Chang, Y. Dai, D. Yu, and D. Chen, "Cell response to carbon nanotubes: size-dependent intracellular uptake mechanism and subcellular fate," Small, vol. 6, no. 21, pp. 2362–2366, 2010.

61. C. L. Lay, H. Q. Liu, H. R. Tan, and Y. Liu, "Delivery of paclitaxel by physically loading onto poly(ethylene glycol) (PEG)-graft-carbon nanotubes for potent cancer therapeutic," Nanotechnology, vol. 21, no. 6, Article ID 065101, 2010.

62. W. Wu, R. Li, X. Bian et al., "Covalently combining carbon nanotubes with anticancer agent: preparation and antitumor activity," ACS Nano, vol. 3, no. 9, pp. 2740–2750, 2009.

63. Z. Liu, K. Chen, C. Davis et al., "Drug delivery with carbon nanotubes for in vivo cancer treatment," The Journal of Cancer Research, vol. 68, no. 16, pp. 6652–6660, 2008.

64. H. Chen, X. Ma, Z. Li et al., "Functionalization of single-walled carbon nanotubes enables efficient intracellular delivery of siRNA targeting MDM2 to inhibit breast cancer cells growth," Biomedicine and Pharmacotherapy, vol. 60, no. 5, pp. 334–338, 2012.

65. P. K. Avti and B. Sitharaman, "Luminescent single-walled carbon nanotube-sensitized europium nanoprobes for cellular imaging," International Journal of Nanomedicine, vol. 7, pp. 1953–1964, 2012.

66. L. Tong, Q. Wei, A. Wei, and J.-X. Cheng, "Gold nanorods as contrast agents for biological imaging: optical properties, surface conjugation and photothermal effects," Photochemistry and Photobiology, vol. 85, no. 1, pp. 21–32, 2009.

67. H. J. Parab, H. M. Chen, T.-C. Lai et al., "Biosensing, cytotoxicity, and cellular uptake studies of surface-modified gold nanorods,"

Journal of Physical Chemistry C, vol. 113, no. 18, pp. 7574–7578, 2009.

68. Albanese and W. C. W. Chan, "Effect of gold nanoparticle aggregation on cell uptake and toxicity,"ACS Nano, vol. 5, no. 7, pp. 5478–5489, 2011.

69. G. Wilson, P. N. Sisco, E. C. Goldsmith, and C. J. Murphy, "Glycosaminoglycan-functionalized gold nanorods: interactions with cardiac cells and type I collagen," Journal of Materials Chemistry, vol. 19, no. 35, pp. 6332–6340, 2009.

70. M. Eghtedari, A. V. Liopo, J. A. Copland, A. A. Oraevsky, and M. Motamed, "Engineering of hetero-functional gold nanorods for the in vivo molecular targeting of breast cancer cells," Nano Letters, vol. 9, no. 1, pp. 287–291, 2009.

71. E. E. Connor, J. Mwamuka, A. Gole, C. J. Murphy, and M. D. Wyatt, "Gold nanoparticles are taken up by human cells but do not cause acute cytotoxicity," Small, vol. 1, no. 3, pp. 325–327, 2005.

72. Y. Xiao, H. Hong, V. Z. Matson, et al., "Gold nanorods conjugated with Doxorubicin and cRGD for combined anticancer drug delivery and Pet imaging," Thernostics, vol. 2, no. 8, pp. 757–768, 2012.

73. S. Kishwar, M. H. Asif, O. Nur, M. Willander, and P.-O. Larsson, "Intracellular ZnO nanorods conjugated with protoporphyrin for local mediated photochemistry and efficient treatment of single cancer cell,"Nanoscale Research Letters, vol. 5, no. 10, pp. 1669–1674, 2010.

74. H. Zhang, B. Chen, H. Jiang, C. Wang, H. Wang, and X. Wang, "A strategy for ZnO nanorod mediated multi-mode cancer treatment," Biomaterials, vol. 32, no. 7, pp. 1906–1914, 2011.

75. C. Wang, J. Chen, T. Talavage, and J. Irudayaraj, "Gold Nanorod/Fe3O4 nanoparticle "nano-pearl- necklaces" for simultaneous targeting, dual-mode imaging, and photothermal ablation of cancer cells,"Angewandte Chemie, vol. 48, no. 15, pp. 2759–2763, 2009.

Chapter 6

Active-targeted Nanotherapy as Smart Cancer Treatment

Katayoun Derakhshandeh[1, 2] and Abbas Hemmati Azandaryani[2]

[1] Department of Pharmaceutics, School of Pharmacy, Hamadan University of Medical Sciences, Hamadan, Iran

[2] Nano Drug Delivery Research Center, Kermanshah University of Medical Sciences, Kermanshah, Iran

ABSTRACT

Drug delivery systems (DDS) can be designed to improve the pharmacological and therapeutic properties of drugs. Targeted drug delivery, sometimes called smart drug delivery, is a method of delivering medication to a patient in a manner that increases the concentration of the medication in infective organs or cells, relative to others. Cancer is one of the major causes of mortality worldwide and innovative methods for cancer therapy are urgently required. Nanoparticles (NPs), by using active targeting strategy, can enhance the intracellular concentration of drugs in cancerous cells while avoiding toxicity in normal cells. Nanoparticles with bioscience are being actively developed for in vivo tumor imaging, bimolecular profiling of cancer biomarkers, and targeted drug delivery. The advantages of the targeted release system are the reduction in the frequency of dosages taken by the patient, having a uniform effect of the drug, reduction of drug side effects, and reduced fluctuation in circulating drug levels. In this chapter, we focus on targeted drug delivery systems integrated from nanobiotechnology.

Keywords: Targeted drug delivery, Nanobiotechnology, Nanocarrier, Active targeting, Cancer therapy

1. INTRODUCTION

Currently, maximizing the safety and efficacy of drug therapy is the main goal of pharmaceutical scientists and physicians. To this end, drug targeting is the best approach. This subject is critical for some diseases such as cancer treatments, which involve a balancing act between the destruction of cancerous and healthy tissues, including damage to the immune system and highly replicating cells.

Newly developed nanotechnological methods as active targeting carrier in the medical treatment have increased attention [1–4].

Active targeting involves attaching different ligands such as antibodies, biological proteins, peptides, sugars, and vitamins or a specific ligand to the drug or drug delivery system, which meet and form a complex with cell receptors and cause the drug to accumulate in the target cells.

Specifically, "targeting" can be categorized into three levels:

- First-order targeting: When the delivery is to a specific organ, for example, drugs may be targeted to the liver because of its leaky or fenestrated vasculature or loose junctions; the drug is not released in other tissues because of their nonleaky vasculature.
- Second-order targeting or cellular targeting: When a drug delivery system releases the drug to a particular cell within an organ or a tissue.
- Third-order or subcellular targeting: When the delivery is to distinct cell types with biological barrier transport, for example, epithelial cells or cells of the lung-associated lymphatic tissue. A good example is the delivery of genes. The delivery system carries the

gene, enters specific cells and releases the gene intracellularly. This is the third order and the most sophisticated type of targeting.

Traditional targeting activities can also be grouped into passive and active targeting [5]. Drug delivery systems that have been developed to be used as targeting carriers include micelles, nanoparticles, polymeric conjugates, and liposomes. NPs protect the drug from premature degradation, prevent drugs from interacting with the biological environment, and enhance the absorption of drugs into a selected tissue. Nanoparticle technologies may improve the therapeutic index of drugs by enhancing their efficacy and/or increasing their tolerability in the body. Nanoparticles could also improve the bioavailability of water-insoluble drugs, carry large payloads, as well as enable the development of novel classes of bioactive macromolecules (e.g., DNA and siRNA) [4–8]. Thus far, over two dozen nanotechnology products have been approved by the US Food and Drug Administration (FDA) for clinical use, and many are under clinical and preclinical development [9].

In our studies, we focused on targeted drug delivery systems integrated from nanobiotechnology. Nanoparticles, by using active targeting strategies such as folate, monoclonal antibodies (mAbs) and aptamer ligands can enhance the intracellular concentration of drugs in cancerous cells while avoiding toxicity in normal cells. Nanoparticles with bioscience are being actively developed for in vivo tumor imaging, biomolecular profiling of cancer biomarkers, and targeted drug delivery. Nanoparticles remain in the blood circulation for a longer time and can passively accumulate at target sites after the systemic administration because of leaky tumor vasculature and poorly developed lymphatic drainage (the enhanced permeation and retention (EPR) effect).

In this chapter, we focus on explaining anticancer agents loaded in different nanoparticles and how they could be targeted to different tissues especially to solid tumors by attaching specific ligands [6–8].

2. NANO DRUG DELIVERY

Drug delivery systems such as lipid-, polymer-, liposome-, dendrimeric-, or biomacromolecule-based nanoparticles can be designed to improve the pharmacological and therapeutic properties of drugs administered parenterally or by other routes of administration. There are considerable interests in exploiting the advantages of DDS for in vivo delivery of new drugs and for their use in targeted therapeutics. Drug targeting can improve the efficacy of therapy and reduce side effects associated with drugs and therapeutic agents [10–12]. Various carriers can be used to deliver a drug in a stable and protective form for conventional or targeted shape (Figure 1); however, it is nanotechnology that offers the most unique and intriguing approach in the field of nanomedicine.

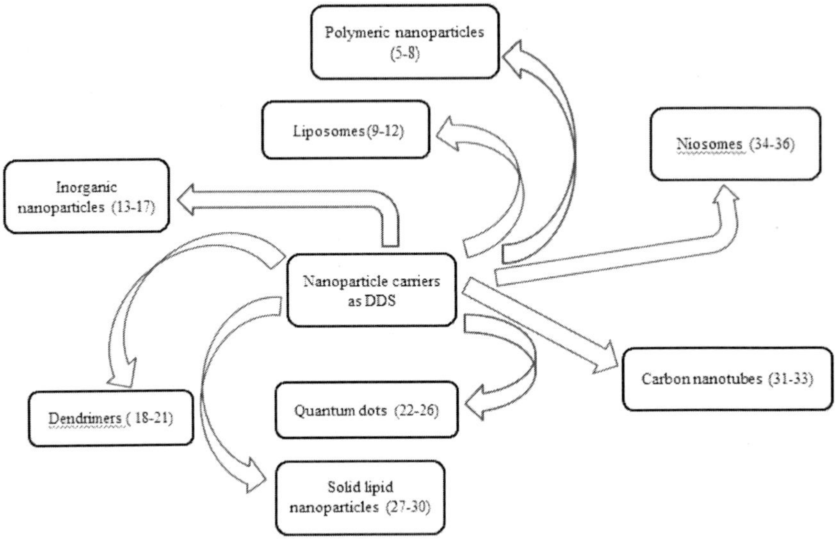

Figure 1. The different types of nanocarriers

Nanobiotechnology, defined as biomedical applications of nano-sized biomacromolecular systems or nano-sized materials with biomaterials, is a rapidly developing area within nanoscience. We define nanomedicines as delivery systems in the nanometer size range (preferably 1–100 nm) containing encapsulated, dispersed, adsorbed, or conjugated drugs and imaging agents. They can also facilitate the important advances in detection, diagnosis, and treatment of diseases, human cancers, vaccine delivery, etc., and have led to a new discipline of nanobiotechnology [13–16]. Nanoparticles are being actively developed for in vivo tumor imaging, biomolecular profiling of cancer biomarkers, and targeted drug delivery. These nanotechnology-based techniques can be applied widely in the management of different malignant diseases [17, 18].

Nanocarriers have numerous points of interest contrasted with free drugs. They protect the labile drugs from degradation in biological environments, increase uptake of the drugs into a chosen tissue such as solid tumors, facilitate modification of the pharmacokinetics and body distribution, and enhance intracellular infiltration.

Nanotechnology applications in medicine, termed as nanomedicine, have introduced a number of nanoparticles of variable chemistry and architecture in the targeted drug delivery system. Nanotechnology involves engineering multifunctional devices with dimensions on the nanoscale with similar dimensions of large biological molecules in the body, viruses, and other synthesized macromolecules. These devices can carry one or two detection signals and/or therapeutic agents for drug delivery targeting [19, 20].

Nanotechnology is well introduced in drug delivery technology for several advantages such as first passive drug delivery, increasing of drug solubility, increasing of drug half-life in the body, modification of the drug distribution pattern, and improvement of pharmacokinetics, which will result in improved efficacy. With these advantages, the future of drug delivery cannot be predicted and some problems exist such as site cytotoxicity [21–26].

Currently, the fundamental issue with cancer treatment is that they include an exercise in careful control between the destruction of malignant tissue and healthy tissues, such as damage to the immune system and profoundly replicating cells (gastrointestinal epithelia and hair follicles).

It is important to detect the revelation of malignant cells sufficiently early and in a stage that is sensible for convenient treatment. Recently, created nanotechnology drug delivery systems are promising approaches for oncologists.

The use of nanoparticles in medical treatment has increased in recent years. For example, micro- and nanoparticles, such as polymeric nanoparticles (synthetic or natural polymers), polymeric micelles, dendrimer, and solid lipid nanoparticles (SLN) have long been used as drug delivery systems to encapsulate drugs and protect them from extracellular enzymatic degradation, providing vehicles for delivering drugs to the target area, and are now being investigated as powerful platforms for vaccine delivery [27–33]. Figure 2 represents some kind of nanocarrier in drug delivery.

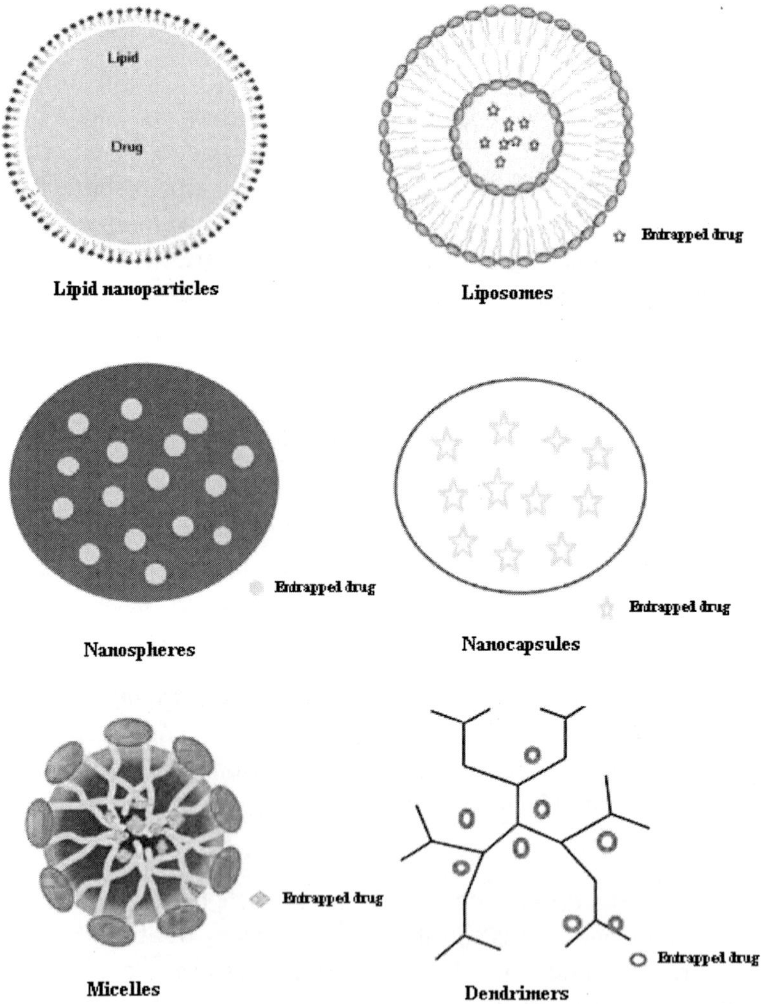

Figure 2. Basic structure of nanoparticles

Being inspired by physiologically existing nanomachines, nanoparticles are designed to safely reach their target and specifically release their therapeutic agent at the site of the disease, thus increasing the drug's tissue bioavailability. Nanoparticles used in this manner for enhanced permeation and retention effect of cancerous cells that are caused by leaky angiogenetic vessels and poor lymphatic drainage has been, in turn, used to explain why macromolecules and nanoparticles are found at higher ratios in tumors compared with normal tissues [29]. Carriers are associated with the drug in a covalent or noncovalent attached mode of targeting materials, and they have been used for the delivery of drug exactly on the target tissue.

In this study, we focus on important nanoparticles such as polymeric nanoparticles and liposomes and their recent results on targeting drug delivery systems for the purpose of biomaterial.

3. BIOCONJUGATION OF NANOCARRIERS FOR TARGET THERAPY

The conjugation of bioagents to nanocarriers is one of the most important functions of the targeted drug delivery system. For this purpose, several methods and works have been performed until now [34–36].

One of the usual methods for attaching biomolecular ligands to nanoparticle's surface is diimide-activated amidation by direct coupling of carboxylic acid to legends using N-ethyl- N-(3-dimethyl aminopropyl) carbodiimide hydrochloride (EDAC) or N,N-dicyclohexyl carbodiimide (DCC) as a coupling agent. The schematic perspective of the connection of proteins to carbon nanotubes (CNTs) by means of diimide-activated amidation is presented in Figure 3. Functionalization of carbon nanotubes was likewise completed using 1-pyrenebutanoic acid, succinimidyl ester for the immobilization of biomolecules, anti-fullerene IgG monoclonal antibody bound to single-wall carbon nanotubes. Proteins and DNA have also been used to modify multiwall carbon nanotubes (MWCNT) [36].

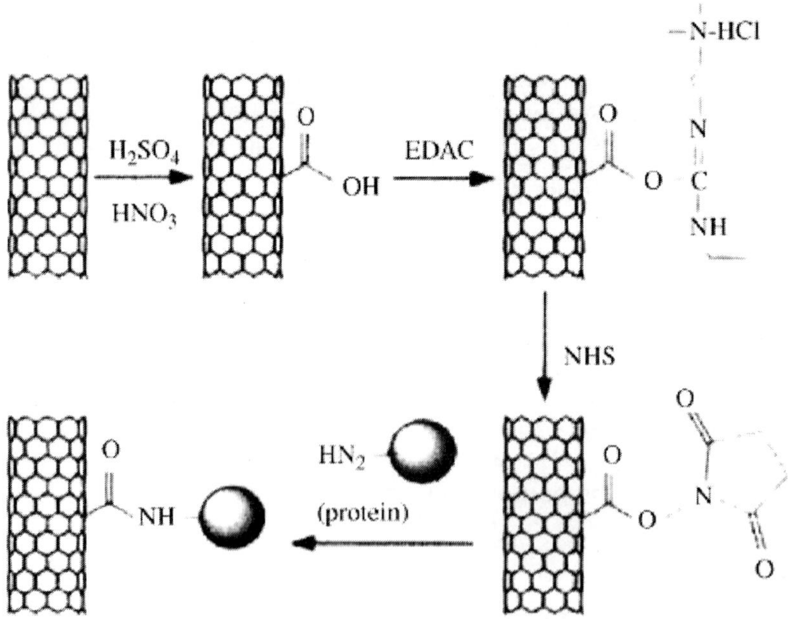

Figure 3. Schematic view of the attachment of proteins to CNTs via diimide activated amidation [51]

Recently, the ubiquitous alkyne–azide Huisgen "click" reaction has been used to attach proteins to NPs (Figure 4). A variety of proteins have been attached in functional form using this method, including lipase, horseradish peroxidase, and luciferase [34]. Hapuarachchige et al. [37] investigated the click reaction for specific internalization of nanotherapeutics. In this study, the pretargeting component, anti-HER2 humanized monoclonal antibody, functionalized with azide groups, labels cancer cells. This group demonstrated high efficacy for targeted nanotherapeutics using the click reaction.

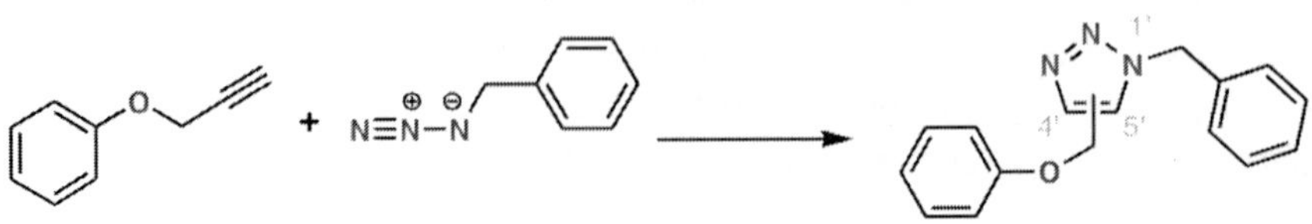

Figure 4. Azide–alkyne Huisgen cycloaddition "click" reaction

The biotin– streptavidin interaction (Figure 5) is widely used for the conjugation of NP systems. The formation of avidin (or streptavidin)–biotin complexes is useful in a wide variety of applications. This specific binding is largely used to immobilize enzymes, antibodies, or DNA. Biotin is a small molecule, which could bind to avidin or streptavidin binding sites with very high affinity (Ka = $10^{15}M^{-1}$).

In addition, avidin and streptavidin are tetrameric proteins that have four known binding sites for biotin (Figure 5). Streptavidin with an isoelectric point equivalent to 5 is accordingly ideally utilized over avidin, which has a PI of 10.5, to maintain a strategic distance from nonspecific interactions [35,38].

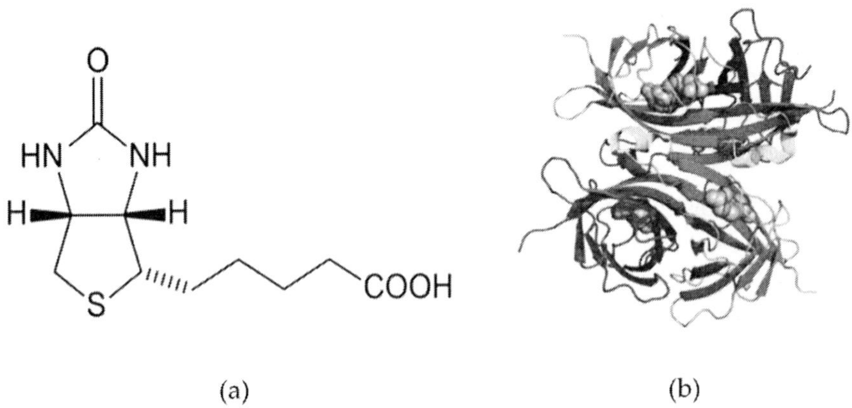

Figure 5. Biotin structure (a) and the simple graph for biotin–avidine binding (b)

4. ACTIVE TARGETING USING POLYMERIC NANOCARRIER

Polymeric nanoparticles with specific recognition ligands bound to the surface have a good potential for site-selective delivery, and offer higher drug carrier capacity than bioconjugates, as well as improved specificity for drug targeting [1, 39–41]. The attached ligands to the surface of nanocarriers can include any molecule that specifically binds to target cells such as peptides, glycoproteins, carbohydrates and polymers, and monoclonal antibodies, which have been the most broadly studied [20, 24].

Kocbek and coworkers developed new active-targeted poly (D,L-lactic-co-glycolic acid) (PLGA) nanoparticles by attaching mAb, which have the ability to target specific antigens on breast epithelial cancer cell lines. Attempts to attach mAb to nanoparticles by covalent bonding were less successful, since the natural action of the bound mAb was inactivated. The specificity of the immunonanoparticles was shown from their selective distribution in a co-culture of MCF-10A neoT and Caco-2 cells, resulting in their final internalization by the former cells [42].

A novel, nonviral, polyethylenimine (PEI)-based, HER2-targeted gene transfer vector has been investigated. The anti-HER2 humanized antibody, trastuzumab (HerceptinR), was used as the targeting moiety to the HER2 overexpressing cancer cells. Subsequently, trastuzumab conjugation of PEI may render PEI a much more selective gene delivery carrier for anticancer gene therapy. The opinion of attaching a targeting ligand, with intrinsic antitumor activity, to a gene transfer vector may be beneficial for further investigations [43].

Recently, poly (butyl cyanoacrylate) (PBCA) NPs coated with polysorbate-80 have been proposed as suitable drug carriers for brain drug delivery. Nerve growth factor (NGF) is important for the survival of peripheral ganglion cells and central cholinergic neurons of the basal forebrain. In spite of its inability to cross the blood–brain barrier (BBB), the NGF activity on these neuronal populaces and its adequacy in avoiding neurodegeneration recommended its potential utilization in the treatment of neurological pathologies, for example, diabetic neuropathies and Huntington's disease. Systemic administration of NGF loaded in P80-coated PBCA NPs successfully reversed scopolamine-induced amnesia and improved recognition and memory in acute amnesia rat model [44].

Yang and coworkers synthesized doxorubicin magnetic PLGA nanoparticles conjugated with well-tailored antibodies for the detection and therapy of breast cancer. They suggested that magnetic nanocrystals embedded in polymeric nanoparticles did not inhibit the nanoparticle formulation or drug release kinetics. The multimodal nanoparticles demonstrated remarkable cancer cell affinity and ultrasensitivity via magnetic resonance imaging. However, the in vivo effects of the NPs were not evaluated [45].

Due to the overexpression of the folate receptor on tumor surface, the folate has been popularly used as a targeting moiety for various anticancer agents to avoid their nonspecific attacks on normal tissues and also to increase their cellular uptake within target cells [46–48]. Derakhshandeh et al. prepared the folate-decorated biodegradable PLGA nanoparticles for tumor targeting. In this study, folate-conjugated PLGA was synthesized and then PLGA-Fol nanoparticles were prepared by nanoprecipitation method, adopting PLGA as a drug carrier, folic acid (FA) as a targeting ligand, and 9-nitrocampthotecin (9-NC) as an anticancer drug model. The in vitro intracellular uptake of nanoparticles showed that the PLGA-Fol nanoparticles have been more efficiently taken up by MCF-7 cells compared with nonfolate-mediated carriers, and also showed greater cytotoxicity than other treated groups [49].

Active-targeted nanocarriers to the special sites and cellular uptake are especially important to therapeutics that is not taken up easily by cells, and they require facilitation by fusion, endocytosis, or other processes to access their cellular active sites. They can also enhance the penetration and distribution of nanomedicine within the tumor interstitium and resistant cancer cells. Active targeting nanocarriers have various points of interest over targeting ligand–drug conjugates [47].

Recently, Wu et al. [50] investigated polymeric nanoparticles for the treatment of metastases. This group studied the ability of micellar nanocarriers incorporating (1,2-diaminocyclohexane) platinum(II) for liver metastases of bioluminescent murine colon adenocarcinoma C-26 treatment, during overt and preangiogenic metastatic stages and thus obtained a novel approach for early diagnosis and treatment of metastases.

5. INORGANIC NANOPARTICLES FOR TARGETED DRUG DELIVERY

Porous inorganic nanoparticles with high specific surface area have recently emerged as attractive material for the development of delivery systems, where various guest molecules could be absorbed into the pores and later released into various solutions [51, 52].

Inorganic nanoparticles, for example, gold and iron oxide, are usually conjugated with the drug, polyethylene glycol (PEG), and the targeting ligands. It gives the idea that the PEG coating and ligand design are common constituents in most types of nanoparticles for anticancer delivery. These carriers have several applications in cancer diagnosis and treatment, and large portions of them have quickly moved into clinical trials. Overall, there is still a space for optimization in the field of nanoparticle pharmacokinetics such as enhanced plasma retention time and tumor bioavailability and understanding the effectiveness of targeting ligands in the cancer treatment. The need to add to a novel and productive legand has never been more noteworthy, and the use of proper conjugation chemistry is essential [20].

Recently, Zhou et al. prepared a surface engineered of NaGd F4:Ce/Tb hybrid nanoparticles with DNA for new type of pH-responsive therapeutic platform to enhance the therapeutic efficiency while minimizing side effects. The introduction of the layer of aptamer molecule on the surface facilitated the cellular uptake of the resulting nanocomposite into specific target cells via receptor-mediated endocytosis. This group proved that the hybrid nanocarrier may serve as a practical and multifunctional probe for cancer therapy [53].

6. LIPOSOMES IN TARGETING DRUG DELIVERY

Dispersion of neutral phospholipids or amphiphilic lipids (i.e., cholesterol, glycolipids) in the aqueous solution leads to the formation of closed vesicular structures, which morphologically resemble cells. These closed vesicles have been called "Liposomes" [54] (fat bodies) and consist of hydrated bilayers. Liposomes not only have the ability to mimic structures of cell membranes but also have the potential either to encapsulate hydrophilic materials in the inner liposome water phase or to associate the lipophilic materials within the lipid bilayer region. Initial studies on the fate of liposomes and entrapped agents started in 1970 [55].

Liposomes were recommended as drug carriers in cancer chemotherapy by Gregoriadis in 1974 and later the interest in liposomes has increased and is currently being widely concentrated on as drug carriers. Three fundamental requirements need to be met if liposomes are to be fruitful in drug delivery, specifically to cancerous tissues: (i) prolonged blood circulation, (ii) adequate tumor accumulation, and (iii) controlled drug release and uptake by tumor cells with a release profile coordinating the pharmacodynamics of the drug [56–60].

Stealth liposomes are suggested to carry the drug in the aqueous core, and they are usually decorated by recognition molecules, being widely studied and applied [61]. The poor outcome of current therapies continuously stimulates the search for new treatment strategies. This includes the activation of the normal vasculature to form tumor blood vessels and the involvement of immune response elements in tumor development proliferation. The hindrance of these procedures introduces an attractive therapeutic strategy and a new class of anticancer therapeutics such as angiogenesis inhibitors and anti-inflammatory drugs [62].

Tumor-associated inflammation has been perceived as an important tumor growth propagator and, therefore, represents an attractive target for anticancer therapy. Glucocorticoids (GCs), a potent class of anti-inflammatory drugs, showed antitumor effects at high daily doses. Unfortunately, this dose leads to severe side effects, including morbidity and mortality, attributable to severe immunosuppression. Recently, researchers have improved this unfavorable therapeutic index using long circulating liposomes as the glucocorticoid delivery nanocarrier. This vehicle could strongly inhibit tumor growth, after administration of a single weekly dose [63].

The effectiveness of the liposomal formulation was attributed to modification in drug pharmacokinetics such as increased blood circulation and glucocorticoid accumulation in the tumor, and the so-called enhanced permeability and retention effect.

Inspired by recent findings, in the tumor microenvironment, a main mechanism of the antitumor activity of GC is the inhibition of macrophage activity and downregulation of pro-angiogenic factors, which are produced by functional tumor-associated macrophages. In addition, in vitro information proposed a direct cytotoxic and antiproliferative activity to both endothelial and tumor cells [64].

Kluza et al. developed paramagnetic and fluorescent liposomes, encapsulating prednisolone phosphate, to evaluate its antitumor activity and therapeutic response. In this study, cytotoxicity of the new multifunctional liposomes (120 nm diameter) was tested in B16F10 melanoma subcutaneously (20 mg/kg/week) inoculated in C57BL/6 mice and compared with the free drug formulation. It was significantly found to inhibit tumor growth compared with nontreated mice and similarly to free form [63].

PEGylated liposomal doxorubicin (DOX) is approved for the treatment of refractory ovarian cancer and Kaposi sarcoma in the United States. In this carrier, the efficacy of the drug was preserved and a cardiac toxic effect was significantly decreased [18].

Albumin nanoparticle-bound paclitaxel, is also approved in the United States for the treatment of metastatic breast cancer, has greater efficacy compared with the conventional castor oil-based formulation and has lesser side effects [18].

Liposomes can also be used as a nonviral vector to deliver siRNA to target cells for gene therapy. Mokhtarieh and his coworkers developed a novel method of producing asymmetric liposome particles (ALPs) with highly efficient siRNA encapsulation. In their work, liposomes were prepared by the solvent evaporation and dialysis method, composed of ionizable cationic 1,2- dioleoyl-3- dimethyl ammonium-propane and 1,2-dioleoyl-sn-glycero-3-phosphoethanolamine (DOPE), which entrap siRNA, and the outer one is composed of 1,2-distearoyl-sn-glycero-3-phosphocholine, DOPE, polyethylene glycol- 1,2- distearoyl-sn-glycero-3-phosphatidyl ethanolamine (PEG–PE), and cholesterol. Ninety percent of siRNA was entrapped in negatively charged surface liposomes. The surface-modified ALPs with a polyarginine peptide (R12) induced nonspecific cell penetration, while naked liposome has almost no uptake into cells. The modification of ALP's surface by the antihuman epidermal growth factor receptor antibody (anti-EGFR) induces an EGFR-mediated uptake into the nonsmall cell lung cancer cell lines and did not take up NIH-3T3 cell line without the receptor [65].

The triggered release of pH-sensitive liposomes is probably the most biocompatible method for releasing drugs directly in the cytoplasm of cells. When liposomes are internalized to endosomes, they enter an acidic environment. Reddy and Low prepared the pH-sensitive lipid formulation from DOPE and citraconic anhydride and used them to prepare liposomes. They observed that the resulting liposomes were stable at neutral pH but fusogenic at pH 5 [66]. Figure 6 shows the schematic diagram of the liposome in targeted drug delivery.

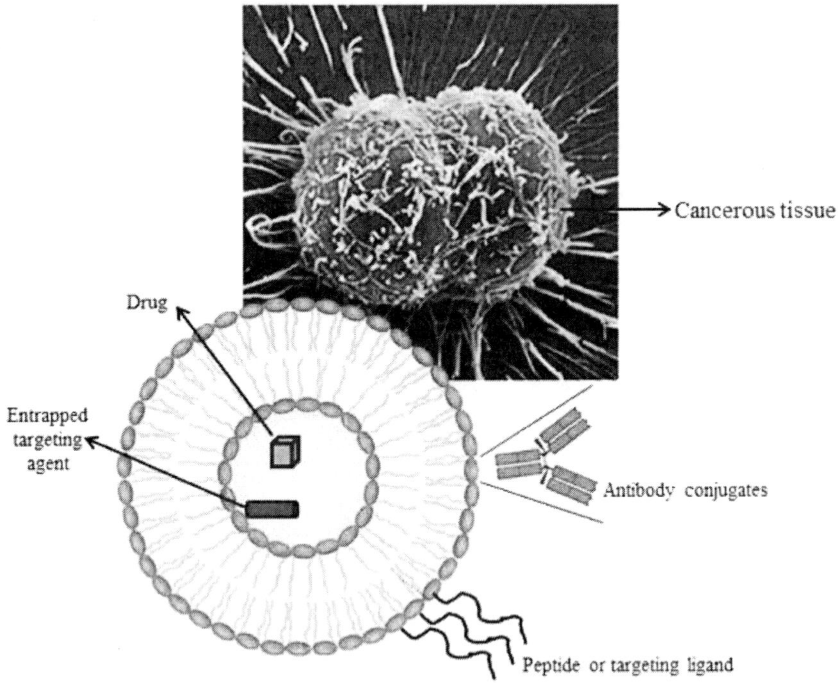

Figure 6. Liposome in target drug delivery

Choi and coworkers synthesized an amphiphilic DNA hybrid duplex by using Watson–Crick base pairing and DNA bioconjugation with cholesterol or tLyp-1 tumor-homing peptide. The resultant amphiphilic DNA hybrid duplexes can self-assemble in an aqueous solution into nanoliposome with the outer ligand of tLyp-1 peptides. This nanocarrier can efficiently entrap doxorubicin and also has the pH-dependent structure, which can release the drug in the acidic environment of cytosol of tumor cells [67]. These results provide an alternative approach to specifically deliver doxorubicin into targeted cells for cancer therapy as well as controlling drug release under acidic conditions such as endosomes or lysosomes.

Chiang et al. investigated the combination of polymer and liposome in carrier preparation. This group prepared pH-responsive polymer–liposome for intracellular drug transfer and targeted cancer therapy.

From this work, it was obvious that the combination of carrier should be a promising for targeted drug delivery in the future, exactly when this new carrier combines with biotechnology.

7. SOLID LIPID NANOPARTICLES AS A TARGETED DRUG DELIVERY SYSTEM

In the late 1990s, SLNs were proposed for brain drug targeting application independently by two research groups, although the first proof of lipid particle transport across the BBB had already been provided. SLNs are colloidal carrier systems, which provide controlled–release profiles for many substances [68–72]. Kashanian et al. prepared aqueous dispersions of lipid nanoparticles using a modified, pH-sensitive derivative of phosphatidyl ethanolamine loaded with triamcinolone acetonide as a drug. The SLNs prepared in this study were able to control the release of drug under acidic conditions. This group showed that with increasing pH, the amount of releasing drug is increased due to the burst effect in this condition as well [30].

Studying the pharmacokinetics of two anticancer agents, namely camptothecin and doxorubicin, drug accumulation in the brain was observed after both oral and i.v. administration when loaded into SLN. As previously shown in PACA NPs, better results in brain targeting were achieved when SLN surface characteristics were modified by means of PEG derivatives or PEG-containing surfactants [73].

8. GOLD NANOPARTICLES IN TARGET DRUG DELIVERY

Bactericidal efficacy of gold nanoparticles (GNPs) conjugated with ampicillin, streptomycin, and kanamycin was evaluated. Gold nanoparticles were conjugated with the antibiotics and drugs during the synthesis of nanoparticle utilization [74-76], by functionalizing gold particles, where amino acids, glutathione, polyethylene glycol, etc. were used as linkers [77-79]. The conjugated gold nanoparticles showed greater antibacterial effects and lower MIC compared with the free drug in three bacterial strains, Escherichia coli DH5a, Micrococcus luteus, and

Staphylococcus aureus. In addition, nanoconjugate could increase their heat stability [80,81].

Bergen and coworkers prepared nanoparticle formulations of GNPs with varying particle size, surface charge, and surface hydrophilicity. In this study, the galactose attached to the surface of NPs by conjugation of PEG-thiol and galactose-PEG-thiol to gold colloids. This platform was applied to screen for NP formulations that demonstrate hepatocyte-targeted delivery in vivo. This group investigated that the presence of galactose ligands was found to significantly affect the targeting efficiency [82].

9. NIOSOMES

Nonionic surfactant vesicles (niosomes), are biodegradable, relatively nontoxic, more stable, and inexpensive, and therefore could be an alternative to liposomes [83]. Due to the encapsulation of a wide range of toxic drugs such as antiviral, anticancer, and anti-AIDS drugs in niosomes, this carrier is so valuable in the delivery of proteins and biological medications. Niosome is a promising carrier system in comparison with ionic drug carriers, which are relatively toxic and moderately harmful [84].

Bragagni and coworkers developed a stable and safe niosomal formulation to effectively encapsulate DOX. The developed formulation, in virtue of its relatively high efficiency of drug encapsulation and good stability, could find useful applications as an effective tool for achieving DOX brain delivery, exploiting the brain uptake properties of the glucose-targeted vesicles [85].

Preliminary in vivo studies involved the i.v. administration of a single dose of the developed niosome formulation with respect to the target tissue. This formulation gave rise to stable and nano-sized vesicles, which are able to improve doxorubicin brain delivery. Positive results of preliminary in vivo studies require future pharmacokinetic studies to gain more insight into the mechanism of drug transport of functionalized niosomes [86].

10. QUANTUM DOTS

Quantum dots (QDs), semiconductor fluorescent nanoparticles, ranging from 2 to 10 nm in size has a core of hundreds to thousands of atoms of group II and VI elements (e.g., cadmium, technetium, zinc, and selenide) or group III (e.g., tantalum) and V elements (e.g., indium). This carrier with a cadmium selenide core and a zinc sulfide shell, by a coating of an amphiphilic polymer, is ordinarily utilized for drug delivery systems [87]. QDs greatly expand the possibilities for fluorescence imaging of cells and living animals [88].

QDs have been conjugated to antibodies, allowing for simultaneous labeling and accurate quantification of these target proteins in one target section. Direct conjugation of targeted antibodies to the surface of QDs in a molar ration of four to ten, without the use of secondary antibodies, might be the best approach to achieve multiplex detection of molecular targets.

QDs can be bioconjugated to either the 3′ or 5′ end of an oligo sequence. Xiao and Barker have discussed the ability to control the number of attached oligonucleotides by the use of a streptavidin–biotin quantum dot system [89].

This bioconjugate has a high affinity to target cells and causes minimum nonspecific binding to normal cells. The quantum dot-based assay was developed that could quantitatively detect the estrogen receptor, progesterone receptor, and ERBB2 (e.g., MCF-7, BT474, and MDA-231 cells) in paraffin-embedded human breast cancer cells [90]. These cell lines were overexpressed by these receptors and were stained simultaneously with multiple quantum dots, which were directly bioconjugated to targeting antibodies for these three proteins [91].

Biotinylated DNA probes for labeled cells by streptavidin-coated quantum dots could identify of ERBB2, even at low levels of expression. This information recommends that the use of quantum dot-labeled oligonucleotides for detecting gene amplification especially at low levels of expression may offer points of interest over the standard fluorescence in situ hybridization (FISH) method [91].

11. TARGETING DRUG DELIVERY WITH MAGNETIC NANOPARTICLES

Magnetic nanoparticles (MNPs) offer several advantages when used as a drug carrier, including the large surface area, which can be properly modified to attach to drug molecules. Magnetic NPs can also be used with other carriers for drug delivery. Ensuring biocompatibility and nontoxicity, iron oxide-based particles (magnetite) with superparamagnetic characteristics are commonly used as magnetically responsive components, which can be manipulated by an external magnetic field gradient. Based on these properties, the superparamagnetic nanoparticles could be transported through the vascular system, concentrated in a specific part of the body with the aid of a magnetic field, and used as a carrier [92–94].

Iron oxide nanoparticles have found applications in the so-called magnetic drug targeting. Iron oxide nanoparticles in an external magnetic field are able to deliver particles to the desired target area [95,96] and fix them there while the drug is released to exert a local effect [97]. Although magnetic targeting has been evaluated for a number of tumor-targeting studies, the most recent work is related to brain cancer.

It has been demonstrated that the release of drugs from magnetoliposomes could be controlled by an alternative current magnetic heating [98]. Although magnetoliposomes could be specifically heated to 42°C, the heating was mostly limited inside the thin lipid bi-layers [99].

Hsu and Su developed magnetic lipid nanoparticles with sizes ranging from 5 to 25 mm, composed of multiple drugs controlling their release in a desired pattern. The lipid matrices are solid at body temperature and melt around 45–55°C. In this study, the dissipated magnetic heat liquefied the encompassing lipid networks and resulted in an accelerated release of the encapsulated drugs.

Three accomplishments resulted: (1) Preparation of magnetic lipid nanoparticles with co-encapsulated drugs and heating components; (2) conjugation of surface-modified g-Fe_2O_3 particles that can be remotely energized to activate the heating and rapid drug release; and (3) designing a new nanocarrier, which can accomplish localized heating and pulsative release [99].

Zhu et al. prepared the chitosan-coated magnetic nanoparticles (CS MNPs) as carriers of 5-fluorouracil (CS–5-FuMNPs) through a reverse microemulsion method. It was found that the synthesized CS–5-Fu MNPs were spherical in shape with an average size of 100 ± 20 nm, low aggregation, and good magnetic responsivity. The result of CS–5-Fu MNPs cytotoxicity on K562 cancer cells showed that the nanoparticles have significant antitumor activities, and FITC-labeled nanoparticles could effectively enter into the cancer cells and induce cell apoptosis [74].

Gollavelli and Ling [75] investigated a novel magnetic and fluorescent graphene nanoparticles with a simple noncovalent approach. In this work, a hydrophobic silicon napthalocyanine bis (trihexylsilyloxide) (SiNc4) photosensitizer was adopted to immobilizing onto water-dispersible magnetic and fluorescent graphene (MFG) via pep stacking to yield MFGeSiNc4 functioned as a theranostic nanocarrier. The developed MFGeSiNc4 may thus be utilized as a potential theranostic nanocarrier for phototherapy of cancer cells with a single light source for less time-consuming and cost-effective treatments with a minimal therapy dose.

12. TARGETED DELIVERY FOR VACCINE

The unique properties of nanoparticles, which can be altered by planned application, make excellent approaches for immunization and treatment of different diseases. The use of nanoparticles as vaccine adjuvants and carriers has opened up an entire new field of research. Different materials in the viral (20–200 nm) or bacterial (200–5000 nm) size ranges introduced in vaccine formulations with a stable half-life prevent enzymatic degradation of antigen and increase antigen uptake by specifically targeting specialist antigen-presenting cells (APCs) [76,100]. Some nanoparticle-based vaccines are designed to include ligands that can target APC and hence help trigger immune responses. Some possess internal adjuvants, triggering toll-like receptor (TLR) ligation and local danger signals to potentiate the effective antigen presentation to T cells.

Different designs and compositions of nanoparticle-based vaccines allow for specific tailoring of antigen delivery to the target cell type or specific tissue. In addition, the size of the particles plays a major role in the mechanism of particle uptake by APCs, influencing the type of the resulting immune response [100].

More recently a synthetic nanoparticle vaccine platform that targets lymph node-resident dendritic cells (DCs) has been developed, capable of mounting an immune response to conjugated antigen. The cross-presentation by DCs was demonstrated by direct antibody staining and in vitro stimulation of $CD8^+$ T cells from OT-I mice and was indeed the most efficient with the reduction-sensitive conjugation.

Similarly, interferon (IFN) production by $CD4^+$ T cells from OT-II mice has been observed. Finally, immunization with OVA peptide-bearing nanoparticles resulted in in vivo proliferation and IFN production by adoptively transferred CD8+ OT-I T cells and was also the most efficient with reduction-sensitive linking of the peptide antigen. These results demonstrate the relevance of the poly (propylene sulfide) nanoparticle vaccine platform and antigen conjugation scheme for activating both cytotoxic and helper T-cell responses [101].

13. NONCOVALENT PROTEIN–NANOPARTICLE CONJUGATION USED FOR TARGETED DRUG DELIVERY

Some of the studies have investigated the thermodynamics of binding between proteins and nanomaterials, demonstrating that properly functionalized NPs interact with proteins in an analogous fashion to protein–protein interactions. The biophysical characteristics of these interactions, such as binding affinity, residence time, binding cooperatively of NP, and the common serum proteins such as albumin, have been quantitatively described in the buffer medium to determine the behavior of proteins on NP surfaces [34,102].

Carbon nanotubes have a high surface area for chemical interactions and conjugations. The nonspecific protein–nanotube conjugates contain electrostatic interactions and hydrogen bonding, especially when carbon nanotubes are pretreated with oxidative acids (Figure 7) [103,104].

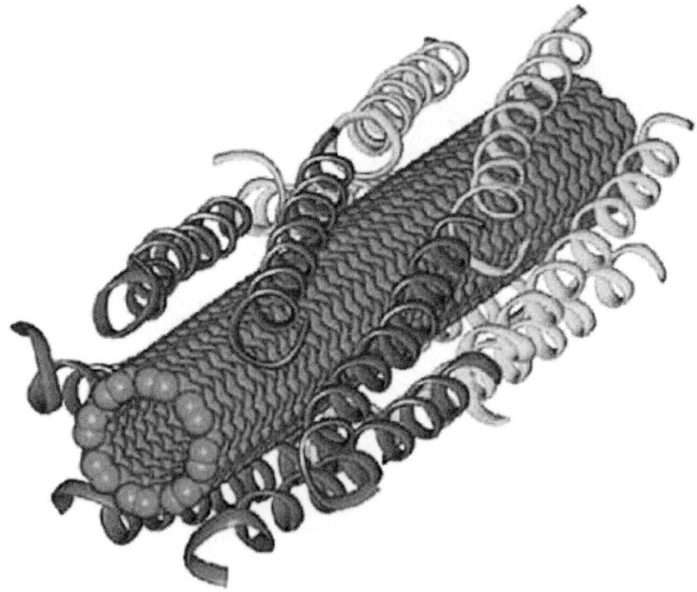

Figure 7. Immobilization of biomacromolecules on carbon nanotube surfaces

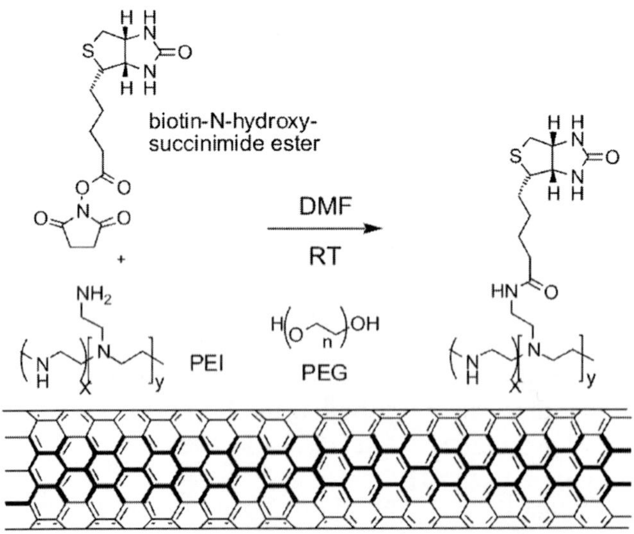

Figure 8. Absorption of polymer on the nanotube surface with the aid of PEG and PEI

In this conjugation reaction, selected chemical reagents are utilized with known chemistry to link proteins to nanotubes in a more controllable manner. Protein surface amino groups of residues, such as lysine and nanotube-bound carboxylic acids, which are exposed by oxidative acid treatments, are widely involved in some of these specific conjugations and form amide linkages [35].

In another report, PEG was co-adsorbed onto single-wall nanotube (SWNT) devices with polyethylenimine. The pendant primary amine groups on PEI were available for subsequent biotin derivatization, and thus streptavidin recognition (Figure 8) [105].

14. CONCLUSIONS

Targeted drug delivery, sometimes called smart drug delivery, is a method of delivering medication to a patient in a manner that increases the concentration of the medication in infective organs or cells, relative to others. The objective of a targeted drug delivery system is to prolong, localize, and concentrate the drug in the target diseased tissue. The advantages of the targeted release system are the reduction in the frequency of the dose administration by the patient, more uniform effect of the drug, reduction of drug side effects, and reduced fluctuation in circulating drug levels. The disadvantage of the system is high cost, which makes profitability more troublesome and productivity difficult.

Nanotechnology plays an important role in therapies of the future as "nanomedicines" by enabling this situation to happen, thus lowering doses required for efficacy as well as expanding the therapeutic windows and safety profiles of new medicines.

Conventional chemotherapeutic agents are distributed nonspecifically in the body where they influence both cancerous and normal cells, thereby limiting the dose achievable within the tumor and also resulting in suboptimal treatment due to excessive toxicities. Molecularly targeted therapy has developed as one way to overcome the problem of nonspecifity of routine anticancer drugs. However, the development of resistance in cancer cells can avoid the cytotoxicity of ordinary chemotherapeutics as well as the more up-to-date targeted therapeutics [105].

Both passive- and active-targeted nanoparticles can enhance the intracellular concentration of drugs in cancer cells while avoiding toxicity in normal cells. Furthermore, when nanoparticles bind to specific receptors and then enter the cell, they are usually enveloped by endosomes via receptor-mediated endocytosis, thereby bypassing the recognition of P-glycoprotein, one of the main drug resistance mechanisms. However, although nanoparticles offer many advantages as drug carrier systems, there are still many limitations to be solved such as poor oral bioavailability, instability in circulation, inadequate tissue distribution, and toxicity.

15. NOMENCLATURE

Phrase	Abbreviation
Blood brain barrier	(BBB)
1,2-dioleoyl-sn-glycero-3-phosphoethanolamine	DOPE
Antigen-presenting cell	APC
Carbon nanotubes	CNT
Dendritic cells	DC
N,N-dicyclohexyl carbodiimide	DCC
Doxorubicin	DOX
Drug delivery systems	DDS
N-ethyl-N-(3-dimethylaminopropyl) carbodiimide hydrochloride	(EDAC)
Epidermal growth factor receptor	EGFR
Enhanced permeation and retention	EPR
Fluorescein isothiocyanate	FITC
Folic acid	FA
Glucocorticoid	GC
Gold nanoparticles	GNP
Murine canin fibroblast	MCF-7
Minimum inhibition concentration	MIC
Magnetic nanoparticles	MNP
Monoclonal antibodies	mAb
Multiwall carbon nanotubes	MWCNT
Poly (D, L-lactic-co-glycolic acid)	PLGA
Quantum dots	QD
Single-wall carbon nanotubes	SWCNT
Solid lipid nanoparticles	SLN
Triggering toll-like receptor	TLR

REFERENCES

1. Allen TM, Cullis PR 2004 Drug delivery systems: entering the mainstream. Science 303: 1818–1822

2. Farokhzad OC, Langer R 2009 Impact of nanotechnology on drug delivery. ACS Nano 3(1): 16–20

3. Petros RA, desimone JM 2010. Strategies in the design of nanoparticles for therapeutic applications. Nat Rev Drug Discov 9(8): 615–627

4. Shi J, Votruba AR, Farokhzad OC, Langer R 2010 Nanotechnology in drug delivery and tissue engineering: from discovery to applications. Nano Lett 10(9): 3223–3236.

5. Dawar S, Singh N, Kanwar RK, Kennedy RL, Veedu RN, Zhou SF, Krishnakumar S, Hazra S, Sasidharan S, Duan W, Kanwar JR 2013 Multifunctional and multitargeted nanoparticles for drug delivery to overcome barriers of drug resistance in human cancers. Drug Discov Today 18: 1292–1300.

6. Derakhshandeh K, Erfan M, Dadashzadeh S 2007. Encapsulation of 9-nitrocamptothecin, a novel anticancer drug, in biodegradable nanoparticles: factorial design, characterization and release kinetics. Euro J Pharm Biopharm 66: 34-41.

7. Afshari M, Derakhshandeh K and Hosseinzadeh L 2014 Characterization, cytotoxicity and apoptosis studies of methotrexate-loaded PLGA and PLGA-PEG nanoparticles. J Microencapsul 31: 239–245.

8. Derakhshandeh K, Fathi S 2012 Role of chitosan nanoparticles in the oral absorption of Gemcitabine. Int J Pharm. 437(1-2): 172–177.

9. Davis ME, Chen Z, Shin DM 2008 Nanoparticle therapeutics: an emerging treatment modality for cancer. Nat Rev Drug Discov 7(9): 771–782

10. Xu Q, Kambhampati SP, Kannan RM 2013 Nanotechnology approaches for ocular drug delivery. Middle East Afr J Ophthalmol 20: 26– 37.

11. Prokop A, Davidson JM2008. Nanovehicular intracellular delivery systems. J Pharm Sci 97: 3518–3590.

12. Kluza E, Yeo SY, Schmid S, van der Schaft DW.J, Boekhoven RW, Schiffelers RM, Storm G, Strijkers GJ, Nicolay K 2011 Anti-tumor activity of liposomal glucocorticoids: the relevance of liposome-mediated drug delivery, intratumoral localization and systemic activity. J Control Release 151: 10–17.

13. Ferrari M 2005 Cancer nanotechnology: opportunities and challenges. Nat Rev Cancer 5: 161–171.

14. Jain K 2005 Nanotechnology in clinical laboratory diagnostics. Clin Chim Acta 358: 37–54.

15. Sutton D, Nasongkla N, Blanco E, Gao J 2007 Functionalized micellar systems for cancer targeted drug delivery. Pharm Res 24: 1029–1046.

16. Xiang SD, Wilson K, Day S, Fuchsberger M, Plebanski M 2013 Methods of effective conjugation of antigens to nanoparticles as non-inflammatory vaccine carriers. Methods 60: 232–241.

17. Gao Z, Zhang L, Sun Y 2012 Nanotechnology applied to overcome tumor drug resistance. J Control Release 162: 45–55.

18. Yezhelyev MV, Gao X, Xing Y, Al-Hajj A, Nie S, O'Regan RM 2006 Emerging use of nanoparticles in diagnosis and treatment of breast cancer. Lancet Oncol 7: 657–667.

19. Vasir JK, Reddy MK, Labhasetwar VD 2005 Nanosystems in drug targeting: opportunities and challenges. Curren Nanosci 1: 47–64.

20. Wang M, Thanou M 2010 Targeting nanoparticles to cancer. Pharmacol Res 62: 90–99.

21. Au JL, Jang SH, Zheng J, Chen CT, Song S, Hu L 2001 Determinants of drug delivery and transport to solid tumors. J Control Release 74: 31–46.

22. Fetterly GJ, Straubinger RM 2003 Pharmacokinetics of paclitaxel containing liposomes in rats. AAPS Pharm Sci 5: E32.

23. Hoarau D, Delmas P, David S, Roux E, Leroux JC 2004 Novel long circulating lipid nanocapsules. Pharm Res 21: 1783–1789.

24. Moghimi SM, Szebeni J 2003 Stealth liposomes and long circulating nanoparticles: critical issues in pharmacokinetics, opsonization and protein-binding properties. Prog Lipid Res 42: 463–478.

25. Wang T, Kievit FM, Veiseh O, Arami H, Stephen ZR, Fang C, Liu Y, Ellenbogen RG, Zhang M 2013 Targeted cell uptake of a noninternalizing antibody through conjugation to iron oxide nanoparticles in primary central nervous system lymphoma. World Neurosurg 80: 134–141.

26. Pissuwan D, Niidome T, cortiemb 2011 The forthcoming applications of gold nanoparticles in drug and gene delivery systems. J Control Release 149: 65–71.

27. Derakhshandeh K, Soheili M, Dadashzadeh S, Saghiri R 2010 Preparation and in vitro characterization of 9-nitrocamptothecin-loaded long circulating nanoparticles for delivery in cancer patients. Int J Nanomed 5: 463–471.

28. Derakhshandeh K, Hochhaus G, Dadashzadeh S 2011 In-vitro cellular uptake and transport study of 9-nitrocamptothecin PLGA nanoparticles across caco-2 cell monolayer model. Iran J Pharm Res 10: 425–434.

29. Parveen S, Misra R, Sahoo SK 2012 Nanoparticles: a boon to drug delivery, therapeutics, diagnostics and imaging. Nanomed Nanotechnol Biol Med 8: 147–166.

30. Kashanian S, Azandaryani AH, Derakhshandeh K 2011 New surface-modified solid lipid nanoparticles using N-glutarylphosphatidylethanolamine as the outer shell. Int J Nanomed 6: 2393–2401.

31. Afshari M, Derakhshandeh K, Hosseinzadeh L 2014 Characterisation, cytotoxicity and apoptosis studies of methotrexate-loaded PLGA and PLGA-PEG nanoparticles. J Microencapsul 31: 239–245.

32. Ramana LN, Sharma S, Sethuraman S, Ranga U, Krishnan UM 2014 Evaluation of chitosan nanoformulations as potent anti-HIV therapeutic systems. Biochimica et Biophysica Acta 1840: 476–484.

33. Shi C, Guo X, Qu Q, Tang Z, Wang Y, Zhou S 2014 Actively targeted delivery of anticancer drug to tumor cells by redox-responsive star-shaped micelles. Biomaterials: 1–12.

34. Rana S, yehyc, Rotello VM 2010 Engineering the nanoparticle–protein interface: applications and possibilities. Curr Opin Chem Biol 14: 828–834.

35. Kumar C 2005 Biofunctionalization of Nanomaterials. Copyright 8. WILEY-VCH Verlag gmbh & Co. Kgaa, Weinheim. ISBN: 3-527-31381-8

36. Daniel S, Rao TP, Rao KS, Rani SU, Naidu GRK, Lee HY, Kawai T 2007 A review of DNA functionalized/grafted carbon nanotubes and their characterization. Sens Actuators B 122: 672–682.

37. Hapuarachchige S, Zhu W, Kato Y, Artemov D 2014 Bioorthogonal, two-component delivery systems based on antibody and drug-loaded nanocarriers for enhanced internalization of nanotherapeutics. Biomaterials 35: 2346–2354.

38. Olejnik M, Krajnik B, Kowalska D, Lin G, Mackowski S 2013 Spectroscopic studies of plasmon coupling between photosynthetic complexes and metallic quantum dots. J Phy Condens Matter 25: 1–12.

39. Yokoyama M 2005 Drug targeting with nano-sized carrier systems. J Artif Organs 8: 77–84.

40. Jia H, Zhu J, Wang X, Cheng H, Chen G, Zhao Y, Zeng X, Feng J, Zhang X, Zhuo R 2014 A boronate-linked linear-hyperbranched polymeric nanovehicle for ph-dependent tumor-targeted drug delivery. Biomaterials 35: 5240e–5249e

41. Kulhari H, Pooja D, Shrivastav S, Mc Naidu VG, Sistla R 2014 Peptide conjugated polymeric nanoparticles as a carrier for targeted delivery of docetaxel. Colloid Surf B 117: 166–173.

42. Kocbek P, Obermajer N, Cegnar M, Kos J, Kristl J 2007 Targeting cancer cells using PLGA nanoparticles surface modified with monoclonal antibody. J Control Release 120: 18–26.

43. Chiu SJ, Ueno NT, Lee RJ 2004 Tumor-targeted gene delivery via anti-HER2 antibody (trastuzumab, herceptinr) conjugated polyethylenimine. J Control Release 97: 357–369.

44. Abdel Wahab BA, Evgenivetch PV, Alyautdin RN 2005 Brain targeting of nerve growth factor using poly(butylcyanoacrylate) nanoparticles. Internet J Pharmacol 3.

45. Yang J, Lee CH, Park J, Seo S, Lim EK, Song YJ, Suh JS, Yoon HG, Huh YM, Haam S 2007 Antibody conjugated magnetic PLGA nanoparticles for diagnosis and treatment of breast cancer. J Mater Chem 17: 2695–2699.

46. Sudimack J, Lee RJ 2000 Targeted drug delivery via the folate receptor. Adv Drug Deliv Rev 41: 147–162.

47. Koo OM, Rubinstein I, Onyuksel H 2005 Role of nanotechnology in targeted drug delivery and imaging: a concise review. Nanomedicine 1: 193–212.

48. Kim JS, Oh MH, Park JY, Park TG, Nam YS 2013 Protein-resistant, reductively dissociable polyplexes for in vivo systemic delivery and tumor-targeting of sirna. Biomaterials 34: 2370–2379.

49. Heidarian S 2012 Folate targeted nanoparticles: preparation, physicochemical characterization and in vitro cytotoxicity effect. Phd thesis. Kermanshah University of Medical Science.

50. Wu H, Cabral H, Toh K, Mi P, Chen YC, Matsumoto Y, Yamada N, Liu X, Kinoh H, Miura Y, Kano MR, Nishihara H, Nishiyama N, Kataoka K 2014 Polymeric micelles loaded with platinum anticancer drugs target preangiogenic micrometastatic niches associated with inflammation. J Control Release 189: 1–10.

51. Tarn D, Ashley CE, Xue M, Carnes EC, Zink JI, Brinker CJ 2013 Mesoporous silica nanoparticle nanocarriers: biofunctionality and biocompatibility. Acc Chem Res 46: 792–801.

52. Chen C, Geng J, Pu F, Yang X, Ren J, Qu X 2011 Polyvalent nucleic acid/mesoporous silica nanoparticle conjugates: dual stimuli-responsive vehicles for intracellular drug delivery. Angew Chem Int Ed 50: 882–886.

53. Zhou L, Chen Z, Dong K, Yin M, Ren J, Qu X 2014 DNA-mediated biomineralization of rare-earth nanoparticles for simultaneous imaging and stimuli-responsive drug delivery. Biomaterials 35(30):8694-6702.

54. Hong JS, Vreeland WN, depaoli Lacerda SH, Locascio LE, Gaitan Mi, Raghavan SR 2008 Liposome-templated supramolecular assembly of responsive alginate nanogels. Langmuir 24: 4092–4096.

55. Gregoriadis G, Ryman BE 1972 Fate of protein-containing liposomes injected into rats. An approach to the treatment of storage diseases. Eur J Biochem 24: 485–491.

56. Andresen TL, Jensen SS, Jorgensen K 2005 Advanced strategies in liposomal cancer therapy: problems and prospects of active and tumor specific drug release. Prog Lipid Res 44: 68–97.

57. Lim SB, Banerjee A, Önyüksel H 2012 Improvement of drug safety by the use of lipid-based nanocarriers. J Control Release 163: 34–45.

58. Kraft JC, Freeling JP, Wang Z, HO RJY 2014 Emerging research and clinical development trends of liposome and lipid nanoparticle drug delivery systems. J Pharm Sci 103: 29–52.

59. Howard MD, Greineder CF, Hood ED, Muzykanto VR 2014 Endothelial targeting of liposomes encapsulating SOD/catalase mimetic EUK-134 alleviates acute pulmonary inflammation. J Control Release 177: 34–41.

60. Ninomiya K, Yamashita T, Kawabata S, Shimizu N 2014 Targeted and ultrasound-triggered drug delivery using liposomes co-modified with cancer cell-targeting aptamers and a thermosensitive polymer. Ultrason Sonochem 21: 1482–1488

61. Yuan F, Leunig M, Huang SK, Berk DA, Papahadjopoulos D, Jain RK 1994 Microvascular permeability and interstitial penetration

of sterically stabilized (stealth) liposomes in a human tumor xenograft. Cancer Res 54: 3352–3356.

62. Immordino ML, Dosio F, Cattel L 2006 Stealth liposomes: review of the basic science, rationale, and clinical applications, existing and potential. Int J Nanomed 1: 297–315.

63. Kluza E, Yeo SY, Schmid S, van der Schaft DWJ, Boekhoven RW, Schiffelers RM, Storm G, Strijkers GJ, Nicolay K 2011 Anti-tumor activity of liposomal glucocorticoids: the relevance of liposome-mediated drug delivery, intratumoral localization and systemic activity. J Control Release 151: 10–17.

64. Cho K, Wang X, Nie S, Chen Z, Shin DM 2008 Therapeutic nanoparticles for drug delivery in cancer. Clinical Cancer Res 14: 1310–1316.

65. Mokhtarieh AA, Cheong S, Kim S, Chung BH, Lee MK 2012 Asymmetric liposome particles with highly efficient encapsulation of sirna and without nonspecific cell penetration suitable for target-specific delivery. Biochim Biophys Acta 1818: 1633–1641.

66. Reddy JA, Low PS 2000 Enhanced folate receptor mediated gene therapy using a novel ph-sensitive lipid formulation. J Control Release 64: 27–37.

67. Choi K, Kwon IC, Ahn HJ 2013 Self-assembled amphiphilic DNA-cholesterol/DNA-peptide hybrid duplexes with liposome-like structure for doxorubicin delivery. Biomaterials 34: 4183–4190

68. Muller RH, Mader K, Gohla S 2000 Solid lipid nanoparticles (SLN) for controlled drug delivery – a review of the state of the art. Eur J Pharm Biopharm 50: 161–177.

69. Rostami E, Kashanian S, Hemati Azandaryani A 2014 Preparation of solid lipid nanoparticles as drug carriers for levothyroxine sodium with in vitro drug delivery kinetic characterization. Mol Biol Rep. 41(5): 3521-3527.

70. Rostami E, Kashanian S, Hemati Azandaryani A, Faramarzi H, Ezzati J, Omidfar K 2014 Drug targeting using solid lipid nanoparticles. Chemis Phys Lipids 181: 56–61.

71. Bondi ML, Craparo EF 2010 Solid lipid nanoparticles for applications in gene therapy: a review of the state of the art. Expert Opin Drug Del 7: 7–18.

72. Mehnert W, Maeder K 2012 Solid lipid nanoparticles: production, characterization and applications, Adv Drug Deliv Rev 64: 83–101.

73. Jin SE, Kim CK 2012 Long-term stable cationic solid lipid nanoparticles for the enhanced intracellular delivery of SMAD3 antisense oligonucleotides in activated murine macrophages. J Pharm Pharm Sci 15: 467–482.

74. Zhu L, Ma J, Jia N, Zhao Y, Shen H 2009 Chitosan-coated magnetic nanoparticles as carriers of 5-fluorouracil: preparation, characterization and cytotoxicity studies. Colloids Surf B Biointerfaces 68: 1–6.

75. Gollavelli G, Ling YC 2014 Magnetic and fluorescent graphene for dual modal imaging and single light induced photothermal and photodynamic therapy of cancer cells. Biomaterials 35: 4499–4507.

76. Mishra D, Mishra H, Mishra PK, Nahar M, Dubey V, Jain NK 2010 Evaluation of solid lipid nanoparticles as carriers for delivery of hepatitis B surface antigen for vaccination using subcutaneous route. J Pharm Pharm Sci 13: 495–509.

77. Groneberg DA, Giersig M, Welte T, Pison U 2006 Nanoparticle-based diagnosis and therapy. Curr Drug Targets. 7: 643–648.

78. Gu YJ, Cheng J, Man CW, Wong WT, Cheng SH 2012 Gold-doxorubicin nanoconjugates for overcoming multidrug resistance. Nanomed 8: 204–211.

79. Bhattacharya D, Saha B, Mukherjee A, Ranjan Santra C, Karmakar P 2012 Gold nanoparticles conjugated antibiotics: stability and functional evaluation. Nanosci Nanotechnol 2: 14–21.

80. Paciotti GF, Kingston DGI, Tamarkin L 2006 Colloidal gold nanoparticles: a novel nanoparticle platform for developing

multifunctional tumor-targeted drug delivery vectors. Drug Develop Res 67: 47–54.

81. Saha B, Bhattacharya J, Mukherjee A, Ghosh AK, Santra CR, Dasgupta AK, Karmakar P 2007 In vitro structural and functional evaluation of gold nanoparticles conjugated antibiotics. Nanoscale Res Lett 2: 614–622.

82. Bergen JM, von Recum HA, Goodman TT, Massey AP, Pun SH 2006 Gold nanoparticles as a versatile platform for optimizing physicochemical parameters for targeted drug delivery. Macromolecular Biosci 6: 506–516.

83. Uchegbu IF, Vyas SP 1998 Non-ionic surfactant based vesicles (niosomes) in drug delivery. Int J Pharm 172: 33–70.

84. Dufes C, Schatzlein AG, Tetley L, Gray AI, Watson DG, Olivier JC, Couet W, Uchegbu IF 2000 Niosomes and polymeric chitosan based vesicles bearing transferrin and glucose ligands for drug targeting. Pharm Res 17: 1251–1258.

85. Bragagni M, Mennini N, Ghelardini C, Mura P 2012 Development and characterization of niosomal formulations of doxorubicin aimed at brain targeting. J Pharm Pharm Sci 15: 94–102.

86. Bragagnia M, Menninia N, Ghelardinib C, Muraa P 2012 Development and characterization of niosomal formulations of doxorubicin aimed at brain targeting. J Pharm Pharm Sci 15: 184–196.

87. Medintz IL, Uyeda HT, Goldman ER, Mattoussi H 2005 Quantum dot bioconjugates for imaging, labelling and sensing. Nature Mater 4: 435–446.

88. Howarth M, Takao K, Hayashi Y, Ting A 2005 Targeting quantum dots to surface proteins in living cells with biotin ligase. Proc Natl Acad Sci U S A 102: 7583–7588.

89. Xiao Y, Telford WG, Ball JC, Locascio LE, Barker PE 2005 Semiconductor nanocrystal conjugates, FISH and ph. Nature Methods 2: 723–732.

90. Yezhelyev M, Morris C, Gao X 2005 Simultaneous and quantitative detection of multiple biomarkers in human breast cancers using semiconductor multicolor quantum dots breast cancer research and treatment. Breast Cancer Res Treat 94: 48–57.

91. Yezhelyev M, Gao X, Markus A 2005 Multiplex molecular diagnostic of tumor tissue using quantum dots. Am Soc Clin Oncol 23: 843–849.

92. Neuberger T, Schopf B, Hofmann H, Hofmann M, Rechenberg B 2005 Superparamagnetic nanoparticles for biomedical applications: possibilities and limitations of a new drug delivery system. J Magn Magn Mater 293: 483–496.

93. Chen JP, Yang PC, Ma YH, Wu T 2011 Characterization of chitosan magnetic nanoparticles for in situ delivery of tissue plasminogen activator. Carbohydr Polym 84: 364–372.

94. Cole AJ, Yang VC, David AE 2011 Cancer theranostics: the rise of targeted magnetic nanoparticles. Trends Biotechnol 29: 323–332.

95. Alexiou C, Jurgons R, Schmid R. Hilpert A, Bergemann C, Parak F, Iro H 2005 In vitro and in vivo investigations of targeted chemotherapy with magnetic nanoparticles. J Magn Magn Mate 293: 389–393.

96. Mahmoudi M, Sant S, Wang B, Laurent S, Sen T2011 Superparamagnetic iron oxide nanoparticles (spions): development, surface modification and applications in chemotherapy. Adv Drug Deliv Rev 63: 24–46.

97. Liu X, Guan Y, Liu H, Ma Z, Yang Y, Wu X 2005 Preparation and characterization of magnetic polymer nanospheres with high protein binding capacity. J Magn Magn Mate 293: 111–118.

98. Babincova M, Cicmanec P, Altanerova V, Altaner C, Babinec P 2002 AC-magnetic field controlled drug release from magnetoliposomes: design of a method for site-specific chemotherapy. Bioelectro Chem 55: 17–25.

99. Hsu MH, Su YC 2008 Iron-oxide embedded solid lipid nanoparticles for magnetically controlled heating and drug delivery. Biomed Microdevices 10: 785–793.

100. Xiang SD, Wilson K, Day S, Fuchsberger M, Plebanski M 2013 Methods of effective conjugation of antigens to nanoparticles as non-inflammatory vaccine carriers. Methods 60: 232–241.

101. Hirosue S, Kourtis IC, van der Vlies AJ, Hubbell JA, Swartz MA 2010 Antigen delivery to dendritic cells by poly(propylene sulfide) nanoparticles with disulfide conjugated peptides: cross-presentation and T cell activation. Vaccine 28: 7897–7906.

102. Fu K, Huang W, Lin Y, Zhang D, Hanks TW, Rao AM, Sun YP 2002 Functionalization of carbon nanotubes with bovine serum albumin in homogeneous aqueous solution. J Nanosci Nanotechnol 2: 457–461.

103. Monteiro-Riviere, NA, Nemanich RJ, Inman AO, Wang YY, Riviere JE 2005 Multi-walled carbon nanotube interactions with human epidermal keratinocytes. Toxicol Lett 155: 377–384.

104. Chengqun Chen, Huijuan Zhang, Lin Hou, Jinjin Shi, Lei Wang, Chaofeng Zhang, Mingyue Zhang, Hongling Zhang, Xiufang Shi, Huixiang Li, Zhenzhong Zhang 2013 Single-walled carbon nanotubes mediated neovascularity targeted antitumor drug delivery system. J Pharm Pharm Sci 16(1):40-51.

105. Star, A, Gabriel JCP, Bradley K, Gruner G 2003 Electronic detection of specific protein binding using nanotube FET device. Nano Lett 3: 459–463.

106. Xiao Y, Barker PE 2004 Semiconductor nanocrystal probes for human metaphase chromosomes. Nucleic Acids Res 32: 28–33.

Chapter 7

Modelling of a Targeted Nanotherapeutic 'Stroma' to Deliver the Cytokine LIF, or XAV939, a Potent Inhibitor of Wnt–B-Catenin Signalling, for use in Human Fetal Dopaminergic Grafts in Parkinson's Disease

Jing-Wei Zhao[1], Sean C. Dyson[1], Christina Kriege[2], Pam Tyers[1], Xiaoling He[1], Tarek M. Fahmy[2], Su M. Metcalfe[1], Roger A. Barker[1]

[1]*John van Geest Centre for Brain Repair, Addenbrookes Hospital, University of Cambridge, Cambridge, CB2 0PY, UK.*

[2]*Department of Biomedical Engineering, Yale University, Malone Engineering Center, 55 Prospect Street, New Haven, CT 06511, USA.*

ABSTRACT

The endogenous reparative capacity of the adult human brain is low, and chronic neurodegenerative disorders of the central nervous system represent one of the greatest areas of unmet clinical need in the developing world. Novel therapeutic strategies to treat them include: (i) growth factor delivery to boost endogenous repair and (ii) replacement cell therapy, including replacing dopaminergic neurons to treat Parkinson's disease (PD). However, these approaches are restricted not only by rapid degradation of growth factors, but also by the limited availability of cells for transplant and the poor survival of implanted cells that lack the necessary stromal support. We therefore hypothesised that provision of a transient artificial stroma for paracrine delivery of pro-survival factors could overcome both of these issues. Using leukaemia inhibitory factor (LIF) – a proneural, reparative cytokine – formulated as target-specific poly(lactic-co-glycolic acid) (PLGA) nano-particles (LIF-nano-stroma), we discovered that attachment of LIF-nano-stroma to freshly isolated fetal dopaminergic cells improved their survival fourfold: furthermore, *in vivo*, the number of surviving human fetal dopaminergic cells tended to be higher at 3 months after grafting into the striatum of nude rats, compared with controls treated with empty nanoparticles. In addition, we also analysed the effect of a novel nano-stroma incorporating XAV939 (XAV), a potent inhibitor of the developmentally important Wnt–β-catenin signalling pathway, to investigate whether it could also promote the survival and differentiation of human fetal dopaminergic precursors; we found that the numbers of both tyrosine-hydroxylase-positive neurons (a marker of dopaminergic neurons) and total neurons were increased. This is the first demonstration that LIF-nano-stroma and XAV-nano-stroma each have pro-survival effects on human dopaminergic neurons, with potential value for target-specific modulation of neurogenic fate in cell-based therapies for PD.

INTRODUCTION

The prevalence of neurodegenerative disease is increasing as the population ages. After Alzheimer's disease, Parkinson's disease (PD) is the second commonest neurodegenerative disorder of the central nervous system (CNS). In PD, the disease process critically involves the nigrostriatal dopaminergic (DA) neurons, resulting in their loss and subsequent decreased dopamine levels in the dorsal striatum. The concept of replacing lost DA neurons with healthy cells of the same lineage underpins one major clinical approach that uses allografts of human fetal ventral mesencephalic (hfVM) tissue. This strategy has shown significant long-term benefits in some patients with PD (reviewed by Barker et al., 2013). However, the approach has a number of ethical and practical problems inherent to it and, thus, for the future, the derivation of DA precursors from embryonic stem cells or induced pluripotent cells will be an essential key research goal for clinical translation. But, as is the case for all cellular therapeutic approaches, two challenges arise: first, the need to deliver appropriate numbers of cells to the right site(s) and, second, to promote their survival long-term. In this latter respect, therapeutic support of the transplanted cells is required, raising the question, can the delivery of neurogenic growth factors or small molecules improve the efficacy and efficiency of cell therapy? The simplicity of such an approach has been hampered by the problem of delivering sufficient concentrations of factors in a sustained paracrine-type manner locally at the site of implantation. As a potential solution, we have been exploring the development of a biodegradable, surrogate stroma preloaded with a defined cargo of growth factor(s) or small molecules, the stroma itself being created by cargo-loaded solid-phase nano-particles of some 100 nM diameter, attached to the cell surface by cell-specific targeting antibody. Our prototype uses poly(lactic-co-glycolic) acid (PLGA), which is already approved by the FDA for therapeutic devices (Danhier et al., 2012). *In vivo*, PLGA slowly degrades by hydrolysis to lactic acid and glycolic acid, monomeric derivatives that feed into metabolic pathways for eventual release as carbon dioxide and water. PLGA allows for the creation of 'designer' particles for delivery; these particles can be modified for specific targeting as well as the type of cargo (which can be multiple) and the release kinetics of that cargo. Other approaches that have used synthetic biomaterials to mimic the extracellular microenvironment include bioengineered fibrillar matrices (reviewed by Lutolf and Hubbell, 2005), or adhesive micro-particles to deliver nerve growth factor (Mahoney and Saltzman, 2001). In the current study, we use nano-particles functionalised to bind directly to individual cells, testing cargos able to influence development in addition to cargos that support neurogenesis.

RESOURCE IMPACT

Background

Neurodegenerative diseases of the brain represent a large and increasing area of unmet clinical need. After Alzheimer's disease, Parkinson's disease (PD) is the second commonest neurodegenerative disorder. In PD, the disease process critically involves nigrostriatal dopaminergic (DA) neurons, resulting in their loss and decreased dopamine levels in the dorsal striatum. For individuals affected by PD, the development of tremor, rigidity and cognitive decline are compounded by an increased risk of early dementia and postural instability. The concept of replacing lost DA neurons with healthy cells of the same lineage underpins one current clinical approach that uses allografts of human fetal ventral mesencephalic (hfVM) tissue. However, many fetuses are required to graft a single individual, owing to the loss of harvested DA neurons denuded of their natural stromal microenvironment.

Results

In this study, the authors pioneer the use of nanotechnology to model a surrogate 'nano-stroma' engineered to deliver proneural growth factors to targeted cells. They report that LIF-nano-stroma, a prototype biodegradable poly(lactic-co-glycolic acid) (PLGA)-based nanoparticle matrix (PLGA is FDA approved for therapeutic devices) loaded with leukaemia inhibitory factor (LIF; a proneural and reparative factor) provided fourfold increased survival when targeted to DA neurons maintained *ex vivo*. Moreover, human fetal DA neurons pre-coated with LIF-nano-stroma outnumbered cells pre-coated with empty-nano 12 weeks after transplantation into the striatum of nude rats. Notably, DA cells showed the greatest benefit from LIF-nano-stroma pre-coating. The authors also developed a nano-stromal construct using the small molecule XAV939 (XAV) as cargo. XAV is a potent inhibitor of the Wnt–β-catenin signalling pathway, which is involved in neural development. XAV-nano-stroma retained bioactivity and promoted the survival of hfVM *ex vivo*, including that of DA precursors.

Implications and future directions

These findings provide the first demonstration that LIF-nano-stroma and XAV-nano-stroma both have pro-survival effects on human DA neurons. Moreover, they show that, to work, the nanoparticles must be attached physically to their target cells and must include a cargo – simple attachment of empty nano-stroma was not beneficial. More generally, these findings have implications for the application of nanotechnology to healthcare. Nano-medicine is a rapidly expanding field, and modelling the outcome of treatment is crucial for its progress. Notably, these findings highlight the potential of using surrogate nano-stromal niches to modulate the fate-determination pathways of precursor cells towards a desired phenotype. This approach might in future be used to support the translation of cell therapies derived from embryonic stem cells or induced pluripotent cells for neurodegenerative disease into clinical practice.

Leukaemia inhibitory factor (LIF) is an IL-6 family member; LIF-specific activity is endowed by the LIF-specific receptor subunit gp190. LIF is attractive as a therapeutic agent in cell therapy for PD, being both proneural and reparative (Laterza et al., 2013; Deverman and Patterson, 2012; Ling et al., 1998) as well as anti-inflammatory and tolerogenic through suppressing IL-6-linked TH17-mediated inflammatory immunity (Gao et al., 2009; Cao et al., 2011). To overcome the problem of the rapid degradation of LIF and its excretion *in vivo*, we previously developed LIF formulated as PLGA-nanoparticles (LIF-nano) and demonstrated that LIF-nano is superior to soluble LIF in being able to provide a stable source of low-dose LIF, mimicking paracrine delivery (Park et al., 2011), with activation of the STAT-3 signalling pathway (Anna Williams and S.M.M., unpublished observations). As such, LIF-nano met our aims to provide stromal support when attached to targeted cells by antibody and has been used successfully in the past for manipulation of T cell lineage differentiation (Gao et al., 2009;Park et al., 2011). Likewise, LIF-nano is known to support mouse embryonic stem cells in the absence of soluble LIF (Corradetti et al., 2012) as well as promote the survival of transplanted pancreatic β-cell islets (Dong et al., 2012). Therefore, we now asked, can a surrogate stroma provided by LIF-nano be targeted to primary neural precursor cells, and, by so doing, increase cell survival? Compared with other cell types, DA cells are highly susceptible to stress but nevertheless are the obvious candidate for neural grafting in PD. Thus, we looked at the response of these cells to LIF-nano and found that it had pro-survival effects on both rodent and human fetal nigral cells, and also *in vivo* for primary hfVM cells transplanted into the striatum of nude rats.

In addition to LIF-nano, we generated and tested a range of other novel nano-therapeutics as stromal candidates, including the small molecule XAV939 (XAV). XAV is a potent inhibitor of tankyrase (Huang et al., 2009), and this inhibition stabilises Axin1 and Axin2. Axin2 is known to bind β-catenin – the mediator of Wnt signalling (Moon et al.,

2002; Vacik et al., 2011) – and increased levels of Axin2 are able to retain β-catenin in the cytoplasm, preventing its nuclear translocation where it binds to T cell factors (TCFs) that regulate Wnt-controlled gene expression: these include genes required in neural development (Patapoutian and Reichardt, 2000). We therefore reasoned that the use of XAV-nano might modulate the Wnt–β-catenin signalling pathway and promote plasticity during neural lineage development, with the potential to manipulate lineage differentiation to give more neurons, including, for example, more DA cells, which is especially relevant to future stem-cell-based approaches to treating PD. We now show that XAV-nano retains XAV-mediated bioactivity and is strongly pro-survival when targeted to hfVM-derived cells, including the neural precursors of human DA cells.

RESULTS

Neurogenic 'stromal' nanoparticles

PLGA formulation of the neurogenic factors was based on the successful LIF-nano construct with proven bioactivity in guiding T lymphocyte lineage differentiation (**Fig. 1**). In the current study, novel cargo-carrying nanoparticles with the potential to influence neurogenic cell fate were created, including those carrying brain-derived neurotrophic factor (BDNF-nano), glial-derived neurotrophic factor (GDNF-nano), 7,8-dihydroxyflavone (a TrkB agonist; DHF-nano) (Jang et al., 2010) and XAV939 (XAV-nano). Encapsulation of each cargo within the avidin-coated nanoparticles was successful, although GDNF-nano proved to be relatively unstable, requiring several preparations before incorporation with good bioactivity was achieved. Cargo incorporation was around 1/1000 as measured by ELISA so that 1 mg of nanoparticles was estimated to correspond to 1 ng of cargo. In fact, the potency of the nano-formulated growth factor when compared with the soluble growth factor was increased in the order of 100- to 1000-fold as previously shown for LIF-nano (Park et al., 2011) and mathematically modelled by Labowsky and Fahmy (Labowsky and Fahmy, 2012). A fully detailed procedure for creating the PLGA-nano-stromal constructs used in this study is provided in the Materials and Methods section.

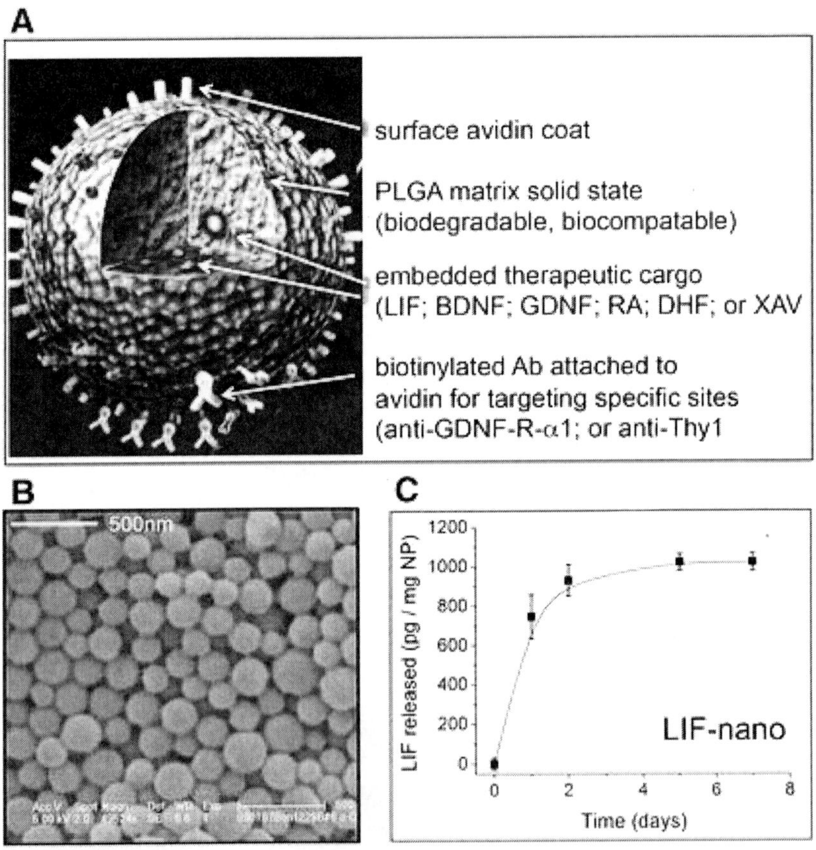

Figure 1. Design and cargo release rate of nanoparticle constructs. (A) Cartoon of PLGA nanoparticle functionalised with avidin for binding of biotinylated targeting antibody. Cargo for delivery is embedded within the solid PLGA matrix. Cargo abbreviations of LIF, BDNF, GDNF, DHF and XAV are detailed in the main text; RA, retinoic acid. (B) Scanning electron micrograph of nanoparticles showing tight size distribution: average diameter is 120 nm. (C) Cargo release rate from PLGA nanoparticles (NP) as exemplified by LIF after suspending LIF-nano in aqueous medium and sampling using ELISA measurements.

Nano-LIF-stroma is pro-survival for E14 rat DA neurons

We first asked, do primary fetal rat E14 ventral mesencephalon (VM) cells, known to include DA precursors, benefit from stromal support provided by LIF-nano? Because LIF signalling requires the heterodimeric receptor consisting of gp190 (LIF-specific subunit) and gp130 (common signalling subunit), we needed to confirm that the tyrosine-hydroxylase-positive (TH^+) cells co-express gp190 and gp130. **Fig. 2A** shows adherent cells at 3 days *in vitro* (DIV), with co-staining for TH plus gp190, and TH plus gp130. Unexpectedly, gp190 staining was nuclear. This subcellular stain is seen in the Human Protein Atlas (HPA) database (insert to **Fig. 2A**). The presence of nuclear receptors could indicate an intracrine signalling capacity for fetal VM cells, as has been shown for arcuate neurons expressing nuclear receptor for the IL-6 family cytokine member ciliary neurotrophic factor (Couvreur et al., 2012).

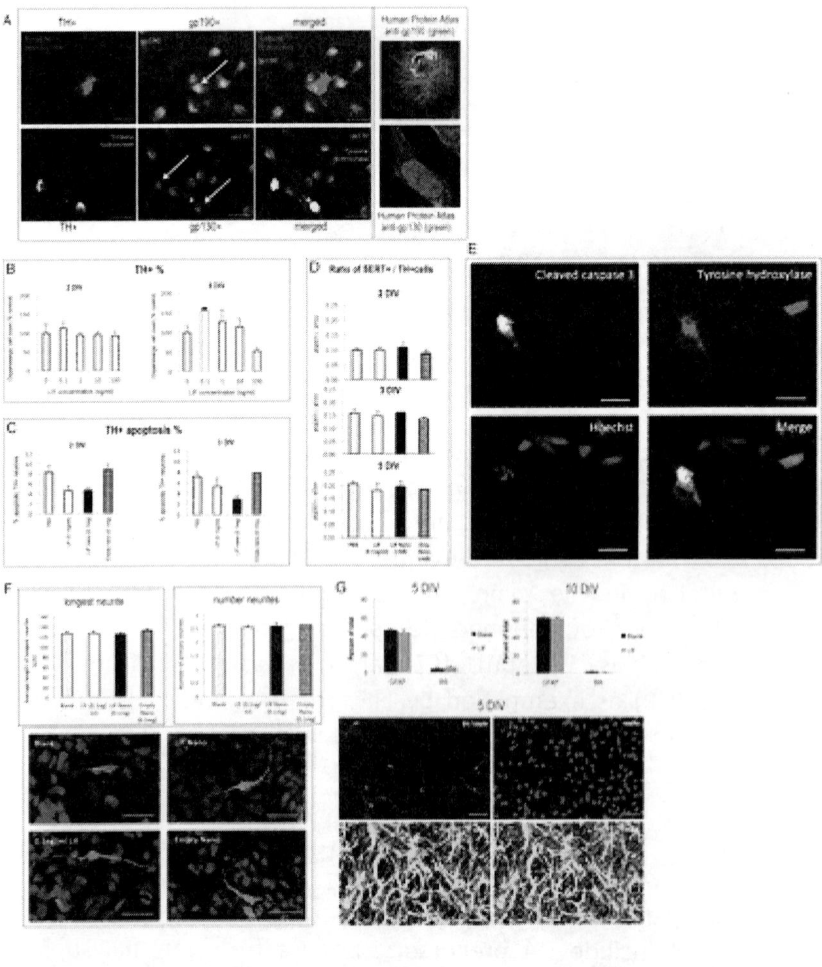

Figure 2.Rat fetal VM DA cells respond to LIF with increased survival and normal differentiation. (A) Immunocytochemistry of primary E14 rat VM cells after 3 days in culture in differentiation growth medium: staining for tyrosine hydroxylase (TH) and co-staining for the LIF-R subunits, gp130 or gp190, revealed co-expression in TH^+ cells. Upper left three panels: TH (red) and gp190 (white) staining showed, unexpectedly, gp190 to be nuclear in the rat VM cells, a location also seen in the human glioblastoma astrocytoma cell line U-251 stained with rabbit anti-gp190 HPA00478 (green, upper right insert). Lower left three panels: TH (blue) and gp130 (white) staining showed gp130 at the plasma membrane; for reference, the human U-2 OS cell line stained with rabbit anti-gp130, CAB025784, is shown (lower right insert). Arrows indicate double-positive DA cells. Scale bars: 25 μm for rat VM cells; 10 μm for human cells. For publically available Human Protein Atlas (HPA) details seehttp://www.proteinatlas.org/ENSG00000113594/subcellular (gp190) andhttp://www.proteinatlas.org/ENSG00000134352/subcellular (gp130). HPA stains: green=antibody; red=tubulin; blue=nucleus. (B) Effects of soluble LIF on the percentage of TH^+ cells in primary E14 rat VM tissue grown as monolayer cultures in differentiation medium supplemented with a range of LIF doses from 0.1 to 100 ng/ml for 2 (left panel) or 3 (right panel) days. At 2 DIV, no significant effect of LIF treatment was seen (one-way ANOVA, $F_{4,14}=0.31$, $P>0.05$); at 3 DIV, 0.1 ng/ml LIF significantly increased the DA cell count as compared with untreated controls (one-way ANOVAs, $F_{4,14}=4.55$, post-hoc Tukey tests, $P<0.05$). (C) Replicate cultures of primary E14 rat VM were treated with soluble LIF, LIF-nano or empty-nano and fixed at 2 DIV (left panel) or 3 DIV (right panel). Apoptotic DA neurons were identified as cells immunopositive for both tyrosine hydroxylase (TH) and cleaved caspase-3. Both soluble and nanoparticle LIF reduced the proportion of apoptotic DA neurons at 2 DIV (one-way ANOVA, $F_{3,11}=14.13$, $P<0.01$, post-hoc Tukey tests, $P<0.05$). No treatments had a significant effect on levels of dopaminergic apoptosis at 3 DIV (one-way ANOVA, $F_{3,10}=4.33$, $P>0.05$). (D) LIF treatment does not alter the serotonergic to DA ratio in E14 rat VM cultures. Monolayer cultures of E14 VM tissue were treated with soluble LIF (0.1 ng/ml), LIF-nano (0.1 mg/million cells) or empty-nano (0.1 mg/million cells). After 2, 3 or 5 DIV, the cultures were fixed and stained for TH and SERT. One-way ANOVA demonstrated that there was no effect of treatment on the serotonergic to DA cell ratio at 2 DIV ($F_{3,13}=0.45$, $P>0.05$), 3 DIV ($F_{3,10}=0.68$, $P>0.05$) or 5 DIV ($F_{3,12}=0.36$, $P>0.05$). Thus, LIF therapy does not alter rat fVM composition. (E) Photomicrographs of a single group of fixed cells co-stained at 2 DIV for cleaved caspase-3, TH and Hoechst to identify apoptosis of TH^+ cells. (F) LIF treatment has no effect on the morphological development of DA neurons *in vitro*. Monolayer cultures of rat E14 VM tissue in differentiation medium were treated with soluble LIF (0.1 ng/ml), LIF-nano (0.1 mg/million cells) or empty-nano (0.1 mg/million cells). At 5 DIV, cultures were fixed and stained for TH. Representative images of individual TH^+ DA neurons from each treatment group are shown in red. The development of DA neurons was quantified as the length of the longest neurite and the absolute number of primary neurites per neuron (see histograms). Neither measure was found to be affected by LIF treatment, with the average length of the longest neurite being 125 μm ($F_{3,12}=0.32$, $P>0.05$) and average number of primary neurites per neuron being 2.5 ($F_{3,12}=0.17$, $P>0.05$). Scale bars: 50 μm. (G) Expansion of E14 VM neural progenitor cells in the presence of 0.1 ng/ml LIF did not alter the neuronal:glial ratio. E14 VM precursor cells were expanded as neurospheres for 7 days in proliferation medium containing 10% FCS with, or without, 0.1 ng/ml LIF before plating in differentiating medium for 5 or 10 DIV. GFAP and βIII-tubulin staining respectively identified cells of glial and neuronal lineages: cell counts showed no significant effect (two-way Student's *t*-tests, $P>0.05$ at either 5 or 10 DIV) as shown in the histograms, and illustrated for 5 DIV staining. Scale bars: 50 μm. Quantification was based on five independent repeats (i.e. five litters of embryos) enumerated as detailed in the Materials and Methods together with the protocol for morphological analyses and statistical analysis.

We next tested responsiveness by adding soluble LIF to primary cultures of differentiating E14 VM cells. After 2 DIV – when the cells had become stably adherent – no effect of LIF was seen but, after 3 DIV, it induced a significant increase in TH^+ cells (**Fig. 2B**). Reasoning that increased numbers of TH^+ cells reflected either increased survival or increased lineage amplification, we looked for early effects on apoptosis by staining for caspase-3 cleavage and here included LIF-nano targeted to GFRα-1, having first confirmed dual staining for GFRα-1 plus TH. Both soluble LIF and LIF-nano halved the rate of apoptosis seen in the TH^+ cell population at 2 DIV as revealed by co-staining for cleaved caspase-3 (**Fig. 2C,E**). Importantly, empty nanoparticles (empty-nano) targeted to GFRα-1 had no effect (**Fig. 2C**) and extended controls showed that both targeting of the nanoparticles plus delivery of a cargo was required for the nano-stromal effect, as detailed by Dyson et al. (Dyson et al., 2014). Because apoptosis was recorded at 2 DIV, when no difference in TH^+ cell numbers was apparent, we surmise that some of the TH^+ cells seen at 2 DIV in untreated control cultures were already in the early stages of apoptosis. The data implies a pro-survival property of LIF for DA precursors, including when delivered as a nano-stroma targeted to GFRα-1.

We also investigated potential effects on neural lineage composition in the context of growth factor delivery during development of precursor cell populations. For example, high serotoninergic to DA cell counts in hfVM grafts in PD patients has been linked to the development of graft-induced dyskinesias (GID). Because serotoninergic ($SERT^+$) cells express GFRα-1 (Dyson et al., 2014), we measured the ratio of $SERT^+$ to TH^+ cells in rat fVM cultures. **Fig. 2D** shows that neither soluble LIF nor LIF-nano altered the serotoninergic to DA cell ratio measured at 2, 3 and 5 DIV. **Fig. 2F** shows maturing DA cells with equivalent differentiation in the presence of soluble LIF, LIF-nano and empty-nano: this was confirmed by analysing neurite numbers and length.

To address the possibility that LIF might influence glial versus neuronal differentiation, we investigated primary E14 VM tissue expanded in proliferation medium as neurospheres in the presence, or absence, of 0.1 ng/ml soluble LIF. Following a week of expansion, tissue was plated as monolayer cultures in differentiation medium without further LIF treatment and grown for either 5 or 10 days. Quantification of βIII-tubulin-positive neurons and glial fibrillary acidic protein (GFAP)-positive astrocytes (**Fig. 2G**) demonstrated that LIF exposure during neurosphere expansion had no effect on subsequent neural versus glial differentiation at either of these two time points. The relatively high proportion of glia reflects expansion as neurospheres when precursors decline in the ability to make neurons.

Nano-stromal-induced activation of Trk-B is pro-survival

Because soluble BDNF has been reported to support DA cells (Hyman et al., 1991) and increase the morphological development of DA neurons as assessed by the number and length of their primary neurites (Beck et al., 1993; Kontkanen and Castrén, 1999), we went on to explore the effect of BDNF in nano-formulation on these neuronal features. In contrast to LIF, which signals through the LIF-receptor complex of gp130-gp190, BDNF signals through the neurotrophic tyrosine kinase receptor type 2 (TrkB). It was therefore of interest to include, in parallel to BDNF, a recently published small-molecule agonist of TrkB, namely 7,8-dihydroxyflavone (7,8-DHF) (Jang et al., 2010). We asked: (i) does BDNF-nano retain bioactivity and (ii) is the potency for TrkB signalling comparable between BDNF-nano versus DHF-nano? By determining the percentage of TH^+ cells as a function of total cell counts, then counting the number of primary neurites per TH^+ cell and measuring the longest neurite, the effect of signalling through TrkB was recorded as detailed in **Fig. 3A–C**: this is summarised in **Table 1**. **Fig. 3D** illustrates the observed effect of 50 ng/ml soluble BDNF on DA cell maturation. At this dose there was a selective increase in the number of DA cells, to a level that was equivalent to that seen with 7,8-DHF at 100 nM. When in nano-formulation, both BDNF-nano and 7,8-DHF-nano showed maximal equivalent bioactivity at 0.1 mg nanoparticles per million cells.

Unexpectedly, 7,8-DHF treatment did not mimic the effect of BDNF in enhancing the morphological development of primary DA neurons (compare the relevant **Fig. 3B,C** histogram sets). In fact, treatment with 1 μM 7,8-DHF induced a small but significant 7% reduction in the average length of the longest primary neurite from DA neurons. The basis of this effect is unclear.

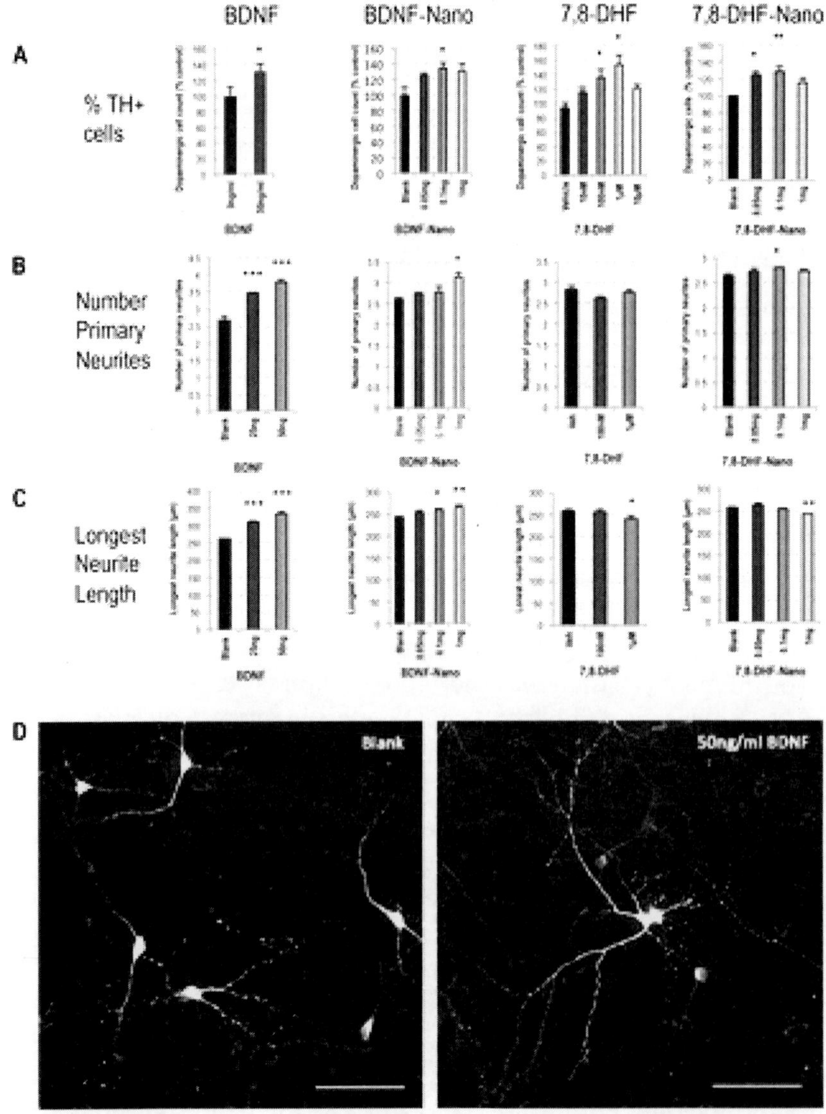

Figure 3. Comparison of BDNF versus 7,8-DHF, each in soluble and nano formulation, showed effects on rat E14 VM DA neuron survival and maturation. (A) The sets of histograms show % TH^+ cells in rat E14 VM cultures at 7 days post-plating in differentiation growth medium. In these same cultures, the histograms in B show the average number of primary neurites per DA TH^+ cell, and C shows the average length of the longest neurite per TH^+ cell: results for each set are detailed below. Total cell counts of Hoechst-stained nuclei in each culture were made and the effect of therapy on total cell number is stated in the relevant figure legend text. The four treatment groups were BDNF, BDNF-nano, 7,8-DHF and 7,8-DHF-nano: the overall data are summarised in **Table 1**. The nanoparticles were targeted to Thy-1. No toxicity was observed in any of the culture conditions. (A) BDNF primary E14 VM cells cultured in 50 ng/ml BDNF showed significantly enhanced survival of the DA neurons (one-tailed Student's *t*-test, $*P<0.05$): the total cell count was unchanged (two-tailed Student's *t*-test,$P>0.05$). BDNF-nano primary E14 VM cells cultured in Thy-1-targeted BDNF nanoparticles at 0.1 mg/million cells showed significantly enhanced DA cell survival (one-way ANOVA, $F_{3,29}=3.73$, $P<0.05$, post-hoc Tukey tests, $*P<0.05$): the total cell count was unchanged (one-way ANOVA, $F_{3,18}=0.54$, $P>0.05$). 7,8-DHF primary E14 VM cells cultured in 7,8-DHF showed a dose-dependent enhancement of DA cell survival at 100 nM and 1 µM (one-way ANOVA, $F_{4,27}=3.65$, $P<0.05$, post-hoc Tukey tests, $*P<0.05$): treatment had no effect on total cell count (one-way ANOVA, $F_{4,17}=0.28$, $P>0.05$). 7,8-DHF-nano primary E14 VM cells cultured with Thy-1-targeted 7,8-DHF nanoparticles showed significantly enhanced DA cell survival at doses of both 0.05 and 0.1 mg/million cells (one-way ANOVA, $F_{3,11}=8.34$, $P<0.01$, post-hoc Tukey tests, $*P<0.05$, $**P<0.01$): treatment had no effect on total cell count at any of the doses tested (one-way ANOVA, $F_{3,15}=0.85$, $P>0.05$). (B,C) BDNF primary E14 VM cells cultured in BDNF showed a significant increase in the average number of primary neurites per DA neuron (one-way ANOVA, $F_{2,8}=62.45$, $P<0.001$, post-hoc Tukey tests, $***P<0.001$) and BDNF also increased the average length of the longest neurite (one-way ANOVA, $F_{2,8}=51.87$, $P<0.001$, post-hoc Tukey tests, $***P<0.001$). BDNF-nano at 1 mg of Thy-1-targeted BDNF nanoparticles per million cells significantly enhanced the average number of primary neurites per DA neuron (one-way ANOVA, $F_{3,11}=6.63$, $P<0.05$, post-hoc Tukey tests, $*P<0.05$) and BDNF-nano at this dose significantly increased the length of the longest neurite in DA neurons (one-way ANOVA, $F_{3,11}=7.45$, $P<0.05$, post-hoc Tukey tests, $*P<0.05$, $**P<0.01$). 7,8-DHF shows that, although 7,8-DHF had no significant effect on the average number of primary neurites per DA neuron (one-way ANOVA, $F_{2,7}=1.74$, $P>0.05$), 7,8-DHF at 1 µM significantly reduced the average length of the longest neurite (one-way ANOVA, $F_{2,7}=8.85$, $P<0.05$, post-hoc Tukey tests, $*P<0.05$). 7,8-DHF-nano shows that Thy-1-targeted 7,8-DHF nanoparticles at 0.1 mg per million cells induced a small but significant increase in the average number of primary neurites per DA neuron (one-way ANOVA, $F_{3,14}=3.91$, $P<0.05$, post-hoc Tukey tests, $*P<0.05$), whereas 7,8-DHF-nano treatment at 1 mg per million cells caused a significant decrease in the average length of the longest primary neurite (one-way ANOVA, $F_{3,14}=18.28$, $P<0.001$, post-hoc Tukey tests, $**P<0.01$). Quantification was based on five independent repeats (i.e. five litters of embryos) as detailed in the Materials and Methods. (D) Treatment with 50 ng/ml BDNF enhanced maturation of DA neurons in rat E14 VM cultures. Representative images of control and 50 ng/ml BDNF-treated E14 VM cultures at 7 days post-plating in differentiation growth medium with or without 50 ng/ml soluble BDNF. Tyrosine hydroxylase staining is shown in white. Scale bars: 200 µm.

Table 1. Comparisons of (i) BDNF and the TrkB agonist 7,8-dihydroxyflavone, and (ii) soluble factor versus nano-formulated factor, on numbers of DA cells in primary rat E14 VM cultures at 7 DIV

Treatment*	Dose	TH^+ cells/total cells ×100%	Significance**	Notes
Control	Vehicle only	100%	–	–
BDNF soluble	50 ng/ml	136%	$P<0.05$	A
BDNF-nano	0.1 mg/10^9 cells	136%	$P<0.05$	A
7,8-DHF soluble	100 nM	140%	$P<0.05$	B
7,8-DHF-nano	0.1 mg/10^9 cells	130%	$P<0.01$	B

*BDNF-nano and 7,8-DHF-nano were targeted to Thy-1 antigen.
**One-way ANOVA.
A: Increased DA cell maturation evident by significant increases in both the number and length of neurites. Number of primary neurites comparing untreated to treated BDNF soluble $P<0.001$; BDNF-nano $P<0.05$. Length of longest neurite comparing untreated to treated BDNF soluble $P<0.001$; BDNF-nano $P<0.05$.
B: DA cell morphology unchanged from control cultures except for a significant increase in the number of primary neurites in 100 nM soluble 7,8-DHF, $P=0.05$.

The BDNF and 7,8-DHF experiments established that different types of cell surface receptor are accessible to nanotherapeutic formulations, and that different types of molecule acting on the same cell surface receptor retain potency in nano-formulation. Of note, the cost of 7,8-DHF is some thousand-fold less than recombinant BDNF – an important consideration in the context of potential therapeutic application.

hfVM-derived DA cells benefit from nano-stromal support

When preparing donated primary human fetal tissue for cell transplantation into a recipient PD patient, loss of cells – already a scarce resource – is substantial throughout the procedure from harvest to grafting. This means that many fetuses are required to graft a single patient and there is a need to store the fetal tissues at +4°C in hibernation media for several days to allow for the accrual of sufficient fetal material for transplantation. If the yield of DA cells per donated hfVM could be increased, the benefits would be great because fewer donors would be required per patient. Accordingly, we went on to ask, can the nano-stromal approach protect and improve the yield of healthy human DA cells under conditions used for transplantation?

Here, in addition to LIF-nano, we included nano-stromal cargos to target delivery of BDNF, GDNF and XAV, reasoning firstly that BDNF and GDNF are already known to be pro-survival for DA neurons (Hyman et al., 1991; Villadiego et al., 2005), and secondly that XAV might provide in the future a means to modulate neuronal fate. **Fig. 4A** outlines the process of hfVM harvest prior to cell preparation and nano-stromal treatment. For most of the experiments multiple stored hfVM tissues were dissociated into single-cell suspensions that were pooled prior to aliquoting: each aliquot was coated with nano-stroma targeted to Thy-1 by overnight incubation at 37°C in proliferation medium. Thy-1 was selected as a target antigen because it is expressed on both human fetal DA cells – confirmed in preliminary work here – and on T cells, where LIF-nano is known to be tolerogenic (Gao et al., 2009; Park et al., 2011), a desirable property in the context of cell transplantation. For adherent cultures, the nano-stromal-coated cells were seeded in differentiation medium and cultured for 4 days using five replicate coverslips per treatment group. After staining for TH, βIII tubulin and DAPI, the different cell phenotypes in each culture were counted.

Because proliferation medium (PM) is used to prepare hfVM cells for clinical transplantation, whereas use of differentiation medium (DM) is required for the *in vitro* experiments, we first asked, does the type of growth medium (PM versus DM) influence the response of hfVM cells to nano-stromal delivery of cargo? Responses to the tested nano-stromal types were unaffected by PM versus DM, and **Fig. 4B**illustrates the results for GDNF-nano and BDNF-nano. Next, the dose of nanoparticle used to provide the nano-stroma was optimised for each cargo type. For LIF-nano, 1/100 dilution had the greatest effect on increasing both the percentage of TH^+ cells (**Fig. 4C**, upper panels) and the total cell number. However, unexpectedly, although XAV-nano increased total cell number, the percentage of TH^+ cells was reduced (**Fig. 4C**, lower panels). This is illustrated in **Fig. 4D**. It therefore became of interest to ask, firstly, what was the actual number of TH^+ cells following XAV-nano and how did these compare to treatment with LIF-nano, BDNF-nano or GDNF-nano? Secondly, is the effect of XAV-nano dominant over LIF-nano, or vice versa? Using a single pool of donor cells, the comparative experiment in **Fig. 4E**shows total βIII-tubulin-positive ($βIII^+$) neuronal cell numbers (left panel), total TH^+ cell numbers (centre panel) and percent TH^+ cells (right panel). Only XAV-nano had a selective effect, in that

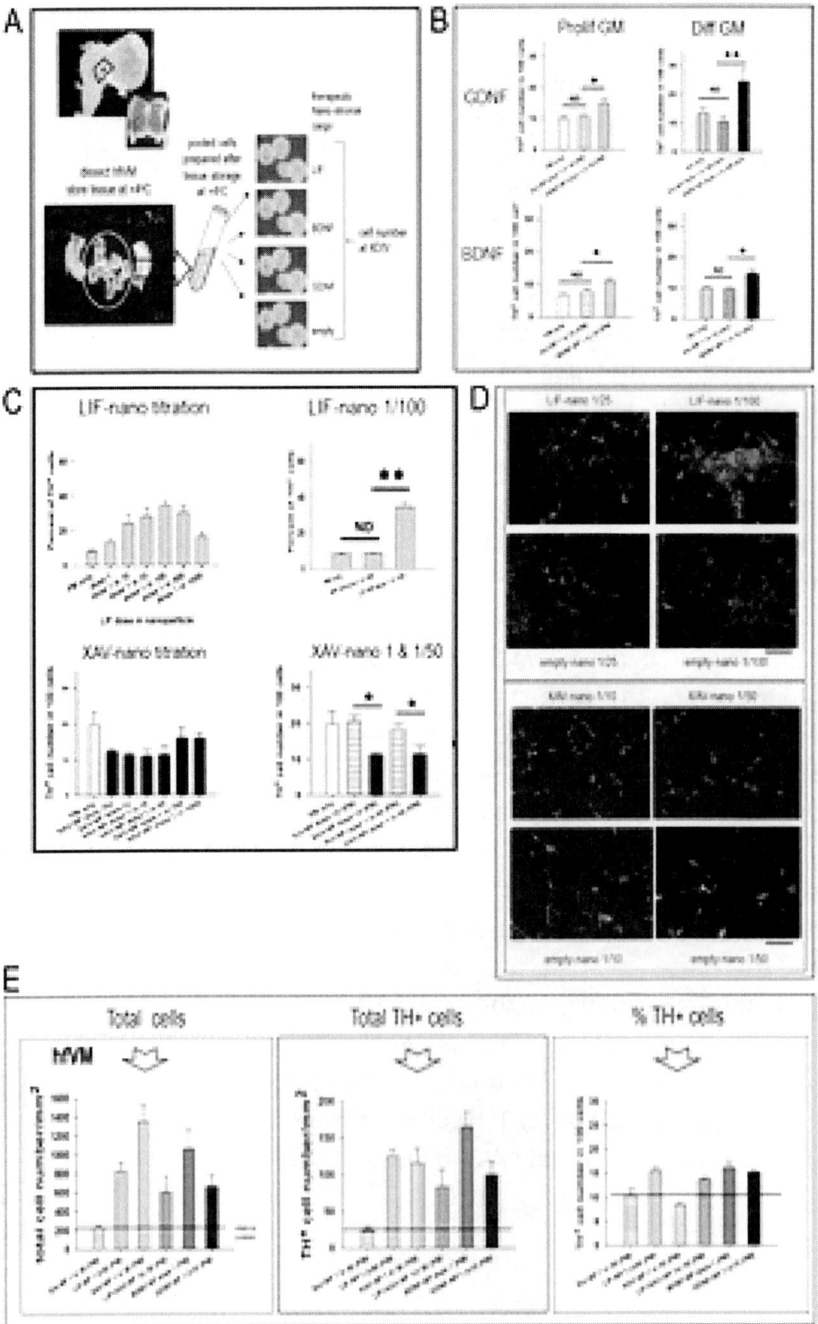
A
B
Prolif GM
Diff GM
GDNF
BDNF
C
LIF-nano titration
LIF-nano 1/100
ND
XAV-nano titration
XAV-nano 1 & 1/50
D
E
Total cells
Total TH+ cells
% TH+ cells
hVM

Figure 4. Nano-stromal-mediated pro-survival effects might be uncoupled from pro-differentiation effects. (A) Illustrates the procedure for setting up human fetal ventral mesencephalon (hfVM) cultures: the nano-stroma are exemplified for LIF, BDNF and GDNF, with empty-nano as control. hfVM material was obtained at the time of routine termination of pregnancy: fetal age was determined based on crown/rump length. Following dissection, the hfVM was stored at +4°C in HibE for up to 4 days prior to dissociating the cells and coating with nano-stroma. Being of primary human source, no truly identical biological replicates between experiments was possible, but repeat experiments using material from different donors gave similar results for each of the treatments used. Within each experiment there were five replicates per treatment condition. When different treatments were directly compared – as in E – a single batch of donated tissue was used: in some cases cells from multiple donors were pooled prior to aliquoting for treatment to ensure direct comparability. Data are presented as percentage of TH^+ cells in the total BIII-tubulin$^+$ cell population. (B) Histograms showing the percentage of TH^+ cells in hfVM cultures comparing treatment in either proliferation or differentiation medium (PM or DM, respectively), with or without GDNF-nano (top panels) or BDNF-nano (bottom panels). The experiments shown used either 48-day or 49-day hfVM tissue stored overnight in HibE at +4°C: this was then dissociated into single cells, incubated at 37°C for 16 hours with the various nanoparticle treatments in either PM or DM. The cells were then cultured in DM for 4 days prior to fixing and staining for TH (DA cells) and βIII tubulin (neurons). Both GDNF-nano and BDNF-nano treatment increased the percentage of TH^+ cells in the culture when compared with empty-nano controls at equivalent dilution, regardless of treatment in either PM or DM. GDNF-nano/PM one-way ANOVA, $F_{2,11}$=5.479, *P*=0.028; GDNF-nano/DM one-way ANOVA, $F_{2,10}$=5.599,*P*=0.030; BDNF-nano/PM GDNF-nano/PM one-way ANOVA, $F_{2,11}$=7.261, *P*=0.013; GDNF-nano/DM one-way ANOVA, $F_{2,11}$=9.862, *P*=0.005. EmNP, empty-nano; ND, no difference; **P*<0.05; ***P*<0.01. (C) Histograms showing the dose response curve based on the percentage of TH^+ cells in hfVM cell cultures treated with LIF-nano ranging from 1:1 to 1:1000 in PM for 14 hours prior to growth in DM for 4 days (top left). The donor age was 50 days and the VM cells were prepared freshly prior to treatment. Top right compares the LIF-nano dose that had maximum effect (1:100), resulting in a significantly increased percentage of TH^+ cells compared with untreated controls, or cells treated with empty-nano at equivalent dilution. The lower left histogram shows that treatment with XAV-nano decreased the percentage of TH^+ cells: in this experiment, the decrease was not significant (*P*=0.060: lower right histogram). The donor age was 42 days and the tissue had been stored overnight in HibE prior to cell preparation and treatment in PM for 18 hours, then culture in DM 4 days. **P*<0.05; ***P*<0.01. (D) Images of the hfVM experiment described in C, comparing the effects of LIF-nano versus empty-nano at equivalent dilution (left panel) and XAV-nano versus empty-nano at equivalent dilution (right panel). Scale bars: 200 µm. (E) Histograms showing total numbers of βIII-tubulin$^+$ neurons (left panel), and total TH^+ cells (centre panel), after the culturing of hfVM cells treated with Thy-1-targeted: LIF-nano; XAV-nano; LIF-nano combined with XAV-nano; BDNF-nano; or -GDNF-nano. The number of TH^+ cells, as a percentage of the total number of βIII-tubulin$^+$ neurons is shown in the right hand panel. *n*=4 in each treatment group where cell counts were taken from five random areas of 1 mm^2per coverslip. Error bars show s.e.m.; pairwise multiple comparison procedures post hoc (Holm-Sidak method). Arrow points to the column for XAV-nano-treated cells, where total cell numbers were increased sixfold (left panel), whereas the percentage of TH^+ cells was decreased (right panel): the overall total number of TH$^+$ cells compared with empty-nano controls was fourfold in the presence of XAV-nano. Combined treatment with both LIF-nano and XAV-nano (fourth column) reduced the selective effect of XAV-nano monotherapy on total cell number, and on % TH$^+$ cells.

there was a greater increase in total neuronal cell numbers (sixfold) but the percentage TH$^+$ cells decreased when compared with empty-nano controls (see arrow in histogram **Fig. 4E**). In contrast, **Fig. 4E** shows that LIF-, BDNF- and GDNF-nano each increased both total cell numbers and percent TH$^+$ cells. We conclude that XAV-nano treatment might support the increased expansion of neuronal precursors while also offering some support to the TH$^+$ cell population. Interestingly, the selective effect of XAV-nano was lost in the presence of LIF-nano (fourth column in histograms, **Fig. 4E**), where the percent TH$^+$ cells was similar to hfVM treated with mono-LIF-, BDNF- or GDNF-nano: this suggests dominance of LIF-induced effects over XAV.

Ex vivo stromal coating of hfVM cells provides long-term benefits *in vivo*

Having established a pro-survival effect for hfVM *in vitro*, we next wanted to know, does coating of hfVM cells with a nano-stroma increase TH cell survival following transplantation into the adult rat brain. Using the xenograft model outlined in **Fig. 5A**, hfVM cells were prepared as in **Fig. 4A**, but, instead of being put into culture after coating with the nano-stroma, were implanted into the left striatum of nude rat recipients following the procedures detailed previously (Lopez et al., 2013). Two treatment groups were established from a single stock of hfVM cells, where each recipient received 200,000 cells coated with either empty-nano, or LIF-nano, targeted to Thy-1. Animals were sacrificed at 12–13 weeks, when any increased rate of maturation due to the therapy could realistically first be detected. The brains were removed and sectioned. **Fig. 5B** shows grafts that had been pretreated with either empty-nano or LIF-nano, stained for human nuclear antigen (HuNu) (upper panels) or human-specific tau (HuTau) (lower panels): LIF-nano treatment seemed to improve the viability and integration of the grafted cells. **Fig. 5C**shows human TH$^+$ cells co-stained for HuNu in a

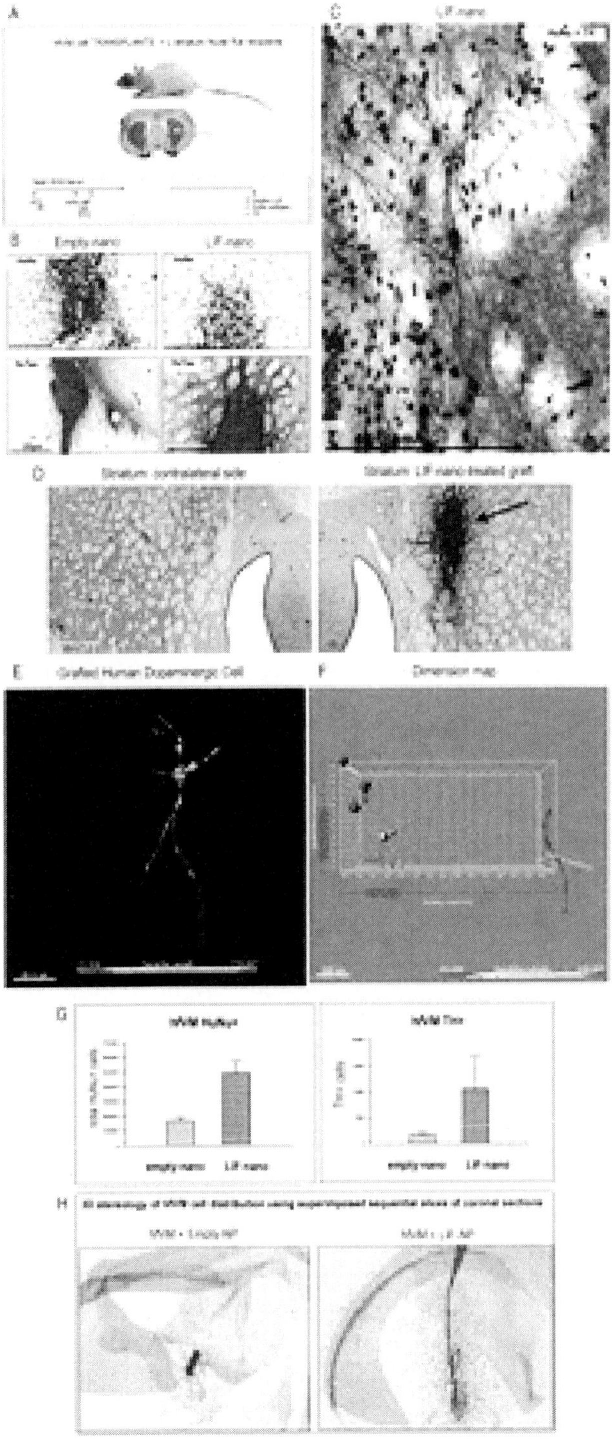

Figure 5. LIF-nano treatment supports the survival and integration of transplanted hfVM cells into the striatum of the nude rat brain.(A) Outlines the protocol for transplantation of hfVM cells into the striatum of nude rat recipients following the procedure described previously (Baker et al., 2000). Briefly, hfVM tissue was stored at +4°C in HibE for 4 days prior to cell preparation and treatment with nanoparticles for 24 hours, then grafted into the striatum. At 12 weeks, recipients were culled and coronal brain sections stained. (B) Low-power photomicrographs of recipient striatum 12 weeks post-grafting with hfVM cells treated *ex vivo* with either empty-nano (left panels) or LIF-nano (right panels): sections were stained either for human nuclear antigen (HuNu: black nuclei show living cells, yellow/brown nuclei are dead cells) or for human tau (HuTau, dark grey). Dead cells were more apparent in empty-nano-treated grafts, which also had fewer $HuTau^+$ neurites extending within the host tissue compared with the LIF-nano-treated grafts. (C) High-power photomicrograph showing double-positive TH and HuNu human DA cells that have matured in the rat striatum. (D) Low-power photomicrographs comparing graft site with contralateral striatum stained for HuTau. Note HuTau positivity extending beyond the main graft area (arrow). Scale bar: 500 μm. (E) High-power image of a TH^+HuNu^+ cell in a graft where the image has been processed using Imaris Filament Tracer software: colours relate to the dimensions of neurites and the cell body. (F) Dimension map of the human DA cell shown in E, using Imaris XT analysis of cell body and neurite diameter, size and shape. (G) Histograms comparing numbers of total $HuNu^+$ cells (left panel, P=0.058) and double-positive TH^+HuNu^+ cells (right panel, P=0.362) 13 weeks after transplantation into the striatum of nude rats. Each recipient animal was analysed. Some 2% of the $HuNu^+$ cells were DA based on co-staining for TH. (H) Three-dimensional stereology using superimposed sections to show the distribution of $HuNu^+$ cells throughout the recipient brain. Cell staining images were taken with a Leica fluorescence microscope with a 20× lens and saved with digital ID. Cells were counted manually using ImageJ software (US National Institutes of Health) with cell counter Plugin. All counting was performed blindly and recorded with ID: total TH^+HuNu^+neurons and total $HuNu^+$ neurons were calculated in each recipient animal. For stereology, quantification used Neurolucida 10.

graft pretreated with LIF-nano. **Fig. 5D**, right panel, shows HuTau expression in a LIF-nano treated graft, where extension of fibres into the host tissue is clear: the left panel shows the contralateral side. **Fig. 5E,F** show the processed image of a grafted human DA neuron using Imaris Filament Tracer and Imaris XT software to reveal dimensions of the cell body and neurites. The cell counts shown in **Fig. 5G** revealed a trend for increased numbers of $HuNu^+$cells in the LIF-nano-treated group compared with empty-nano controls, but this failed to reach statistical significance (P=0.058; **Fig. 5G**, left panel). Some 2% of the $HuNu^+$ cells were DA based on co-staining for TH, but again the apparent higher numbers in the LIF-nano group failed to reach statistical significance (P=0.362). The stereology included recording $HuNu^+$ cell distance from the needle tract, where there was evidence for increased migration in the LIF-nano-treated group (**Fig. 5H**).

Overall, the data suggest that LIF-nano treatment of primary hfVM cells not only supported their survival *in vivo*, but also promoted their integration within the host striatum, with neurites extending well beyond the graft boundary.

DISCUSSION

Here, we investigated whether the use of a surrogate nano-stroma attached to freshly isolated human, or rat, fetal VM cells promotes their survival by delivery of growth factors or small molecules. Significant benefits were found and two critical determinants identified: (1) the need for a cargo to be delivered: simple nano-stromal cross-linking of cell surface antigen by targeting antibody did not constitute a pro-survival signal in the absence of cargo; and (2) the need to physically attach the stromal nanoparticles to the target cell: unbound cargo-carrying nanoparticles failed to have an effect.

The versatility of using nano-spheres to create a local stroma enables cells to be treated individually, a major advantage for *ex vivo* treatment of therapeutic cells prior to grafting. Notably, we found no adverse effects following treatment of primary embryonic VM cells: indeed the more vulnerable DA population showed preferential survival following nanotherapy targeted to GFRα-1, or Thy-1. The technology platform used to prepare the nano-therapeutic particles is the same as that of BIND Therapeutics (http://www.bindtherapeutics.com), where clinical efficacy and safety are already established: notably, BIND technology is being used in ongoing clinical trials for non-small cell lung cancer, and for prostate cancer.

Our experiments showed that a pro-survival effect can be achieved by nano-stromal delivery of either a biologic or a small molecule, and also when subcellular targets differ. Of the small molecules tested, 7,8-DHF acts at the plasma membrane as an agonist of TrkB; in contrast, XAV acts intracellularly, inhibiting tankyrase enzyme activity. Such versatility of specifically targeted cargos provides potential advantages when considering, for example, a multiplicity of agents to create a favourable niche during transplantation of neural precursor cells. Here, our finding of apparent stromal-derived interactions when XAV-nano is combined with LIF-nano is of interest: firstly, recent work has shown that XAV induces cytoplasmic retention of β-catenin/Axin2 (Kim et al., 2013); and, secondly, evidence suggests that cytoplasmic β-catenin interacts with the LIF-receptor plus E-cadherin to maintain intact cell-cell adhesion and pluripotency (del Valle et al., 2013). Accordingly, we hypothesise that crosstalk between signalling pathways might arise during combined nano-stromal treatment with XAV and LIF. Overall, our data imply that surrogate stromal-induced lineage manipulation might be possible using nano-scale paracrine-type delivery of factors in stromal form to manipulate developmental pathways.

A further point of note was the finding that the pro-survival effect of LIF-nano on TH^+ cells was detectable in rat E14 VM at 2 DIV, as evidenced by cells expressing cleaved caspase-3, before overt cell death within the TH^+ population. This suggests that DA cells are especially vulnerable to stress at an early stage of differentiation. *In vivo*, the sustained benefit over 12 weeks gained by a single *ex vivo*treatment of primary hfVM cells demonstrates long-lasting effects, including early integration within the host tissue. These preliminary findings using hfVM support the use of LIF-nano in cell-based therapies, with the added value of tolerogenic properties. Furthermore, conceptually, future developments would include tailored nano-stromal support to provide a surrogate, transient, cell-specific stromal niche: for example, nano-stromal combinations using early delivery of factors linked to embryonic development such as LIF and/or XAV to promote precursor cells transiently, followed by delayed release of BDNF-nano or GDNF-nano, to guide lineage differentiation.

SUMMARY

Improved survival of DA neurons in cell-based transplantation therapies for PD is needed for this therapy to become a clinical reality. Here, using the highly relevant, stringent model of primary DA cell survival and maturation, we demonstrate that nanoparticles used to create a nano-stroma designed to deliver developmental growth factors, or small molecules, to single cells provides a simple and effective means to support DA cell survival, including primary hfVM cells.

MATERIALS AND METHODS

Preparation of PLGA nanoparticles for targeted delivery

Cargos of either recombinant growth factor or small molecule included recombinant murine LIF (Santa Cruz; sc-4378) or human LIF (Santa-Cruz; sc-4988); recombinant human BDNF and human GDNF (R&D Systems); 7,8-DHF (Sigma); and XAV939 (Selleckchem). Cargo was encapsulated in avidin-coated PLGA nanoparticles using a modified version of a previously described water/oil/water double emulsion technique (Steenblock and Fahmy, 2008). Briefly, for example for LIF, 50 μg LIF was dissolved in 200 μl PBS and added dropwise with vortexing to 100 mg PGLA in 2 ml dichloromethane. The resulting emulsion was added to 4 ml of aqueous surfactant solution containing 2.5 mg/ml polyvinyl alcohol and 2.5 mg/ml avidin-palmitate bioconjugate and sonicated to create an emulsion containing nano-sized droplets of polymer/solvent, LIF and surfactant. Solvent was removed by magnetic stirring at room temperature; hardened nanoparticles were then washed three times in deionised water and lyophilized for long-term storage. Nanoparticle size and morphology were analysed via scanning electron microscopy and a Nanosight imaging/sizing system. Release of LIF was measured by incubating particles in phosphate buffered saline (PBS) at 37°C and measuring LIF concentrations in supernatant fractions by enzyme-linked immunosorbent assay (ELISA). Total encapsulation was approximated as the amount of LIF released over a 7-day period and percent encapsulation efficiency calculated as total encapsulation divided by maximum theoretical encapsulation. For cell attachment, biotinylated rabbit anti-GFR-α1 antibody (Acris) or biotinylated anti-Thy-1 was incubated with the avidin-coated nano-particles and free unbound antibody was removed after centrifuging out the nanoparticles, which were then washed once immediately prior to use. Dose was optimised according to dose-response curves (see text): for rat E14 VM this was 0.1 mg/million cells (LIF-, BDNF- and DHF-nano); for hfVM, this was 0.01 mg/million cells (LIF- and XAV-nano) and 0.1 mg/million cells (BDNF- and GDNF-nano).

Rat ventral mesencephalon cell cultures and staining

Culture medium was either for proliferation (PM), consisting of Neurobasal A (Invitrogen), 2% B-27 supplement, 100 U/ml penicillin, 100 µg/ml streptomycin, 250 ng/ml amphotericin B, 2 mM L-glutamine, 20 ng/ml epidermal growth factor and 20 ng/ml fibroblast growth factor-2, or for differentiation (DM), which was made up of Dulbecco's Minimal Essential Medium, 10% fetal calf serum, 2% B-27, 100 U/ml penicillin, 100 µg/ml streptomycin and 250 ng/ml amphotericin B.

VM cultures from time-mated Sprague-Dawley rats at E14 followed the protocol described previously (Pruszak et al., 2009). After a single-cell suspension was prepared, the cells were collected as a crude concentrated cell suspension to which the nanoparticles were added and gently mixed. After at least 30 minutes at room temperature, to allow cell attachment of the nanoparticles, the cells were plated on laminin-coated coverslips as 50 µl droplets containing 50,000 cells. After 30 minutes for cell adherence, 500 µl DM was added per well and cultures incubated at 37°C in 5% CO_2 air. Subsequent medium exchanges involved 50% of the medium being removed and replaced but without nanoparticles. Cultures were fixed for analyses of the total βIII-tubulin$^+$ (mouse anti-βIII-tubulin; Sigma-Aldrich; 1/500) and TH$^+$ (rat anti-TH; AbCam; 1/300) cell numbers as well as serotoninergic cells (rabbit anti-SERT; AbCam; 1/500) and glia (rabbit anti-GFAP; Dako; 1/500) cells: apoptosis was assessed using caspase-3 release using standard techniques (Cell Signaling Technology). To measure the time course of any therapeutic effects, replicate cultures were analysed after 1, 2, 3, 4 and 5 DIV.

HfVM cultures and intrastriatal grafting

hfVM was obtained from routine termination of pregnancies at 6–8 weeks of gestational age, subject to full consent being given under full ethical approval. The collected tissues were pooled over a 4-day period, stored at +4°C in Hibernate E (Life Technologies) and processed for culture as outlined in **Fig. 3A**. Tissue pieces were washed and incubated in HibE/TrypIE (Life Technologies) and Pulmozyme (Roche) before trituration, as described previously (Lopez et al., 2013). Specifically, single-cell suspensions were prepared through gentle enzymatic digestion and trituration and were coated with targeted nanoparticles as described for rat VM cells but with treatment in proliferation medium overnight at 37°C. For *in vitro* experiments, nano-stroma-coated hfVM cells were cultured in differentiation medium for 4 days before fixation and staining for HuNu and TH as previously described (Lopez et al., 2013).

For transplantation, unbound nanoparticles were removed by centrifugation prior to transplanting into the left striatum of male Nu-Nu rats aged 12 weeks as described previously (Lopez et al., 2013). Specifically, the cells were collected in PM at a density of 50,000 cells per μl and held at room temperature prior to stereotactic grafting into the striatum, with each graft consisting of 4 μl of the hfVM cell suspension. A common starting pool of cells was used, this being subdivided for nanoparticle treatment, to ensure direct comparison of cargo-related effects. After 12 weeks the rats were culled and the brains removed and processed for immunohistochemistry staining for TH and HuNu. After coronal sectioning, every 6th slice was stained for a given target antigen. Transplant stereology used Neurolucida and cell counting by the Aperio Imagescope according to manufacturer's instructions to give graft volume, cell counts and the spatial distribution of the grafted cells. Three, and two, recipients received grafts treated with LIF-nano, or empty-nano, respectively: each batch of donor tissue was equally divided between each treatment group to ensure equivalence. Numbers were limited owing to human fetal tissue availability.

Immunocytochemistry of human cells grown on coverslips followed standard procedures. Primary antibodies were diluted in blocking solution and applied overnight at 4°C using rabbit anti-TH (1:1000; Merck Millipore) and mouse anti-βIII tubulin (1:500; Merck Millipore) followed by secondary antibodies for 2 hours at 4°C: antibodies were from Millipore Molecular Probes, including anti-rabbit IgG (A11034, A21206) and anti-mouse IgG (A31570, A21235). Cells were counterstained with DAPI (1 μg/ml). Immunohistochemistry of grafted brains used 40-μm coronal sections collected sequentially into 24-well plates. Sections were taken at regular intervals (for example, 1 in 6) and stained for HuNu (1:1000; Merck Millipore; MAB1281) and TH (Merck Millipore; AB152) using standard protocols. Similarly, a further series of sections were stained for human-specific tau. Each *in vitro* experimental treatment was repeated three times using different donor sources. Within each experiment, five replicate counts/coverslip were made with four coverslips/therapy analysed by ANOVA to give standard error of the mean (s.e.m.).

Quantification and statistical analysis

Data are presented as mean ± s.e.m. Multiple comparisons in the same data set were analysed by a one-way ANOVA; pairwise multiple comparison procedures were used for post-hoc analysis. Single comparisons to controls were made using a two-tailed Student's *t*-test. $^{*}P<0.05$; $^{**}P<0.01$; $^{***}P<0.001$. Further statistical information is provided in the figure legends.

ACKNOWLEDGEMENTS

The authors acknowledge the expert assistance from Leigh-Anne McDuffus (CRUK, Cambridge) and Richard Butler (The Gurdon Institute, Cambridge) for imaging and image quantification. We are also most grateful to Delisa Ibanez Garcia of Bitplane (http://www.bitplane.com) who kindly ran the analyses shown in **Fig. 5E,F**.

COMPETING INTERESTS

No conflict of interest occurred during this study: S.M.M. and T.M.F. declare themselves as co-founders of LIF-NanoRx Ltd UK.

AUTHOR CONTRIBUTIONS

R.A.B. and S.M.M. conceived the project and designed the experiments; J.-W.Z. and S.C.D. performed and analysed the experiments on hfVM (J.-W.Z.) or rat fVM (S.C.D.); T.M.F. and C.K. prepared the nano-therapeutics; P.T. and X.H. assisted in tissue preparations; S.M.M. and R.A.B. wrote the manuscript.

REFERENCES

1. Baker, K. A. M., Hong, M., Sadi, D. and Mendez, I.. (2000). Intrastriatal and intranigral grafting of hNT neurons in the 6-OHDA rat model of Parkinson's disease. Exp. Neurol. 162, 350-360.

2. Barker, R. A., Stacy, M. and Brundin, P. (2013). A new approach to diseasemodifying drug trials in Parkinson's disease. J. Clin. Invest. 123, 2364-2365.

3. Beck, K. D., Knusel, B. and Hefti, F. (1993). The nature of trophic action of brainderived neurotrophic factor, dess(1-3)-insulin-like growth factor 1, and basic fibroblast growth factor on mesencephalic dopaminergic neurons developing in culture. Neuroscience 52, 855-866.

4. Cao, W., Yang, Y., Wang, Z., Liu, A., Fang, L., Wu, F., Hong, J., Shi, Y., Leung, S., Dong, C. et al. (2011). Leukemia inhibitory factor inhibits t helper 17 cell differentiation and confers treatment effects of neural progenitor cell therapy in autoimmune disease. Immunity 35, 273-284.

5. Corradetti, B., Freile, P., Pells, S., Bagnaninchi, P., Park, J., Fahmy, T. M. and de Sousa, P. A. (2012). Paracrine signalling events in embryonic stem cell renewal mediated by affinity targeted nanoparticles. Biomaterials 33, 6634-6643.

6. Couvreur, O., Aubourg, A., Crepin, D., Degrouard, J., Gertler, A., Taouis, M. and Vacher, C.-M. (2012). The anorexigenic cytokine ciliary neurotrophic factor stimulates POMC gene expression via receptors localized in the nucleus of arcuate neurons. Am. J. Physiol. Endocrinol. Metab. 302, E458-E467.

7. Danhier, F., Ansorena, E., Silva, J. M., Coco, R., Le Breton, A. and Préat, V. (2012). PLGA-based nanoparticles: an overview of biomedical applications. J. Control. Release 161, 505-522.

8. del Valle, I., Rudloff, S., Carles, A., Li, Y., Liszewska, E., Vogt, R. and Kemler, R. (2013). E-cadherin is required for the proper activation of the Lifr/Gp130 signaling pathway in mouse embryonic stem cells. Development 140, 1684-1692.

9. Deverman, B. E. and Patterson, P. H. (2012). Exogenous leukemia inhibitory factor stimulates oligodendrocyte progenitor cell proliferation and enhances hippocampal remyelination. J. Neurosci. 32, 2100-2109.

10. Dong, H., Fahmy, T. M., Metcalfe, S. M., Morton, S. L., Dong, X., Inverardi, L., Adams, D. B., Gao, W. and Wang, H. (2012). Immuno-isolation of pancreatic islet allografts using pegylated nanotherapy leads to long-term normoglycemia in full MHC mismatch recipient mice. PLoS ONE 7, e50265.

11. Dyson, S. C., Fahmy, T. M., Metcalfe, S. M. and Barker, R. A. (2014). Biological considerations in design of a nanotherapeutic for cell-based therapy to treat Parkinson's Disease. J. Nanomater. Mol. Nanotechnol. (in press).

12. Gao, W., Thompson, L., Zhou, Q., Putheti, P., Fahmy, T. M., Strom, T. B. and Metcalfe, S. M. (2009). Treg versus Th17 lymphocyte lineages are cross-regulated by LIF versus IL-6. Cell Cycle 8, 1444-1450.

13. Huang, S. M., Mishina, Y. M., Liu, S., Cheung, A., Stegmeier, F., Michaud, G. A., Charlat, O., Wiellette, E., Zhang, Y., Wiessner, S. et al. (2009). Tankyrase inhibition stabilizes axin and antagonizes Wnt signalling. Nature 461, 614-620.

14. Hyman, C., Hofer, M., Barde, Y. A., Juhasz, M., Yancopoulos, G. D., Squinto, S. P. and Lindsay, R. M. (1991). BDNF is a neurotrophic factor for dopaminergic neurons of the substantia nigra. Nature 350, 230-232.

15. Jang, S. W., Liu, X., Yepes, M., Shepherd, K. R., Miller, G. W., Liu, Y., Wilson, W. D., Xiao, G., Blanchi, B., Sun, Y. E. et al. (2010). A selective TrkB agonist with potent neurotrophic activities by 7,8-dihydroxyflavone. Proc. Natl. Acad. Sci. USA 107, 2687-2692.

16. Kim, H., Wu, J., Ye, S., Tai, C. I., Zhou, X., Yan, H., Li, P., Pera, M. and Ying, Q. L. (2013). Modulation of β-catenin function maintains mouse epiblast stem cell and human embryonic stem cell self-renewal. Nat. Commun. 4, 2403.

17. Labowsky, M. and Fahmy, T. M. (2012). Diffusive transfer between two intensely interacting cells with limited surface kinetics. Chem. Eng. Sci. 74, 114-123.

18. Laterza, C., Merlini, A., De Feo, D., Ruffini, F., Menon, R., Onorati, M., Fredrickx, E., Muzio, L., Lombardo, A., Comi, G. et al. (2013). iPSC-derived neural precursors exert a neuroprotective role in immune-mediated demyelination via the secretion of LIF. Nat. Commun. 4, 2597.

19. Ling, Z. D., Potter, E. D., Lipton, J. W. and Carvey, P. M. (1998). Differentiation of mesencephalic progenitor cells into dopaminergic neurons by cytokines. Exp. Neurol. 149, 411-423.

20. Lopez, W. O., Nikkhah, G., Kahlert, U. D., Maciaczyk, D., Bogiel, T., Moellers, S., Schültke, E., Döbrössy, M. and Maciaczyk, J. (2013). Clinical neurotransplantation protocol for Huntington's and Parkinson's disease. Restor. Neurol. Neurosci. 31, 579-595.

21. Lutolf, M. P. and Hubbell, J. A. (2005). Synthetic biomaterials as instructive extracellular microenvironments for morphogenesis in tissue engineering. Nat. Biotechnol. 23, 47-55.

22. Mahoney, M. J. and Saltzman, W. M. (2001). Transplantation of brain cells assembled around a programmable synthetic microenvironment. Nat. Biotechnol. 19, 934-939.

23. Moon, R. T., Bowerman, B., Boutros, M. and Perrimon, N. (2002). The promise and perils of Wnt signaling through β-catenin. Science 296, 1644-1646.

24. Park, J., Gao, W., Whiston, R., Strom, T. B., Metcalfe, S. and Fahmy, T. M. (2011). Modulation of CD4+ T lymphocyte lineage outcomes with targeted, nanoparticlemediated cytokine delivery. Mol. Pharm. 8, 143-152.

25. Patapoutian, A. and Reichardt, L. F. (2000). Roles of Wnt proteins in neural development and maintenance. Curr. Opin. Neurobiol. 10, 392-399.

26. Pruszak, J., Just, L., Isacson, O. and Nikkah, G. (2009). Isolation and culture of ventral mesencaphalic precursor cells and

dopaminergic neurons from rodent brains. Curr. Protoc. Stem Cell Biol. Chapter 2: Unit 2D.5.

27. Steenblock, E. R. and Fahmy, T. M. (2008). A comprehensive platform for ex vivo Tcell expansion based on biodegradable polymeric artificial antigen-presenting cells. Mol. Ther. 16, 765-772.

28. Vacik, T., Stubbs, J. L. and Lemke, G. (2011). A novel mechanism for the transcriptional regulation of Wnt signaling in development. Genes Dev. 25, 1783-1795.

29. Villadiego, J., Méndez-Ferrer, S., Valdés-Sánchez, T., Silos-Santiago, I., Fariñas, I., López-Barneo, J. and Toledo-Aral, J. J. (2005). Selective glial cell line-derived neurotrophic factor production in adult dopaminergic carotid body cells in situ and after intrastriatal transplantation. J. Neurosci. 25, 4091-4098.

Chapter 8

Gold-Silver Alloy Nanoshells: A New Candidate for Nanotherapeutics and Diagnostics

Dana E Gheorghe[1], Lili Cui[1], Christof Karmonik[2], Audrius Brazdeikis[3], Jose M Penaloza[1], Joseph K Young[4], Rebekah A Drezek[4,5] and Malavosklish Bikram[1*]

[1]*Department of Pharmacological & Pharmaceutical Sciences, College of Pharmacy, University of Houston, Texas Medical Center Campus, 1441 Moursund St., Houston, TX 77030, USA*

[2]*The Methodist Hospital, 6565 Fannin, Houston, TX 77030, USA*

[3]*Department of Physics and Texas Center for Superconductivity, University of Houston, 4800 Calhoun Road, Houston, TX 77004, USA*

[4]*Department of Electrical and Computer Engineering, Rice University, 6100 Main Street, MS-366, Houston, TX 77005, USA*

[5]*Department of Bioengineering, Rice University, 6100 Main Street, MS-142, Houston, TX 77005, USA*

ABSTRACT

We have developed novel gold-silver alloy nanoshells as magnetic resonance imaging (MRI) dual T_1 (positive) and T_2 (negative) contrast agents as an alternative to typical gadolinium (Gd)-based contrast agents. Specifically, we have doped iron oxide nanoparticles with Gd ions and sequestered the ions within the core by coating the nanoparticles with an alloy of gold and silver. Thus, these nanoparticles are very innovative and have the potential to overcome toxicities related to renal clearance of contrast agents such as nephrogenic systemic fibrosis. The morphology of the attained nanoparticles was characterized by XRD which demonstrated the successful incorporation of Gd(III) ions into the structure of the magnetite, with no major alterations of the spinel structure, as well as the growth of the gold-silver alloy shells. This was supported by TEM, ICP-AES, and SEM/EDS data. The nanoshells showed a saturation magnetization of 38 emu/g because of the presence of Gd ions within the crystalline structure with r_1 and r_2 values of 0.0119 and 0.9229 mL mg^{-1} s^{-1}, respectively (Au:Ag alloy = 1:1). T_1- and T_2-weighted images of the nanoshells showed that these agents can both increase the surrounding water proton signals in the T_1-weighted image and reduce the signal in T_2-weighted images. The as-synthesized nanoparticles exhibited strong absorption in the range of 600-800 nm, their optical properties being strongly dependent upon the thickness of the gold-silver alloy shell. Thus, these nanoshells have the potential to be utilized for tumor cell ablation because of their absorption as well as an imaging agent.

1. INTRODUCTION

The search for new composite systems consisting of a wide range of metal and semiconductor core materials with an outer inert shell has led to the discovery of novel nanoparticles with a broad range of biomedical applications in areas such as tissue engineering, gene and drug delivery, photo-thermal therapy, cell tracking, and storage systems [1, 2, 3]. Among this broad area of nanometer-sized systems, iron oxide nanocores have gained special attention because of their unique physical properties in which their size, morphology, composition, and surface chemistry can be tailored to many biological and biomedical applications [4, 5]. Tantamount to their physical versatility, these nanocores possess unique magnetic properties that facilitate proton relaxation within specific tissues, which thus make them suitable as T_2 contrast agents for magnetic resonance imaging (MRI) [6, 7]. Typical iron oxides that have extensively been explored for MRI applications include magnetite, Fe_3O_4, with alternating lattices of Fe(II) and Fe(III) ions or maghemite, γ-Fe_2O_3, in which the lattice structure consist of Fe(III) ions only [8]. However, despite their widespread use in the biomedical field, an open challenge for using iron oxide nanoparticles as contrast agents is to improve their magnetic properties, which in turn would lead to higher imaging sensitivity. This can be done by doping them with transition metal ions, in particular lanthanides which have distinctive magnetic and optical properties, associated with their electronic configuration [9, 10].

However, apart from their magnetic properties, these nanocores are unstable both in air and in solution. Iron oxide typically forms aggregates in solution and undergoes oxidation in air [11, 12]. In addition, even though iron oxide nanoparticles are good magnetic materials, the cores are susceptible to corrosion in the presence of water [13, 14] and are more reactive in bulk materials because of their high surface-to-volume ratio [15]. Also, aside from their physical instability and relative biocompatibility [16, 17], iron oxide nanocores have been shown to be toxic [18]. However, these hurdles can be overcome by coating the cores with outer shells, such as inorganic oxides (silica) [19, 20], inert metals (silver, gold, or gold alloys) [11, 21, 22, 23], or bioactive macromolecules such as liposomes and micelles, which can encapsulate a numerous amount of nanoparticles within the structures that then impart an inert physical property to the cores in biological media [2, 24, 25, 26]. Subsequent surface functionalization of the nanocomposite materials with hydrophilic polymers such as poly(ethylene glycols) (PEGs) [27, 28, 29, 30] and dextrans [31, 32] can further increase the physical stability of the nanoparticles particularly in solution. In addition, the coating of the magnetic nanoparticles with inert metals, such as gold, is extremely attractive because the nanocomposite system is resistant to corrosion in biological conditions and can decrease the toxicity of the cores [33, 34, 35].

Moreover, coating of these doped cores with an outer inert shell can sequester toxic metals such as gadolinium within the core of the nanoparticles [12]. Gd(III) ions have to be combined with carrier molecules because of their extreme toxicities, which are strongly associated with a systemic fibrosing disorder that is referred to as nephrogenic systemic fibrosis (NSF) in patients with kidney diseases [36, 37]. The Gd ions are toxic because their ionic radius is almost equal to that of divalent calcium ions, which enable Gd to compete with biological systems including enzymes with a higher binding affinity to alter the kinetics of their systems [38]. In addition, Gd ions are inorganic blockers of voltage-gated calcium channels [39]. Hence, the development of a contrast agent that could completely sequester Gd within the core of the nanoparticle, thereby preventing its release into the body would highly be beneficial as a safe and effective alternative to typical Gd-based contrast agents.

Currently, there is an extensive development of monometallic nanoshells with minor attention given to nanosystems consisting of bimetallic and trimetallic alloy shells [40, 41, 42, 43]. Recent research in this area has shown that gold-silver alloy nanoshells might have additional biomedical applications (e.g., cancer screening), because of their distinct optical properties ranging from visible to the near-IR wavelength region [44]. Our exploratory research aimed at preparing new biocompatible nanoshells for MR imaging that could overcome NSF and can also be utilized for laser ablation of tumor cells has led to the synthesis of novel Gd-doped magnetite cores, Gd:Fe_3O_4, covered with a gold-silver alloy shell.

2. EXPERIMENTAL METHOD

2.1. Materials and synthesis

$FeCl_2\,4H_2O$ (99%), $FeCl_3\,6H_2O$ (97%), $GdCl_3$ (99.9%), $AgNO_3$, HCl (37%), $NaAuCl_4$ (99%), HNO_3 (70%), NaOH (98%), NH_4OH (30%), 3-aminopropyltriethoxysilane (APTES), formaldehyde, and tetrakis(hydroxymethyl)phosphonium (THPC) were purchased from Sigma-Aldrich and used as-received unless otherwise stated. The magnetite nanoparticle cores were doped with a molar ratio of 10% Gd(III) ions that were prepared by a coprecipitation reaction of Fe(III), Fe(II), and Gd(III) salts in NaOH solution at 65°C. The surface of the nanocores was functionalized with $-NH_2$ groups by the addition of 3-aminopropyltriethoxysilane (APTES) [45]. This resulted in surface-terminated $-NH_2$ groups of APTES that were available for covalent coordination to a transition metal through the lone pair of nitrogen. As previously reported in basic medium [46, 47], the terminal amine groups of the amine-functionalized nanocores act as anchoring sites for the gold nanoparticles used in the seeding step by forming covalent Au-N bonds (gold metal being well known for its affinity for binding with amine or thiol terminal groups of organic molecules [48]). A gold seed solution was then prepared by reducing $NaAuCl_4$ with tetrakis(hydroxylmethyl)phosphonium chloride (THPC), as reported by Duff [49, 50]. The gold-seeded method was utilized since the gold nanoparticles can be used as nucleation sites for the growth of a mono or bimetallic shell. Moreover, this method enabled control over shell thickness and composition of the synthesized nanoshells [43]. Finally, the gold-seeded amine-functionalized nanocores were used as nuclei to build up a gold-silver alloy nanoshell formed as a result of a redox reaction, which occurred in the presence of formaldehyde as a reducing agent, when the THPC gold-seeded Gd-doped iron oxide nanoparticles were added to a basic solution of Au(III) and Ag(I) ions corresponding to molar ratios of Au:Ag = 1:1 and 5:1, respectively. Au(III) and Ag(I) ions were simultaneously reduced to metallic gold and silver, forming the alloy-based shell (see Figure 1).

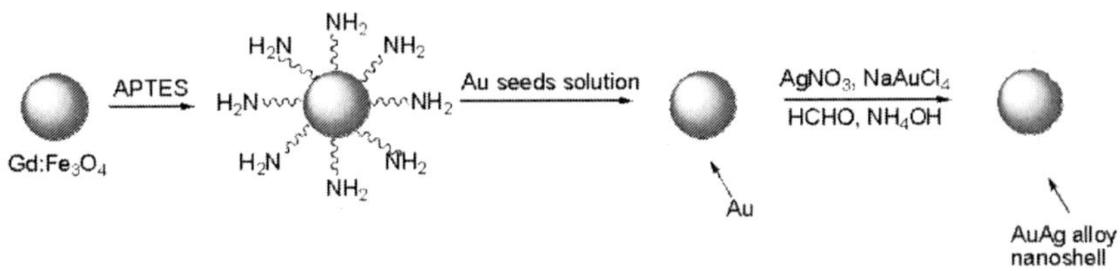

Figure 1. Schematic illustration of the preparation of the Gd-doped iron oxide nanoparticles with gold-silver alloy nanoshells.

2.2 Characterization and measurements

Powder X-ray diffraction analysis was used for the analysis of the synthesized samples. Data were collected at room temperature using a PANanalytical X'Pert PRO diffractometer equipped with Cu Kα radiation (λ = 1.5406 Å). The samples were ground using an agate mortar and pestle to a suitable powder sample. The powder was then placed on a zero background sample holder. The 2θ range was 5-120° with a scan rate of 6.4°/min. Data compilation and analysis were processed using the Diffractometer Management System software package which included a JCPDS powder diffraction database [51]. The composition of the samples was analyzed using a sequential Thermo Jarrell Ash Atomscan 25 inductively coupled plasma (ICP) emission spectrometer. Measurements were made using the following selected lines: 230.562 for Fe, 328.068 for Ag, 242.795 for Au, and 342.347 for Gd. The instrument drift was corrected by running a quality control solution every two to three analyses. The nanoparticles were dissolved in aqua regia and evaporated to dryness. The resulted residues were dissolved in 10% nitric acid and diluted to concentrations in the range of 1-50 ppm for analysis. Standard solutions with concentrations ranging from 0 to 50 ppm were used for calibration curves. Chemical analyses of the samples by means of SEM/EDS were performed on a Jeol JSM 8330 F scanning electron microscope equipped with an energy-dispersive spectrometer (EDS) by means of 15 kV accelerating voltage and 12 μA emission current from a cold-field emission gun. Small volumes of water-dispersed nanoparticles were deposited on a copper disk and allowed to evaporate at room temperature. The copper disk was subsequently attached to a brass sample holder using carbon tape. All the analyses were carried out at approximately 4×10^{-4} Pa. Elemental analysis was used for all our samples. These results complemented the results from XRD and ICP-AES analyses. The size and morphology of the nanoparticles were determined with transmission electron microscopy (TEM) on a JEOL JEM-2000 FX instrument. Statistical analysis and average size distribution of the particles were determined by evaluating a minimum of 100 nanoparticles per sample. The mean standard deviation σ, defined as $\sigma = ((1/(N - 1))*\Sigma_i (x_i - x)^2)^{1/2}$, was also determined for each size distribution. The nanoparticles were dispersed in water and cast on a carbon-coated grid (Pelco® No. 160). The sample was allowed to settle on the grid for approximately 1 min in a humidified atmosphere. The carbon-coated grid was then washed with water, followed by another addition of nanoparticles onto the carbon-coated grid. The grids were then left for another 1 min before gently removing excess liquid with a filter paper. The absorption of the nanoparticles in the ultraviolet-visible-near infrared region (UV-Vis-NIR) was determined with a Beckman Coulter DU 800 spectrophotometer using a 0.1-mm quartz cuvette. The spectra were collected in the range of 190-1100 nm at a resolution of 0.5 nm, and the concentration of the nanoparticles was adjusted so that the maximum absorbance did not exceed 1 absorbance unit. The magnetic susceptibility of the synthesized nanoparticles was measured by a superconducting quantum interference device magnetometer (Quantum Design MPMS). The saturation magnetization measurements were performed at 300 and 5 K. Once the desired measurement temperature was reached at zero field, field cycling from 5 to -5 T back and forth was applied followed by data collection for each M(H) measurement curve. In addition, the zero-field-cooled (ZFC) and field-cooled (FC) measurements were performed by cooling the sample from 300 to 5 K at zero field and then applying 200 Oe field for the warming up scan. Longitudinal and traverse relaxation times were measured in a 1.5-T magnet on a Siemens Avanto, full body clinical scanner (Siemens AG Healthcare) at 37°C. The coil used was standard 12 channel head coil and the samples prepared were dispersed in 1% agarose gel at the following nanoparticle concentrations: 0.005, 0.01, 0.02, 0.03, and 0.04 mg/mL. In brief, solutions were solidified in test tubes of 10 mm diameter, placed in a sample holder, and simultaneously imaged together with calibration samples of copper sulfate ($CuSO_4\ H_2O$) prepared in a similar fashion for the following concentrations: 6.54, 5.872, 5.538, 5.204, 4.87, 4.536, 3.868, 3.2, 2.08, 0.96, and 0.52 mg/mL. Fast spin echo images (echo train length 16, acquisition matrix = 256 × 128, field of view (FOV) = 220 × 110 mm resolution in an isotropic in-plane resolution of 0.86 mm, slice thickness 5 mm) were acquired in two series. In series 1, the echo time was varied from 10 to 160 ms (in increments of 10 ms) with fixed repetition time (TR = 3000 ms). From the signal intensity curves of these images, the spin-spin relaxation time T_2 was determined for each concentration. In series 2, images were acquired for the following TRs: 170, 350, 700, 1000, 2000, 4000, and 5000 ms while keeping the echo time constant at minimum (TE = 9.9 ms). Gray scale values from the MRI images acquired at different TR and TE times were analyzed as follows: signal intensities were determined as average over regions of interest within the test tube (using Image J, NIH) avoiding image voxel at the test tube wall to minimize partial volume averages. The nonlinear Levenberg-Marquardt fitting method was then used to the fit standard equations for MRI signal intensity for spin echo sequences [52] to both the signal intensities at different TE (series 1) to determine T_2 and to the signal intensities at different TR to determine T_1. These fits were performed for the different concentrations of the Au/Ag alloy-coated nanoparticles, the commercial Omniscan®, and the $CuSO_4\ H_2O$ standards. Relaxivities, r_1 and r_2, were then determined using linear regression analysis assuming a linear relationship between relaxation times T_1 and T_2 and concentration. For Omniscan® and $CuSO_4\ H_2O$, relaxivities were compared to literature values.

3. RESULTS AND DISCUSSION

Previously, experimental data reported for an active bimetallic Au-Ag nanoparticle system on inert supports, such as silica, as well as density functional theory calculations performed on selected model clusters proposed for the Au-Ag bimetallic system, indicated that Au-Ag alloy shells formed through adsorption of positively charged Ag^+ ions on negatively charged Au^{3+} ions followed by their reduction with $NaBH_4$[53]. These interactions take place via electrostatic attractions as well as strong Au-Ag metallic interactions in which the later was found to be more predominant. Elemental analysis of the as-synthesized nanoshells by ICP-AES (Table 1) confirmed the presence of Gd ions, which gave molar ratios of Gd:Fe = 0.17:1 and 0.11:1 for the theoretical molar ratios of Au:Ag = 1:1 and 5:1, respectively. Thus, it was estimated that 17 and 11% of Gd(III) ions used in the preparation of the doped nanocores were incorporated into the final Au:Ag = 1:1 and 5:1 nanoparticles, respectively, which gave core compositions of $Gd_{0.17}Fe_{2.83}O_4$ and $Gd_{0.11}Fe_{2.89}O_4$. The crystallinity and structure of the Gd:Fe_3O_4 nanocores, as well as the gold-silver alloy nanoshells, were studied by means of XRD. As shown in Figure 2B, the X-ray powder diffraction pattern confirmed the formation of a single phase of the Gd-doped magnetite nanocores, which had the cubic spinel structure of the well-studied Fe_3O_4 (Figure 2A) [54]. The broad peak at approximately 20° in the diffraction powder pattern corresponds to the sample holder because of difficulties in the preparation of well-packed samples.

Table 1. Compositions obtained by ICP-AES for the analysis of Fe_3O_4, Gd:Fe_3O_4, Au-seeded functionalized Gd:Fe_3O_4, and gold-silver alloy nanoshells on gold-seeded amine-functionalized Gd:Fe_3O_4

Sample	Gd ppm	Fe ppm	Au ppm	Ag ppm	Gd:Fe	Au:Ag
Fe_3O_4	0	70.1	0	0	-	-
Gd: Fe_3O_4	11.6	57.7	0	0	0.2	-
Au-seeded Gd: Fe_3O_4	12.2	62.6	1	0	0.2	-
Au-Ag alloy = 1:1 nanoshells on Au-seeded amine-functionalized Gd: Fe_3O_4	7.0	40.4	6.8	19.5	0.2	0.4
Au-Ag alloy = 5:1 nanoshells on Au-seeded amine-functionalized Gd: Fe_3O_4	7.7	67.6	24.0	4.5	0.1	5.3

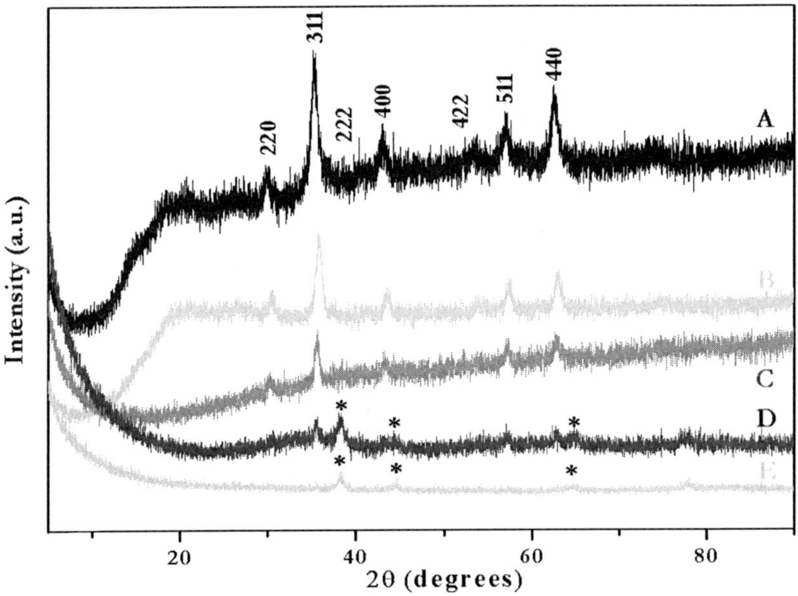

Figure 2. XRD patterns of Fe_3O_4 (A), Gd:Fe_3O_4 (B), gold-seeded Gd:Fe_3O_4 (C) and gold-silver alloy (*) deposited on gold-seeded Gd:Fe_3O_4 nanocores, Au:Ag = 1:1 (D) and Au:Ag = 5:1 (E). Miller indices are indicated for Fe_3O_4.

There was no significant change in the X-ray powder pattern of the Gd:Fe_3O_4 nanoparticles compared to the parent compound, Fe_3O_4, which was prepared as a reference by a coprecipitation reaction of Fe(III) and Fe(II) in NaOH at 65°C (see Figure 2A, B). These results are consistent with nanoparticles previously synthesized by the coprecipitation of the Fe(II), Fe(III), and Gd(III) salts in the same basic solution, which did not result in a mixed oxide system, Gd_2O_3-Fe_3O_4, but a doped Gd:Fe_3O_4[55]. The powder pattern of the as-synthesized nanoparticles indicated a smaller unit cell for the doped nanocores that was confirmed by the shift of the diffraction peaks characterized by Miller indices shown in Figure 2A (220, 311, 222, 400, 422, 511, and 440) toward bigger Bragg angles. Indexing of the powder patterns presented in Figure 2A, B indicated for Gd:Fe_3O_4 a cubic unit cell with lattice parameter a = 8.308 Å, which is approximately 0.8% smaller than the unit cell of the parent compound, Fe_3O_4, a = 8.373 Å, respectively (reported data for Fe_3O_4: cubic unit cell, space group *Fd-3m, a* = 8.384 Å) [56]. It was also suggested that in such doped system, the Gd(III) ions might occupy the octahedral sites [57]. The average particle size of the nanocores was estimated by applying the Debye-Scherrer model, written as $d = 0.9\lambda/ß_d \cos\theta$, where d is the crystallite diameter, λ = 1.540562 Å for Cu Kα line, $ß_d$ is the full width at half maximum of the strongest reflection peak, and θ is the corresponding Bragg angle [58]. This formula was applied for the (311) reflection in the powder pattern shown in Figure 2B in which an average crystallite size of 3.5 nm for the nanocores was calculated. The gold seeding step of the Gd:Fe_3O_4 nanocores had as a result--a decrease in the intensities characteristic to the doped spinel structure (Figure 2C). The X-ray powder diffraction was also used as a tool to verify the formation of the gold-silver alloy nanoshells on the gold-seeded Gd:Fe_3O_4 nanocores. As can be seen from Figure 2D, apart from the weak peaks which corresponded to the (311), (422), (511), and (440) reflections of the Gd:Fe_3O_4, three extra peaks positioned at 2θ values of 38.4°, 44.6°, and 64.7° that corresponded to the gold-silver alloy (molar ratio Au:Ag = 1:1) were observed. In Figure 2E, peaks corresponding to the gold-silver alloy (Au:Ag = 5:1) only are observed. These data indicated the formation of a layer of gold-silver alloy on the nanocores and not the formation of discrete gold and silver nanoparticles, which would have shown six individual peaks: 38.2°, 44.4°, and 64.6° corresponding to (111), (200), and (220) planes for gold [59] and 38.4°, 44.3°, and 64.7° corresponding to (111), (200), and (220) planes for silver [60], respectively. Moreover, the XRD patterns of gold and silver are completely overlapped in Figure 1D, E; therefore, the gold-silver alloy cannot be distinguished from the powder patterns of gold and silver as monometallic phases [61]. In addition, the absence of any diffraction peaks for Gd-doped magnetite cores in Figure 2E is because of the heavy atom effect from gold; it was observed that gold shells dominate the powder pattern because of its high electron density, which is consistent with previously reported data [58]. Our observation is consistent with data reported for gold nanoshells deposited on magnetite cores by others [62, 63, 64], as well as with ICP-AES results (Table 1) which indicated a molar ratio of Au:Ag = 0.4 (theoretical ratio 1:1) and 5.3, respectively (theoretical ratio 5:1). In addition, Liu et al. showed that the powder pattern of gold-silver alloy shells deposited on silica cores exhibited only the peaks characteristic to the gold or silver monometallic phase, whereas the peaks corresponding to the silica support were found to be absent [53].

Thus, our findings from the TEM, ICP-AES, and SEM/EDS data together with previously published one suggested that the Gd:Fe_3O_4 nanocores were completely covered with the gold-silver alloy and hence the formation of the nanoshells. Consistent with these findings was the optical absorption data for the nanoshells, which exhibited only one plasmon band that further supported the suggested nanoshell structure (discussed later). Therefore, we have shown that the reduction of gold and silver salts in the presence of gold-seeded Gd:Fe_3O_4 cores successfully led to the formation of gold-silver alloy nanoshells. However, the gold-silver shell is very thin when Au:Ag = 1:1 since the diffraction from gold and silver does not dominate the powder pattern, but a decrease of the intensity of the reflection peaks for the Gd:Fe_3O_4 nanocores was observed (Figure 1D) [1, 64]. As the ratio of Au:Ag was increased to 5:1, the reflections of gold and silver started to dominate the powder pattern and most of the characteristic peaks of the nanocore disappeared (Figure 2E).

Statistical analysis and average size distribution of the particles were determined by evaluating a minimum of 100 nanoparticles per sample set of Gd:Fe_3O_4, Au:Ag = 1:1, and Au:Ag = 5:1 nanoparticles. A representative set of TEM micrographs of the Gd:Fe_3O_4 nanoparticles, gold-seeded Gd:Fe_3O_4, and gold-silver alloy nanoshells (Au:Ag = 1:1 and 5:1) used for characterization in all studies is shown in Figure 3. There are two major findings from the morphological comparison of the images. First, the nanoparticles exhibited ovoid features with a high degree of crystallinity and an average size diameter of 8.0 ± 2.8 nm for the Gd:Fe_3O_4 nanocores, 8.2 ± 0.4 nm for the gold-silver alloy nanoshells (Au:Ag = 1:1), and 18.6 ± 3.6 nm for the gold-silver alloy nanoshells (Au:Ag = 5:1) (Figure3A-C, respectively). In addition, the nanoshells corresponding to Au:Ag = 5:1 showed a much lighter coat surrounding the dark Gd:Fe_3O_4 core (Figure 3C) (average thickness of the coating = 5.0 ± 2.8 nm) compared to the gold-silver alloy nanoshells at a 1:1 ratio (Figure 3B). Additional TEM micrographs of this sample are shown in "Figure S1 in Additional file 1". In addition, these nanoshells are unique since the alloy shell surrounding the core (Figure 3C) was clearly observed in the TEM images even though it has previously been considered impossible to observe an additional metal shell deposited on the surface of magnetite nanocores [65]. Most probably the lighter color was because of the presence of silver metal within the alloy shell. This observation was consistent with published reports for gold-palladium shells deposited on silica nanocores [43]. In these nanoshells, the lighter color of the surrounding shells around the cores was attributed to the gold-palladium alloy [43]. However, in the case of Au:Ag = 1:1 ratio the alloy shell was not apparently visible (Figure 3B) because of much thinner shell. In this case, the formation of the gold-silver shell was clearly confirmed by XRD (see Figure 2D) as well as semi-qualitative SEM/EDS analysis (see Figure 4A,B). Moreover, the measurement of the surface plasmon resonance band (discussed later) of these nanoparticles provided an indirect piece of evidence supporting the formation of the alloy nanoshells. Another important observation for the Au:Ag = 1:1 ratio nanoshells was that the dispersion of the nanoparticles was not as pronounced as in the case of the 5:1 ratio when the shell was clearly visible and implicitly thicker (see "Figures S1 and S2 in Additional file 1").

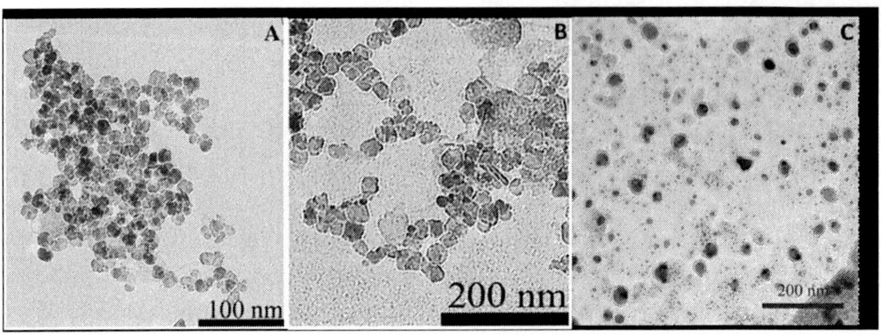

Figure 3. Representative TEM images of as-synthesized (A) Gd:Fe_3O_4 nanocores; (B) gold-silver alloy (Au:Ag = 1:1) nanoparticles; and gold-silver alloy (Au:Ag = 5:1) nanoparticles.

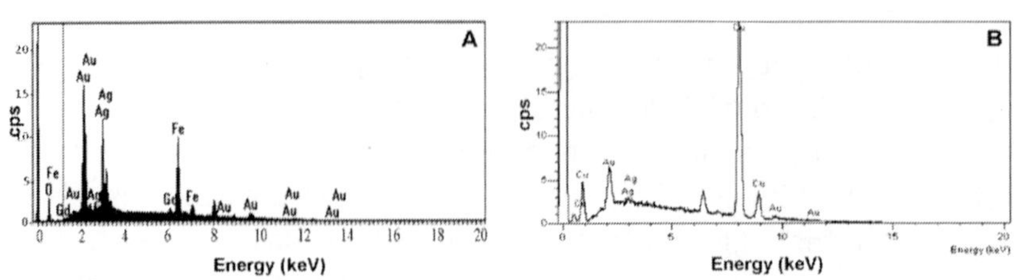

Figure 4. SEM/EDS spectra of as-synthesized gold-silver alloy nanoshells. Theoretical ratio of **(A)** Au:Ag = 1:1, experimental ratio Au:Ag = 3:1, and **(B)** Au:Ag = 5:1, experimental ratio Au:Ag = 3.6:1.

The optical properties of the as-synthesized nanoshells were studied with UV-Vis-NIR spectroscopy over the wavelength range of 190-1100 nm. Systematic studies with reaction times and absorption of nanoparticles (data not shown) indicated that the optimum reaction time for the deposition of the gold-silver alloy was 7 days (see "Figure S3 in Additional file 1"). This was further confirmed by high absorption intensity for the 7 days reaction time; based on Beer-Lambert law this might indicate the complete formation of the alloy nanoshells [64]. The UV-Vis-NIR spectra of the as-synthesized alloy nanoshells for 7 days reaction time for both Au:Ag = 1:1 and 5:1 ratios, respectively, are depicted in Figure 5. As can be seen, maximum absorption peaks were observed at approximately 700 nm for 1:1 ratio (Figure 5A) and approximately 600 nm for 5:1 ratio (Figure 5B), which fell in between those of silver nanoparticles (420 nm) and gold nanoshells (approximately 800 nm) [65]. These data also confirmed that the mixture of the reduced gold and silver ions (Au:Ag = 5:1) in the alloy did not produce two distinctive bands in the spectrum and that the surface plasmon resonance property of the synthesized nanoshells was dependent on the thickness, as reported in the literature [66, 67, 68, 69, 70]. Furthermore, when the ratio Au:Ag was 1:1, two distinctive plasmon bands were observed in the UV-Vis-NIR spectra for 1, 7, and 14 days reaction time (see "Figure S3 in Additional file 1"); for 7 days reaction time one band was centered at 480 nm and the second one at 700 nm, the first band being attributed to the initial stage of the Au-Ag nanoshell grow [53, 65]. The absence of the second plasmon band for a ratio of Au:Ag = 5:1 may be because of a higher concentration of gold in the gold-silver alloy. The 1:1 ratio spectra (Figure 5A) exhibit a broad plasmon band that extends out toward 1100 nm. It is believed that the observed spectral shoulder that extends out from 850 toward 1100 nm can be attributed to particle aggregation. Nonetheless, the bulk of the sample consist of individual particles where the width of the extinction peak, centered at 700 nm, can be attributed to a combination of line broadening and inhomogeneous broadening where inhomogeneous broadening is a result of the nanoparticle size and shape distributions and makes up the bulk of the peak width. This inhomogeneous broadening effect was observed and reported by others for simular metallic shell configurations [69, 70, 71, 72, 73, 74]. Thus, our findings are in a good agreement with reported surface plasmon resonance data for gold-silver alloy nanoshells when the absorption was tuned from 430 to 780 nm. Since we were interested in using these nanoparticles for both MR imaging and as a therapeutic tool for thermal ablation, we selected the gold-silver alloy at the 1:1 ratio for subsequent analysis and physical characterization.

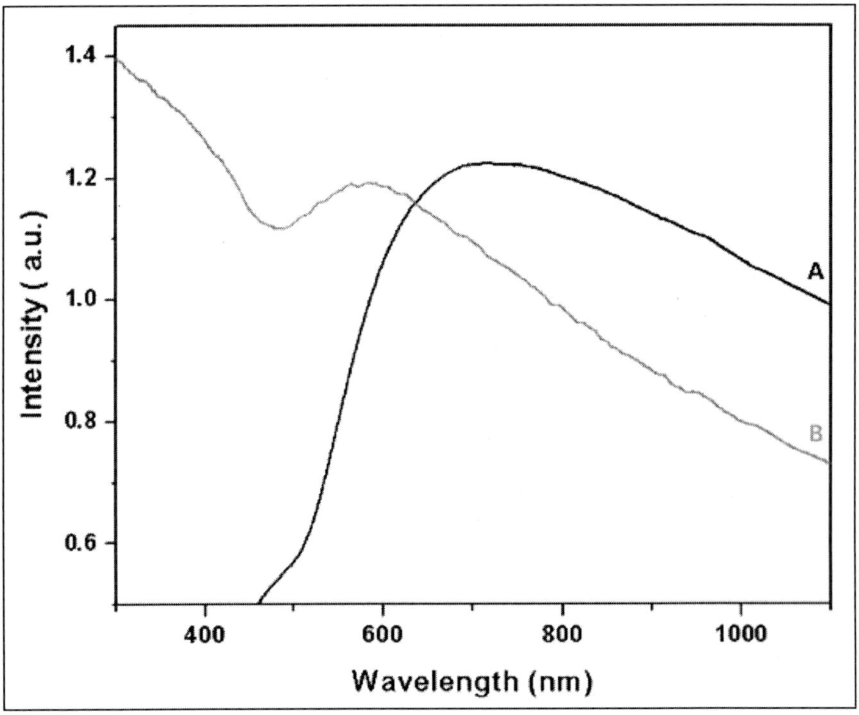

Figure 5. UV-Vis-NIR spectra of as-synthesized gold-silver alloy nanoshells deposited on gold-seeded Gd:Fe_3O_4 nanocores for (A) Au:Ag = 1:1 and (B) Au:Ag = 5:1 nanoparticles.

A common feature of magnetization curves *M*(*T*) is the occurrence of a maximum in ZFC curves at a temperature, associated with the blocking temperature of Gd:Fe_3O_4 nanocores. Analysis of the blocking temperatures (250-280 K) of the as-synthesized Au-Ag alloy = 1:1 nanoshells was found to be consistent with Stoner-Wohlfarth theory and average sizes of Gd:Fe_3O_4 nanocores. Moreover, the variation of the magnetization in the ZFC and FC measurements indicated a superparamagnetic behavior for the Au-Ag alloy (1:1) nanoshells despite the presence of the metallic shell. From the *M*(*H*) measurements (Figure 6), the normalized saturation magnetization at 300 K was 30 emu/g and approached 38 emu/g Gd:Fe_3O_4 for the Au-Ag alloy = 1:1

nanoshells. Owing to the Gd ions occupying the octahedral sites in Gd-doped Fe_3O_4, the magnetization value was found to be slightly reduced compared to undoped Fe_3O_4, consistent with observation by others [75]. Thus, the above magnetic characterization data support the use of Au-Ag alloy nanoshells as superparamagnetic MR contrast agents.

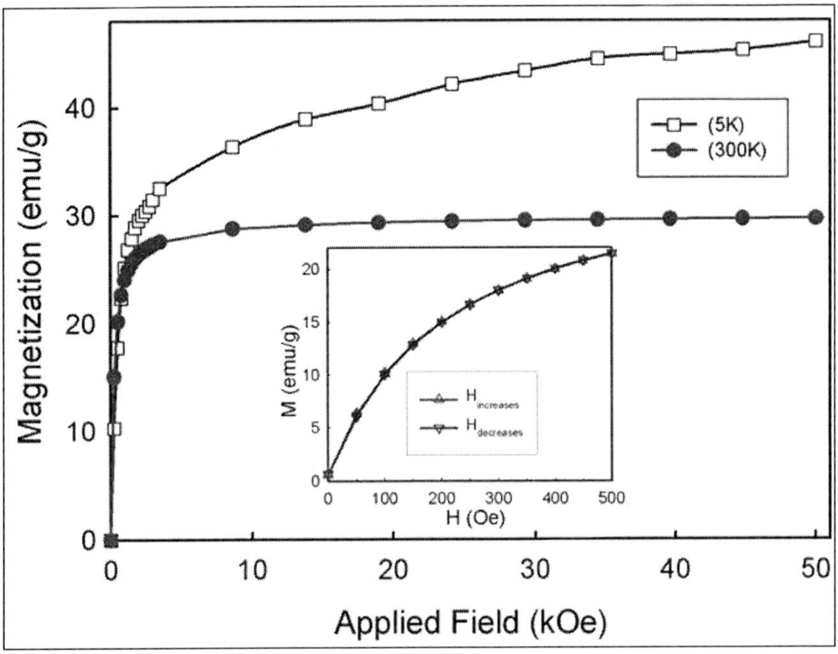

Figure 6.Magnetization versus applied magnetic field plots for the Au-Ag alloy (1:1) nanoshells sample at 300 and 5 K. The inset shows an expanded view of the low magnetic field behavior at 300 K.

The relaxivity rates r_1 (T_1 relaxivity) and r_2 (T_2 relaxivity) were calculated from $1/T_1$ after subtracting $1/T_{10}$ ($T_{10}$of agarose gel from measurement: 3333.333 ms) and from $1/T_2$ after subtracting $1/T_{20}$ (T_{20} of agarose gel from measurement: 144.5 ms), respectively. The r_1 and r_2 values of $CuSO_4$ were calculated to be 0.0039 and 0.0037 mL mg^{-1} s^{-1}, respectively (Figures 7C and 8C), which were found to be similar to values published in the literature (r_1: 0.94 mM^{-1} s^{-1}) [76]. The r_1 and r_2 values of Omniscan® were calculated to be 0.0057 and 0.0079 mL mg^{-1} s^{-1}, respectively (Figures 7B and 8B). The ratio

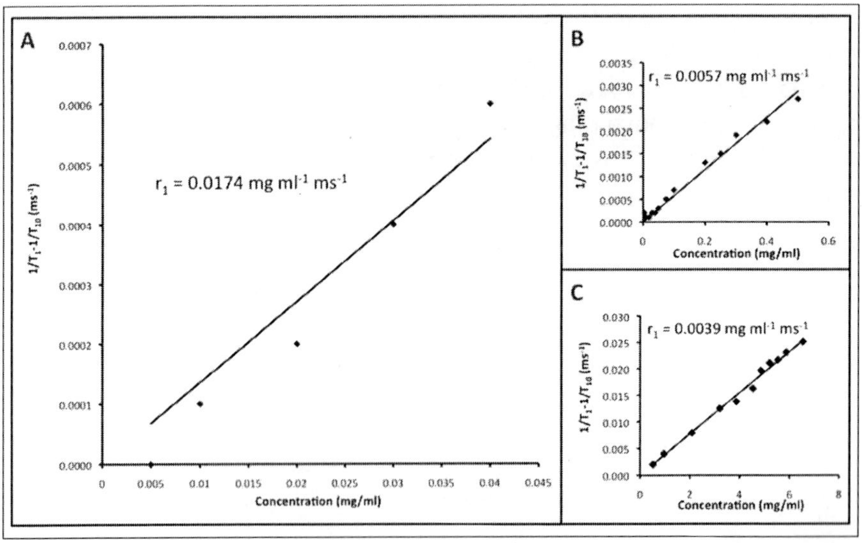

Figure 7. T_1 relaxation rates for (A) Au/Ag alloy-coated nanoparticles, (B) commercial Omiscan®, and (C) $CuSO_4H_2O$.

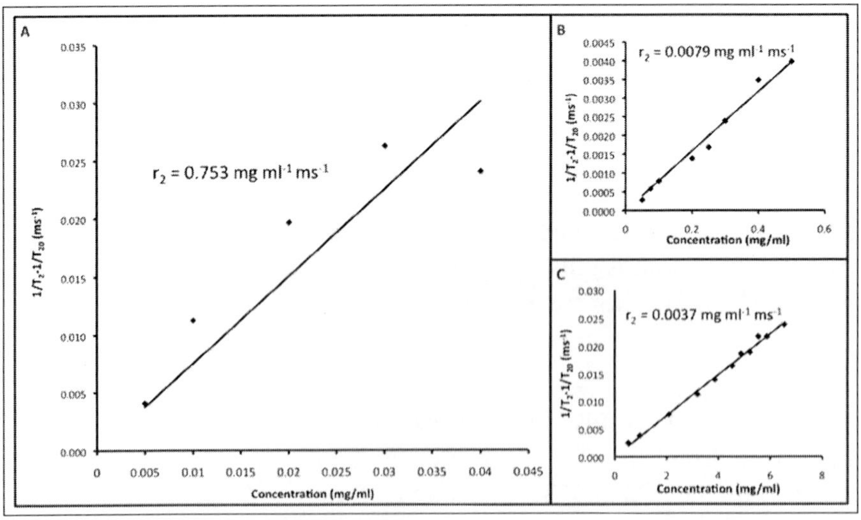

Figure 8. T_2 relaxation rates for (A) Au/Ag alloy-coated nanoparticles, (B) commercial Omniscan®, and (C) $CuSO_4H_2O$.

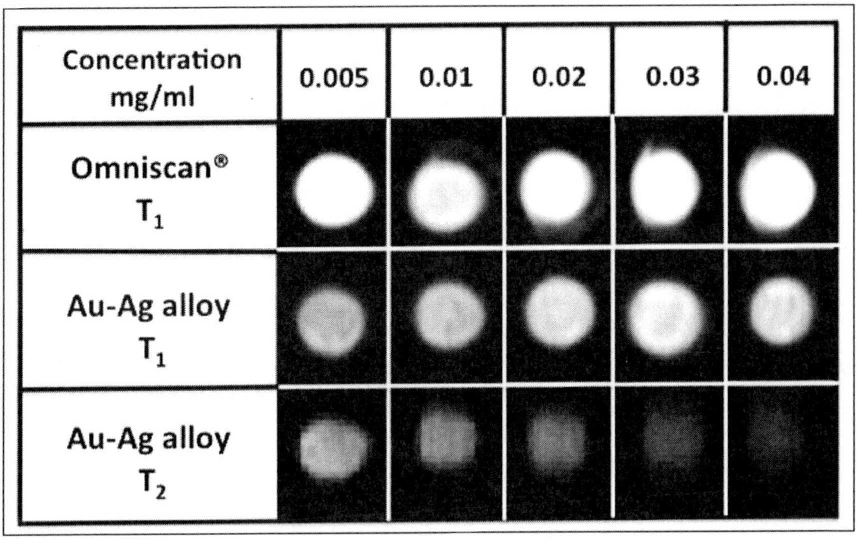

Figure 9. MR images of (A) $\boldsymbol{T_1}$ and (B) $\boldsymbol{T_2}$-weighted Au/Ag alloy-coated nanoparticles at different concentrations.

of r_1 and r_2 was 0.72 which is close to the value published in the literature (4.1/4.7 = 0.87) [77]. The r_1 and r_2 values of the as-synthesized Au-Ag alloy = 1:1 nanoshells were found to be 0.0174 and 0.7532 mL mg^{-1} s^{-1}, respectively (Figures 7A and 8A). A nonlinearity for $1/T_1$ and $1/T_2$ at higher concentrations was noted for the as-synthesized Au-Ag alloy = 1:1 nanoshells (Figures 7A and 8B). Even though this nonlinearity of the data was unexpected it is assumed, potentially that particle clustering occurred, which effectively reduced the coordination number for the water molecules surrounding the as-synthesized nanoshells. Carrying out the above-described analysis for the linear range only, the following values for r_1 and r_2 were obtained: r_1 = 0.0119 and r_2 = 0.9229 mL mg^{-1} s^{-1}. In order to validate the potential of Au-Ag alloy nanoshells as both T_1 and T_2 MR contrast agents, we acquired T_1- and T_2-weighted images as a function of nanoshell concentration. As shown in Figure 9, the alloy-coated nanoshells produced increasingly bright images that corresponded to increasing concentrations of the nanoshells for the T_1-weighted MR images, which resembled lighter images typical of T_1 contrast agents rather than T_2 contrast agents such as iron oxide. In addition, the T_2-weigted images for the alloy-coated nanoshells produced increasingly darker images as a function of concentration that corresponds to the reduction of the MR signal characteristic of iron-oxide-based MR contrast agents. Therefore, these images support the use of Au-Ag alloy nanoshells as dual T_1 and T_2 contrast agents.

4. CONCLUSION

Based on previous investigations [44, 64, 78] as well as our experimental observations, we anticipate that the optical properties of the nanoshells can be tailored in a controlled manner by adjusting the volume of the gold seed solution as well as the amounts of gold and silver salts used as precursors in the formation of the nanoshells. Studies regarding this matter, the optimization of the synthesis conditions of the nanoshells as well as the investigation of their biocompatibility are currently under way. Thus, our findings have shown the successful synthesis of a gold-silver alloy shell on composite magnetite nanocores. In addition, these nanosystems hold great promise for medical applications since based on their composition, the nanoparticles should be able to overcome corrosion and toxicity issues as well as aggregation. Furthermore, the magnetic properties of the nanocores and the thickness of the alloy shell may be systematically investigated and exploited. Complete structural characterizations and measurements of these relevant physical properties of these novel nanoshells are currently underway as well as the evaluation of the nanoshells in biological assays including in-depth cytotoxicity studies and ablation studies in various cell lines.

More details of the sample characterization including results from TEM, UV-Vis-NIR, and $M(T)$ measurements are given in "Figure S4 in Additional file 1."

ACKNOWLEDGEMENTS

We thank Dr. Irene Rusakova for assistance with TEM analysis. We also gratefully acknowledge the financial support of this study that was made available from the Department of Defense (DOD) (OC073093) and Texas Higher Education Coordinating Board-ARP Award (003652-0217-2007).

COMPETING INTERESTS

The authors declare that they have no competing interests.

AUTHORS' CONTRIBUTIONS

DG participated in the study design, synthesized the nanoparticles, performed the physical characterization (XRD, ICP-AES, TEM, SEM/EDS, UV) of the nanoparticles, and drafted the manuscript. LC prepared MRI samples and assisted in the analysis of the MRI data. CK designed MRI studies and analyzed MRI data. AB designed magnetization studies and analyzed magnetization data. JP assisted in the synthesis and characterization of the nanoparticles. RB and JY assisted in the study design and interpretation of the UV data. MB conceived of the study, participated in the design and coordination of the study, and assisted in the drafting of the manuscript.

REFERENCES

1. Xu Z, Hou Y, Sun S: Magnetic core/shell Fe 3 O 4 /Au and Fe 3 O 4 /Au/Ag nanoparticles with tunable plasmonic properties. J Am Chem Soc 2007, 129: 8698–8699.

2. Shubayev VI, Pisanic TR, Jin S: Magnetic nanoparticles for theragnostics. Adv Drug Del Rev 2009, 61: 467–477.

3. O'Neal DP, Hirsch LR, Halas NJ, Payne JD, West JL: Photo-thermal tumor ablation in mice using near infrared-absorbing nanoparticles. Cancer Lett 2004, 209: 171–176.

4. Tartaj P, Morales MDP, Veintemillas-Verdaguer S, Gonzalez-Carreno T, Serna CJ: The preparation of magnetic nanoparticles for applications in biomedicine. J Phys D Appl Phys 2003, 36: R182-R197.

5. Gupta AK, Gupta M: Synthesis and surface engineering of iron oxide nanoparticles for biomedical applications. Biomaterials2005, 26: 3995–34021.

6. Mulder WJM, Strijkers GJ, van Tilborg GAF, Griffioen AW, Nicolay K: Lipid-based nanoparticles for contrast-enhanced MRI and molecular imaging. NMR Biomed 2006, 19: 142–164.

7. Bumb A, Brechbiel MW, Choyke PL, Fugger L, Eggeman A, Prabhakaran D, Hutchinson J, Dobson PJ: Synthesis and characterization of ultra-small superparamagnetic iron oxide nanoparticles thinly coated with silica. Nanotechnology 2008, 19: 335601/1.

8. Jolivet J-P, Tronc E, Chaneac C: Iron oxides: from molecular clusters to solid. A nice example of chemical versatility. C R Geoscience 2006, 338: 488–497.

9. Groman EV, Bouchard JC, Reinhardt CP, Vaccaro DE: Ultrasmall mixed ferrite colloids as multidimensional magnetic resonance imaging, cell labeling, and cell sorting agents. Bioconjugate Chem 2007, 18: 1763–1771.

10. Park JY, Baek MJ, Choi ES, Woo S, Kim JH, Kim TJ, Jung JC, Chae KS, Chang Y, Lee GH: Paramagnetic ultrasmall gadolinium oxide nanoparticles as advanced T 1 MRI contrast agent: account for large longitudinal relaxivity, optimal particle diameter, and in vivo T 1 MR images. ACS Nano 2009, 3: 3663–3669.

11. Lu A-H, Salabas EL, Schüth F: Magnetic nanoparticles: synthesis, protection, functionalization, and application. Angew Chem Int Ed 2007, 46: 1222–1244.

12. Hasebroock KM, Serkova NJ: Toxicity of MRI and CT contrast agents. Exp Opin Drug Metab Toxicol 2009, 5: 403–416.

13. Cho S-J, Idrobo J-C, Olamit J, Liu K, Browning ND, Kauzlarich SM: Growth mechanisms and oxidation resistance of gold-coated iron nanoparticles. Chem Mater 2005, 17: 3181–3186.

14. Jolivet JP, Tronc E: Interfacial electron transfer in colloidal spinel iron oxide. Conversion of Fe 3 O 4 into γ-Fe 2 O 3 in aqueous medium. J Colloid Interface Sci 1988, 125: 688–701.

15. McBain SC, Yiu HHP, Dobson J: Magnetic nanoparticles for gene and drug delivery. Int J Nanomed 2008, 3: 169–180.

16. Koh I, Wang X, Varughese B, Isaacs L, Erhman SH, English DS: Magnetic iron oxide nanoparticles for biorecognition: evaluation of surface coverage and activity. J Phys Chem B 2006, 110: 1553–1558.

17. Wickline SA, Neubauer AM, Winter PM, Caruthers SD, Lanza GM: Molecular imaging and therapy of atherosclerosis with targeted nanoparticles. J Magn Reson Imaging 2007, 25: 667–680.

18. Nel A, Xia T, Mädler L, Li N: Toxic potential of materials at the nanolevel. Science 2006, 311: 622–627.

19. Yu CH, Tam KY, Lo CCH, Tsang SC: Functionalized silica coated magnetic nanoparticles with biological species for magnetic separation. IEEE Trans Magn 2007, 43: 2436–2438.

20. Yu CH, Al-Saadi A, Shih SJ, Qiu L, Tam KY, Tsang SC: Immobilization of BSA on silica-coated magnetic iron oxide nanoparticle. J Phys Chem C 2009, 113: 537–543.

21. Hu M, Chen JY, Li ZY, Au L, Hartland GV, Li X, Marqueze M, Xia Y: Gold nanostructures: engineering their plasmonic properties for biomedical applications. Chem Soc Rev 2006, 35: 1084–1094.

22. Kumar A, Singhal A: Synthesis of colloidal silver iron oxide nanoparticles--study of their optical and magnetic behavior.Nanotechnology 2009, 20: 295606.

23. Pazos-Perez N, Rodriguez-Gonzalez B, Hilgendorff M, Giersig M, Liz-Marzan LM: Gold encapsulation of star-shaped FePt nanoparticles. J Mater Chem 2010, 20: 61–64.

24. Torchilin VP: Recent advances with liposomes as pharmaceutical carriers. Nat Rev 2005, 4: 145–160.

25. Nasongkla N, Bey E, Ren JM, Ai H, Khemtong C, Guthi JS, Chin SF, Sherry AD, Boothman DA, Gao JM: Multifunctional

polymeric micelles as cancer-targeted MRI-ultrasensitive drug delivery systems. Nano Lett 2006, 6: 2427–2430.

26. Lecommandoux S, Sandre O, Checot F, Perzynski R: Smart hybrid magnetic self-assembled micelles and hollow capsules.Prog Solid State Chem 2006, 34: 171–179.

27. Prencipe G, Tabakman SM, Welsher K, Liu Z, Goodwin AP, Zhang L, Henry J, Dai H: PEG branched polymer for functionalization of nanomaterials with ultralong blood circulation. J Am Chem Soc 2009, 131: 4783–4787.

28. Butterworth MD, Illum L, Davis SS: Preparation of ultrafine silica- and PEG-coated magnetite particles. Colloid Surface A2001, 179: 93–102.

29. Flesch C, Unterfinger Y, Bourgeat-Lami E, Duguet E, Delaite C, Dumas P: Poly(ethylene glycol) surface coated magnetic particles. Macromol Rapid Commun 2005, 26: 1494–1498.

30. Lu Y, Yin YD, Mayers BT, Xia Y: Modifying the surface properties of superparamagnetic iron oxide nanoparticles through a sol-gel approach. Nano Lett 2002, 2: 183–186.

31. Heinze T, Liebert T, Heublein B, Hornig S: Functional polymers based on dextran. Adv Polym Sci 2006, 205: 199–291.

32. Shen T, Weissleder R, Papisov M, Bogdanov A Jr, Brady TJ: Monocrystalline iron oxide nanocompounds (MION): physicochemical properties. Magn Reson Med 1993, 29: 599–604.

33. Arsianti M, Lim M, Lou SN, Goon IY, Marquis CP, Amal R: Bi-functional gold-coated magnetite composites with improved biocompatibility. J Colloid Interface Sci 2011, 354: 536–545.

34. Chen M, Yamamuro S, Farrell D, Majetich SA: Gold-coated iron nanoparticles for biomedical applications. J Appl Phys2003, 93: 7551–7553.

35. Sun Q, Kandalam AK, Wang Q, Jena P, Kawazoe Y, Marquez M: Effect of Au coating on the magnetic and structural properties of Fe nanoclusters for use in biomedical applications: a density-functional theory study. Phys Rev B 2006, 73: 134–409.

36. Zech CJ, Herrmann KA, Reiser MF, Schoenberg SO: MR imaging in patients with suspected liver metastases: value of liver-specific contrast agent Gd-EOB-DTPA. Magn Reson Med Sci 2007, 6: 43–52.

37. Lu ZR, Wang X, Parker DL, Goodrich KC, Buswell HR: Poly(l-glutamic acid) Gd(III)-DOTA conjugate with a degradable spacer for magnetic resonance imaging. Bioconjug Chem 2003, 14: 715–719.

38. Sherry AD, Caravan P, Lenkinski RE: Primer on gadolinium chemistry. J Magn Reson Imaging 2009, 30: 1240–1248.

39. Bellin MF, Van Der Molen AJ: Extracellular gadolinium-based contrast media: an overview. Eur J Radiol 2008, 66: 160–167.

40. Liu J-H, Wang A-Q, Chi Y-S, Lin H-P, Mou C-Y: Synergistic effect in an Au-Ag alloy nanocatalyst: CO oxidation. J Phys Chem B 2005, 109: 40–43.

41. Seo D, Yoo CI, Jung J, Song H: Ag-Au-Ag heterometallic nanorods formed through directed anisotropic growth. J Am Chem Soc 2008, 130: 2940–2941.

42. Radziuk D, Shchukin D, Moehwald H: Sonochemical design of engineered gold-silver nanoparticles. J Phys Chem C 2008, 112: 2462.

43. Kim J-H, Bryan WW, Chung H-W, Park CY, Jacobson AJ, Lee TR: Gold, palladium, and gold-palladium alloy nanoshells on silica nanoparticle cores. ACS App Math Interface 2009, 1: 1063–1069.

44. Kim J-H, Bryan WW, Lee TR: Preparation, characterization, and optical properties of gold, silver, and gold-silver alloy

nanoshells having silica cores. Langmuir 2008, 24: 11147–11152.

45. Caruntu D, Cushing BL, Caruntu G, O'Connor CJ: Attachment of gold nanograins onto colloidal magnetite nanocrystals.Chem Mater 2005, 17: 3398–3402.

46. Ettienne M, Walcarius A: Analytical investigation of the chemical reactivity and stability of aminopropyl-grafted silica in aqueous medium. Talanta 2003, 59: 1173–1188.

47. Howarter JA, Youngblood JP: Optimization of silica silanization by 3-amin-opropyltriethoxysilane. Langmuir 2006, 22: 11142–11147.

48. Daniel M-C, Astruc D: Gold nanoparticles: assembly, supramolecular chemistry, quantum-size-related properties, and applications toward biology, catalysis, and nanotechnology. Chem Rev 2004, 104: 293–346.

49. Duff DG, Baiker A, Edwards PP: A new hydrosol of gold clusters. 1. Formation and particle size variation. Langmuir 1993, 9: 2301–2309.

50. Duff DG, Baiker A, Gameson I, Edwards PP: A new hydrosol of gold clusters. 2. A comparison of some different measurement techniques. Langmuir 1993, 9: 2310–2317.

51. Powder Diffraction File-Inorganic Compounds. JCPDS International Center for Diffraction Data, Philadelphia; 1990.

52. Bernstein MA, King KF, Zhou XJ: Handbook of MRI pulse sequences. Elsevier Academic Press; 2004:1040.

53. Liu X, Wang A, Yang X, Zhang T, Mou C-Y, Su D-S, Li J: Synthesis of thermally stable and highly active bimetallic au-ag nanoparticles on inert supports. Chem Mater 2009, 21: 410–418.

54. De Silva CR, Smith S, Shim I, Pyun J, Gutu T, Jiao J, Zheng Z: Lanthanide(III)-doped magnetite nanoparticles. J Am Chem Soc 2009, 131: 6336–6337.

55. Bartos A, Lieb KP, Uhrmacher M, Wiarda D: Golden book of phase transitions. 2002, 1: 123.

56. Montoro V: Miscibilita fra gli ossidi salini di ferro e di manganese. Gaz Chim Ital 1938, 68: 728–733.

57. Kim TY, Lee MS, Kim YI, Lee C-S, Park JC, Kim D: The enhanced anisotropic properties of the Fe 3-x M x O 4 (M = Fe, Co, Mn) films deposited on glass surface from aqueous solutions at low temperature. J Phys D Appl Phys 2003, 36: 1451–1457.

58. Cullity BD: Elements of X-Ray Diffraction. Addison-Wesley Publishing Company; 1967.

59. Couderc JJ, Garigue G, Lafourcade L, Nguyen QT: Standard X-ray diffraction powder patterns. Zeitschrift für Metallkunde1959, 50: 708–716.

60. Swanson HE, Tatge E: Standard X-Ray Diffraction Powder Patterns. Volume 539. USA: National Bureau of Standards; 1953:26–27.

61. Wang AQ, Liu JH, Liu SD, Lin TS, Mou CY: A novel efficient Au-Ag alloy catalyst system: preparation, activity, and characterization. J Catal 2005, 233: 186–197.

62. Wang L, Luo J, Fan Q, Suzuki M, Suzuki IS, Engelhard MH, Lin Y, Kim N, Wang JQ, Zhong C-J: Monodispersed core-shell Fe 3 O 4 @Au nanoparticles. J Phys Chem B 2005, 109: 21593–21601.

63. Mikhaylova M, Kim DK, Bobrysheva N, Osmolowsky M, Semenov V, Tsakalatos T, Muhammed M: Superparamagnetism of magnetite nanoparticles: dependence on surface modification. Langmuir 2004, 20: 2472–2477.

64. Levin CS, Hofmann C, Ali TA, Kelly AT, Morosan E, Nordlander P, Whitmire KH, Halas NJ: Magnetic-plasmonic core-shell nanoparticles. ACS Nano 2009, 3: 1379–1388.

65. Ma LL, Feldman MD, Tam JM, Paranjape AS, Cheruku KK, Larson TA, Tam JO, Ingram DR, Paramita V, Villard JW, Jenkins JT, Wang T, Clarke GD, Asmis R, Sokolov K, Chandrasekar B, Milner TE, Johnston KP: Small multifunctional nanoclusters (nanoroses) for targeted cellular imaging and therapy. ACS Nano 2009, 3: 2686–2696.

66. Graf C, van Blaaderen A: Metallodielectric colloidal core-shell particles for photonic applications. Langmuir 2002, 18: 524–534.

67. Link S, Wang ZL, El-Sayed MA: Alloy formation of gold-silver nanoparticles and the dependence of the plasmon absorption on their composition. J Phys Chem B 1999, 103: 3529–3533.

68. Oldenburg SJ, Averitt RD, Westcott SL, Halas NJ: Nanoengineering of optical resonances. Chem Phys Lett 1998, 288: 243–147.

69. Zhou L, Yu X-F, Fu X-F, Hao Z-H, Li K-Y: Surface plasmon resonance and field enhancement of au/ag alloyed hollow nanoshells. Chin Phys Lett 2008, 25: 1776.

70. Gellner M, Kuestner B, Schluecker S: Optical properties and SERS efficiency of tunable gold/silver nanoshells. Vibrat Spectros 2009, 50: 43.

71. Hovel H, Fritz S, Hilger A, Kreibig U: Width of cluster plasmon resonances: bulk dielectric functions and chemical interface damping. Phys Rev B 1993, 48: 18178–18188.

72. Averitt RD, Westcott SL, Halas NJ: The linear optical properties of gold nanoshells. J Opt Soc Am B 1999, 16: 1824–1832.

73. Rasch MR, Sokolov KV, Korgel BA: Limitations on the optical tunability of small diameter gold nanoshells. Langmuir 2009, 25: 11777–11785.

74. Schwartzberg AM, Olson TY, Talley CE, Zhang JZ: Synthesis, characterization, and tunable optical properties of hollow gold nanospheres. J Phys Chem B 2006, 110: 19935–19944.

75. Kim Y-Il, Im WB, Jeon MK, Lee Y-H, Kim K-B, Ryu K-S: Preferential site of Gd in Gd-doped Fe 3 O 4 nanopowder. J Nanosci Nanotechnol 2011, 11: 810–814.

76. Furmanski P, Longley C: Metalloporphrin enhancement of magnetic resonance imaging of human tumor xenographs in nude mice. Cancer Res 1988, 48: 4604–4610.

77. Shu C, Crowin FD, Zhang J, Chen Z, Reid JE, Sun M, Xu W, Sim JH, Wang C, Fatouros PP, Esker AR, Gibson HW, Dorn HC: Facile preparation of a new gadofullerene-based magnetic resonance imaging contrast agent with high 1 H relaxivity.Bioconjugate Chem 2009, 20: 1186–1193.

78. Mulvaney P, Giersig M, Henglein A: Surface chemistry of colloidal gold: deposition of lead and accompanying optical effects. J Phys Chem 1992, 96: 10419–10424.

Chapter 9

Green Synthesis of Gold Nanoparticles and Their Anticancer Activity

Ravi Geetha[1], Thirunavukkarasu Ashokkumar[1], Selvaraj Tamilselvan[1], Kasivelu Govindaraju[2], Mohamed Sadiq[3] & Ganesan Singaravelu[1]

[1]*Nanoscience Division, Department of Zoology, Thiruvalluvar University, Vellore 632 115, India*

[2]*Centre for Ocean Research, Sathyabama University, Chennai 600 119, India*

[3]*Department of Biochemistry, Adhiparasakthi College of Arts and Science, Kalavai, Tamilnadu, India*

ABSTRACT

As the nano revolution unfolds, it is imperative to integrate nanoscience and medicine. The secret gleaned from nature have led to the generation of biogenic technologies for the fabrication of advanced nanomaterials. Present investigation discloses the gold nanoparticles biosynthesizing capability of the flower of pharmacologically important tree *Couroupita guianensis*. Rapid, cost-effective, one-step process of synthesis has been achieved. Newly genre gold nanoparticles were characterized by involving UV–vis spectroscopy, FTIR, XRD, SEM, and TEM analysis. Interestingly, as a result of extensive screening on the application of newly synthesized gold nanoparticles their anticancer potential has been discovered using MTT assay, DNA fragmentation, apoptosis by DAPI staining, and comet assay for DNA damage.

Keywords: *Couroupita guianensis* Gold nanoparticles Anticancer DNA fragmentation

1 INTRODUCTION

Metal nanoparticles are of great importance due to their high surface area and a high fraction of surface atoms. The scientific and technological significance of metal nanoparticles has made them the subject of intensive research, given their special chemical and physical properties. In particular, gold nanoparticles are employed in many fields: biosensing (Mirkin et al. 1996), catalysis (Sen et al. 2012), electronics (Rao and Cheetham 2001), enzyme electrodes (Crumbliss et al. 1992), super conductors (Sun and Xia 2002), and cancer therapy (El-Sayed et al. 2006) among others.

Presently, biological nanoscience has drawn increasing attention due to its avant-garde nature and the efficacy of produced nanoparticles in industrial, biomedical, and electronic applications such as catalyst (Hashmi and Hutchings 2006), cancer detection (Huang et al. 2007b), and bioimaging (Wu et al. 2006). Among the loads of metal nanoparticles, gold nanoparticles have an especially wide application in DNA recognition, heredity medicine, and nano-catalysis. It has been pointed out that the divergent capabilities of these nanoparticles are controlled by their size (Alivisatos 1996; Jin et al. 2001; Aizpurua et al. 2003).

Numerous methodologies are developed to synthesize noble metal nanoparticles of particular shape and size depending on specific requirements. Biosynthesis of nanoparticles has an emerging highlight of the intersection of nanotechnology and biotechnology which has received increased attention to a growing need to develop environmentally benign technologies in material syntheses. Biomolecules as reductants are found to have significant advantage over chemical reductants due to their non biocompatible nature (Huang et al. 2007a).

In the present cram, a simple biosynthetic method using flower extract of *Couroupita guianensis* is addressed herein for synthesizing gold nanoparticles. The newly synthesized gold nanoparticles were characterized by employing standard technologies. The plant *C.*

guianensis, commonly known as cannon ball tree, has innumerable medicinal applications including antibiotic, antiseptic, anti-inflammatory activity (Geetha et al. 2004). Indeed, it is expected that gold nanoparticles synthesized using the flower of the tree *C. guianensis* might have medicinal properties. Accordingly, efforts are made to identify the newly generated gold nanoparticles' medicinal value. As a result, their antileukemic cancer activity has been explored. Cancer is the leading cause of death worldwide after cardiovascular diseases (Garrett and Workman 1999). Leukemia is a major type of cancer affecting a significant segment of the population, especially children. In fact, leukemia is the most frequent childhood cancer, with 26 % of all cases, and 30 % mortality (Canadian Cancer Society 2005). Clinical trials in identifying new agents and treatment modalities has been studied and achieved. However, current treatments have many limitations related to their side effects and the development of acquired drug resistance (Robert and Jarry 2003). Thus, the new therapeutic agents needed should be more active and produce fewer side effects and they also should act through a mechanism different from that of cytotoxic agents already used.

2 MATERIALS AND METHODS

2.1 Preparation of flower extract

Fresh flowers of *C. guianensis* were collected, washed thoroughly with double distilled water, air dried, and powdered. About 1 g of powdered flower was transferred into a 100-mL beaker containing 50 mL double distilled water and mixed well. The extract obtained was filtered through Whatmann no. 1 filter paper and the filtrate was collected in a separate flask.

2.2 Synthesis of gold nanoparticles using plant extract

One hundred milliliter solution of 1 mM chloroauric acid at concentration of 10^{-3} M was prepared by dissolving in double distilled water. Different reaction concentrations of *C. guianensis* extract and $HAuCl_4$ solution (1:9, 2:8, 3:7, 4:6, and 5:5) were subjected, respectively. The reduction of gold ions to gold nanoparticles was completed within

5 min. The pale yellow color solution turns to ruby red color indicating the formation of gold nanoparticles. The reduction of metal ions was continuously monitored by visual inspection as well as by measuring with UV–visible spectrometer in the wavelength range 300–800 nm.

2.3 Characterization of gold nanoparticles

UV–visible spectrum was recorded as a function of the reaction time on a Techomp (UV 2300) double beam spectrophotometer.

For FTIR measurements, the newly synthesized gold nanoparticles were centrifuged at 8,000 rpm for 10 min and the resulting suspension was redispersed in distilled water. The purified pellets were dried and smirk with KBr pellets and analyzed by Thermo Nicolet Quator instrument in the diffuse reflectance mode operating at a resolution of 4 cm^{-1}.

XRD measurements of the *C. guianensis*-synthesized gold nanoparticles solution drop coated on to glass substrates was done on a Siefert X-ray diffractometer, operated at a voltage of 40 kV and tube current of 30 mA with Cu-Kα radiation. Surface morphology of newly formed gold nanoparticles was determined using scanning electron microscope (FEI Quanta 200 SEM).

For TEM studies, newly synthesized gold nanoparticles were prepared by placing a drop of nanoparticle solution on carbon-coated copper grids and allowing water to evaporate. TEM measurements were performed on JEOL 3010 UHR TEM equipped with a Gatan Imaging Filter.

2.3.1 Assessment of cell morphology

HL-60 cells were cultured in 24-well plates and incubated at 37 °C for 24 h before each well were individually treated with 0, 60, 90, 120, 150, and 180 µg/mL gold nanoparticles for 48 h. Determination of cell morphology was made using a phase contrast microscope (Lu et al. 2010).

2.3.2 DAPI staining for apoptosis

Cells in 12-well plates were treated with or without 0, 80, 120, 180, and 200 μg/mL gold nanoparticles for 48 h. Cells were then stained by using 4,6-diamidino-2-phenylindole dihydrochloride (DAPI) (Chen et al. 2009a).

2.3.3 Comet assay for DNA damage

Cells in 96-well plates were treated with or without 0, 60, 90, 120, 150, and 180 μg/mL gold nanoparticles for 48 h. Cells were then harvested and DNA damage was determined with the Comet assay (Chen et al. 2009b).

2.3.4 DNA gel electrophoresis for DNA fragmentation

Cells in six-well plates were incubated with 0 and 150 μg/mL gold nanoparticles 48 h. Cells were harvested by centrifugation and DNA was isolated before DNA fragmentation was determined by DNA gel electrophoresis (Lu et al. 2010).

2.3.5 Effect of gold nanoparticles on cytotoxicity

HL-60 cells were obtained from the NCCS, Pune, India, and grown in RPMI1640 medium and supplemented with a 2 mg mL^{-1} sodium bicarbonate, 4.5 mg mL^{-1} glucose, 100 μg mL^{-1} streptomycin sulfate, 40 μg mL^{-1} gentamycin, 100 U mL^{-1} penicillin as well as 10 % heat-inactivated fetal calf serum. An environment of humidified air containing 5 % CO_2 was maintained at 37 °C. Peripheral blood mononuclear cells (PBMC) were obtained from healthy donors and cultured as described. Effects of gold nanoparticles on the proliferation of cells was determined by MTT [3-(4, 5-dimethyl thiazoyl-2-yl)-(2,5-diphenyltetrazolium bromide)] assay. Briefly, the cells were suspended at 3×10^5 Cell mL^{-1}. The cells were placed in 96-well microtiter plates (200 μl $well^{-1}$) and incubated at 37 °C in a CO_2 incubator in the presence of the gold nanoparticles. After 5 days, cell viability was measured by

MTT assay, from which cytotoxic concentration (CC_{50}) was calculated (Premnathan et al. 1996).

3 RESULTS AND DISCUSSION

Design and development of nanomaterials with unusual physico-chemical and optoelectronic features is a corner stone in nanoscience. Present report discloses the bioreduction property of gold ions into gold nanoparticles by ethnopharmacologically important *C. guianensis* flower's extract. Synthesis of gold nanoparticles has been achieved in 5 min of reaction without any experimental protocols like stirring, heating, change in pH. Reduction and capping of newly formed gold nanoparticles was achieved with the flower extract of *C. guianensis*. As a result of extensive screening with different concentrations of auric chloride and flower extract, synthesis was successful with the concentration of 2:8 (2 mL of flower extract and 8 mL of auric chloride). Figure 1 shows the UV–vis spectra of the newly formed gold nanoparticles and the characteristic SPR band occurs at ca. 534 and at 5 min that attained the maximum intensity.

Fourier transform infrared (FTIR) was made in order to identify the possible biomolecules responsible for the reduction of gold ions and capping of the bioreduced gold nanoparticles (Fig. 2 a and b). FTIR spectrum of the aqueous extract of *C. guianensis* (curve a) showed peaks at 3,414 (O–H stretch, H–bonded of alcohols/phenols), 2,133 (–C (triple bond) C– stretch of alkynes), 1,648 (–C=C– stretch of alkynes), 1,383 (C–N stretching vibration of aliphatic amines), 1,288 (C–O stretch of alcohols), and 1,073 cm^{-1} (C–N stretching vibration of aliphatic amines or alcohols/phenols). The intense broad absorbance at 3,414 cm^{-1} is characteristic of the hydroxyl functional group in alcohols and phenolic compounds. The FTIR spectrum of the gold nanoparticles (curve b) showed peaks at 3,615 and 3,547 (O–H stretch, H–bonded of alcohols/phenols), 2,924 and 2,855 (C–H stretch), 2,402 and 2,129 (–C (triple bond) C– stretch of alkynes), 1,744 (C=O stretch of carboxylic acids), 1,378 (C–N stretching vibration of aliphatic amines), and 1,071 cm^{-1} (C–N stretching vibration of aliphatic amines or to

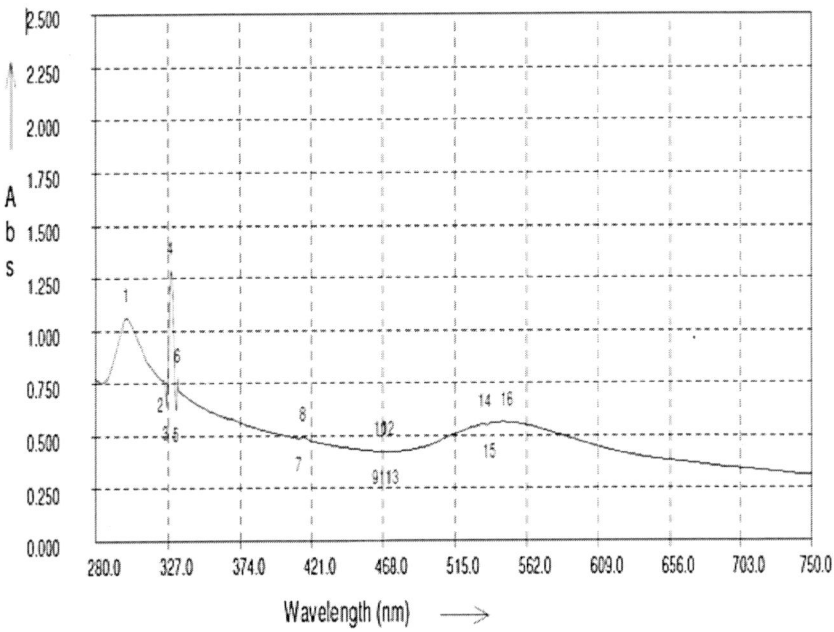

Figure 1. UV–visible absorption spectrum of biosynthesized gold nanoparticles by *Couroupita guianensis* flower extract

alcohols/phenols). Comparing both FTIR spectra it can be identified that the changes in the –COOH group for –OH, i.e., hydroxyl group the peak appeared at 3,414 cm^{-1} in raw material, but after encapsulation of nanoparticles, the peak is narrower and shifted to 3,615 cm^{-1} and also for –C– of carboxylic group the peak intensity reduced after encapsulation of nanoparticles. The peaks at 1,648, 1,383, 1,288, and 1,073 cm^{-1} are reduced and the new peak appeared at 1,744 cm^{-1} which indicates the alcoholic group is converted into aldehyde to reduce Au^{3+} to Au^{0}.

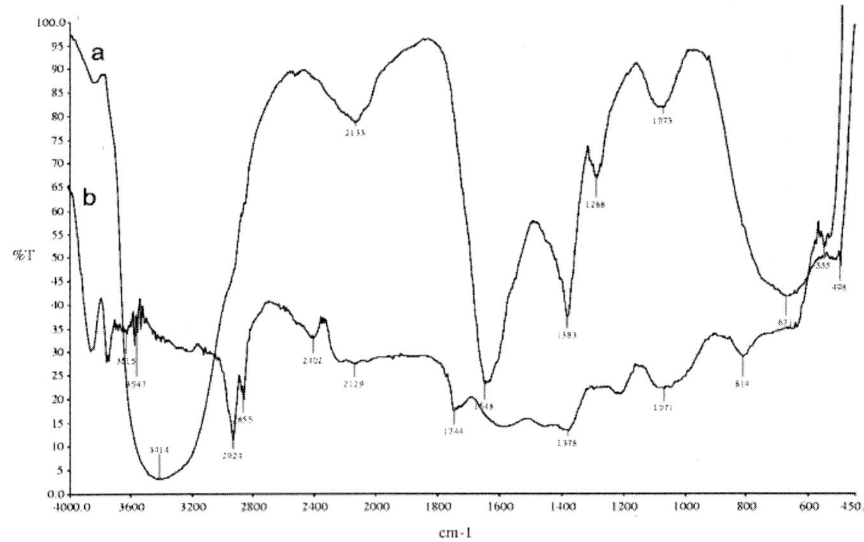

Figure 2. FTIR spectra of **a** *C. guianensis* flower extract, **b** gold nanoparticles synthesized by *C. guianensis* flower extract

A structural analysis of gold nanoparticles prepared from the sample was performed by XRD. Taking into account the angular positions of the Bragg peaks (Fig. 3), a face-centered cubic structure was assigned to the gold nanoparticles. The XRD pattern thus clearly illustrates that the gold nanoparticles synthesized by *C. guianensis* are crystalline in nature.

Figure 4 shows the SEM images of the newly synthesized gold nanoparticles. It was observed that the surface morphology of gold nanoparticles synthesized from flower extract of *C. guianensis* solution clearly indicates that they are in different shapes and well dispersed.

The TEM images confirm the formation of gold nanoparticles and it has been observed that the newly formed nanoparticles are polydispersed consisting of spherical, triangular, tetragonal and pentagonal with irregular contours. The size distribution of gold nanoparticles diameter is located between 7 and 48 nm (Fig. 5). Generation of metal nanoparticles mainly relies on the use of lethal reducing agents. For the development of biocompatible nanoparticles, various biomimetic approaches are being explored. Indeed, a discovery on the application of nanoparticles in medical sciences is exciting which is continually

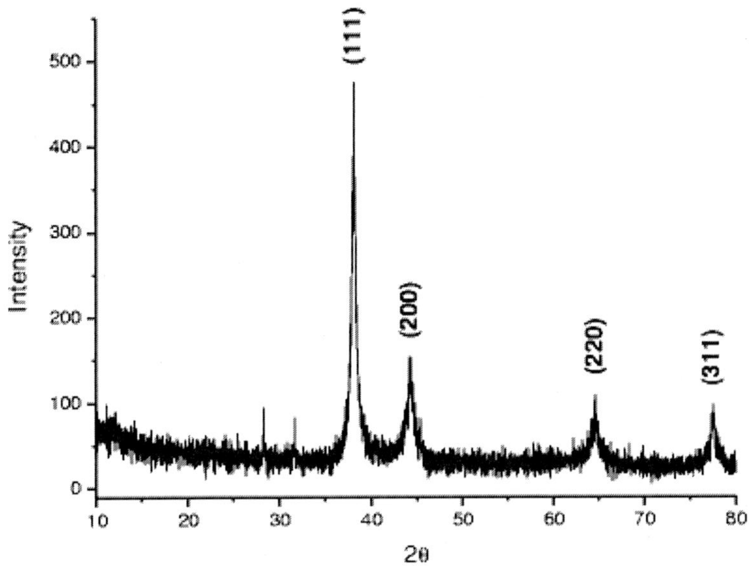

Figure 3. XRD pattern of gold nanoparticles synthesized using *C. Guianensis*

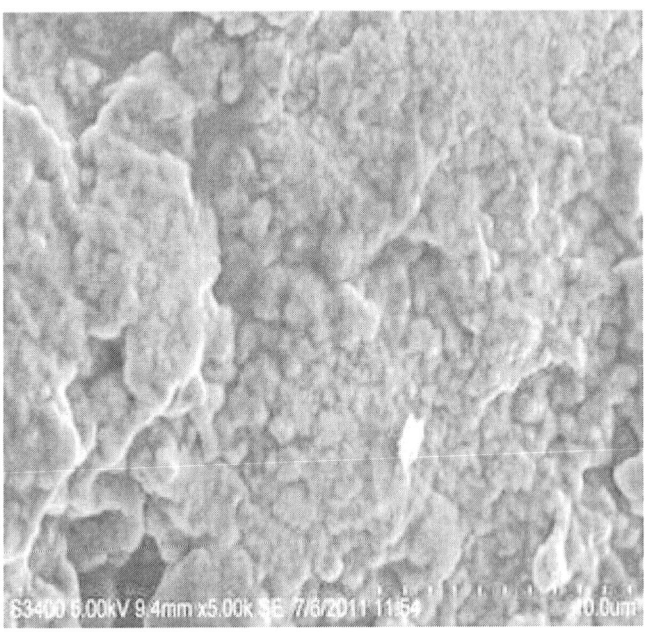

Figure 4. SEM photograph of *C. guianensis* synthesized gold nanoparticles

strengthened by the ever-widening spectrum. This necessitates the need of biologically benign nanoparticles. Biological methods may provide an alternate to the conventional techniques, with emphasis on the production of environmentally benign nanoparticles. However, the limitations such as change in pH and incubation are accountable in the large-scale production. Greener technology on the synthesis of nanoparticles deserves merit to overcome the drawbacks of microbial synthesis of nanoparticles. The result addressed herein is on the biological synthesis of gold nanoparticles using medicinally important tree *C. guianensis* flower extract.

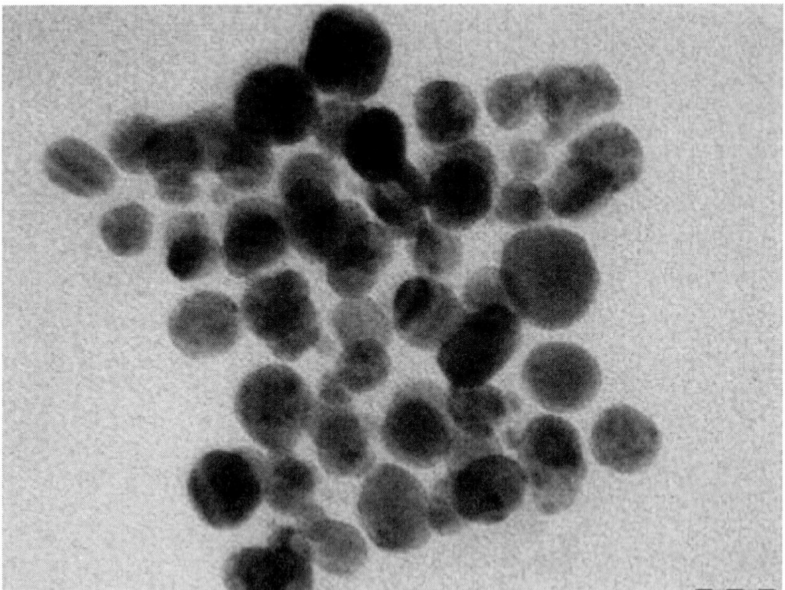

Figure 5. TEM Micrograph of *C. guianensis* synthesized gold nanoparticles

There are reports on the plant-mediated synthesis of gold nanoparticles. Ghoreshi and co-workers (2011) reported on the synthesis of gold nanoparticles using the flower extract of *Rosa damascene*. Studies also demonstrate that the flavanoids and polyphenols of the flower are responsible for the formation of quasi-spherical nanoparticles. Philip (2010) demonstrated *Hibiscus rosa sinensis*-mediated synthesis of gold nanoparticles and it has been reported that carboxylic group of malic acid may be the active principle for the reduction and capping of gold nanoparticles. *Cinnamomum zeylanicum*-mediated synthesis of gold nanoparticles have been reported and possibly the amines of proteins bound the newly formed nanoparticles (Smitha et al. 2009). It has been illustrated that flavanoids of the plant *Syzygium aromaticum* found to have the property of synthesizing irregular-shaped nanoparticles (Deshpande et al. 2010). Pioneering works on nanoparticles synthesis using plant extracts have been carried out by Sastry and co-workers using geranium leaves, neem, *Aloe vera*, and lemon grass are extensively studied (Ankamwar et al. 2005; Shankar et al. 2004; Chandran et al. 2006; Shankar et al. 2005). Singaravelu and co-workers (Singaravelu et al. 2007, Govindaraju et al. 2008, Khaleel et al. 2010) reported on the biological synthesis of gold and silver nanoparticles using *Sargassum wightii*, *Spirulina platensis*, *Psidium guajava* as green chemistry approach.

Foregoing facts discloses that phytochemicals in the synthesis of nanoparticles is an important symbiosis between nanoscience and green chemistry. As a result of our extensive screening on identifying the newly formed gold nanoparticles application, anti leukemic cancer activity has been explored. HL-60 cells were treated with various concentrations of gold nanoparticles for different time-periods. The results shown in Fig. 6a and b indicate the nuclear morphology of dying HL-60 cells due to gold nanoparticles treatment and these effects were dose-dependent. Figure 7a and b indicates that gold nanoparticles induced apoptosis in HL-60 cells, and the results showed less cell number compared to control. Gold nanoparticles induced apoptosis which was consistent with data showing that DNA fragmentation occurred as seen in Fig. 8a and b. Concentrations of gold nanoparticles led to a longer tail (DNA damage), further supporting the fact that gold nanoparticles induced apoptosis in HL-60 cells and data in Fig. 9 show DNA gel electrophoresis of DNA fragmentation which was enhanced with increasing exposure to gold nanoparticles.

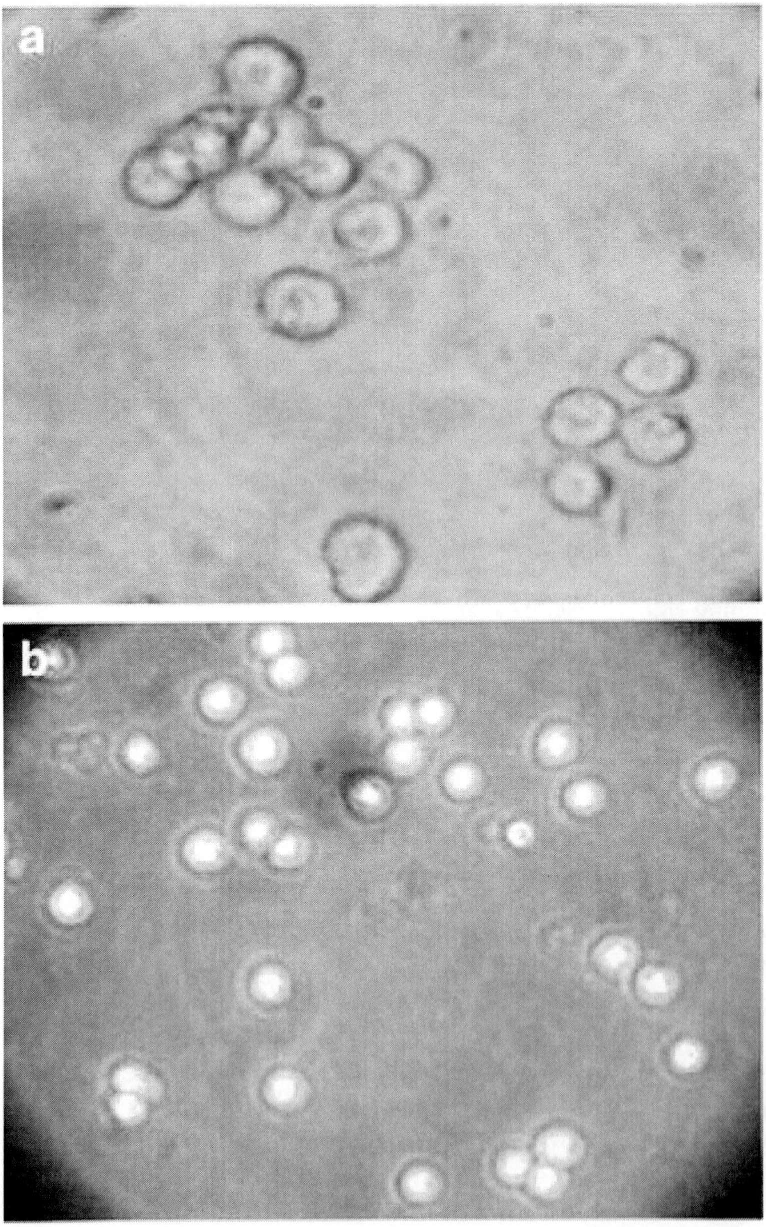

Figure 6. Morphological analysis of HL-60 cells **a** control and **b** *C. guianensis* synthesized gold nanoparticles treated with HL-60 cells

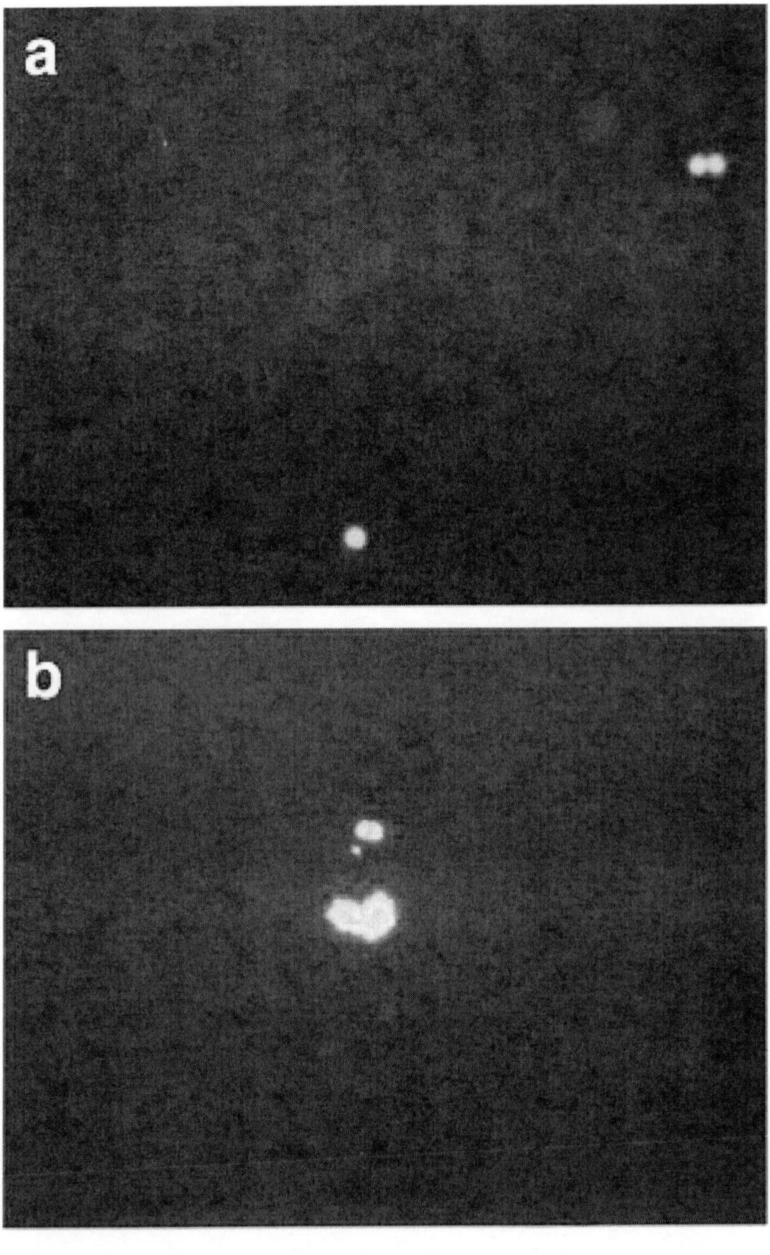

Figure 7. a Control and **b** gold nanoparticles induced apoptosis

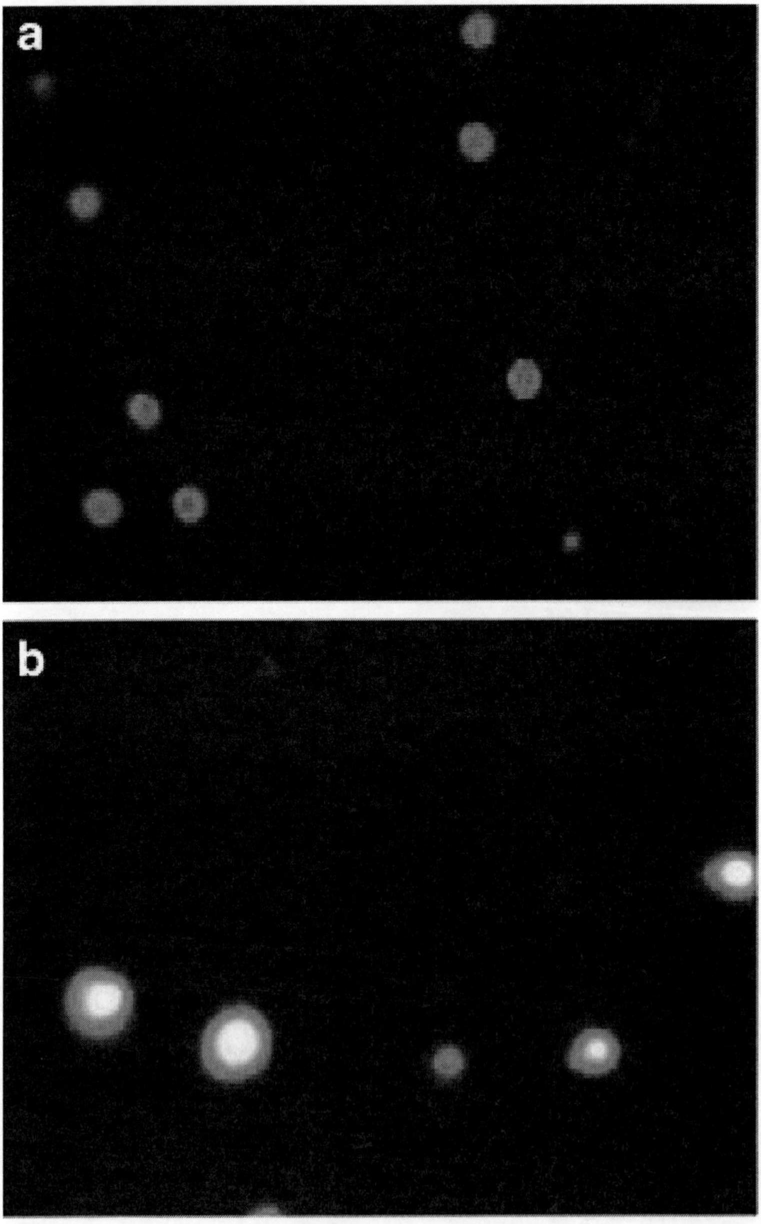

Figure 8. a Control and **b** assessment of DNA damage by comet assay

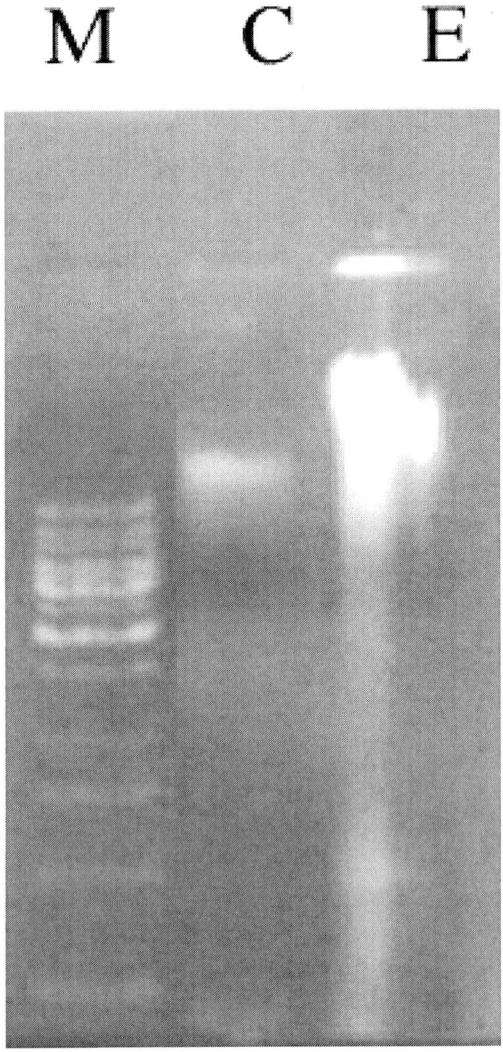

Figure 9. DNA fragmentation analysis using agarose gel electrophoresis. *Lane 1*: marker; *Lane 2*: control (HL-60); *Lane 3*: *C. guianensis*-synthesized gold nanoparticles treated with HL-60 cells

Cell viability determination was made using MTT assay which was conducted for 120 h. *C. guianensis* flower extract-synthesized gold nanoparticles caused a significant cytotoxicity in HL-60 cells in a concentration-dependent manner with the CC_{50} value of 5.14 µM whereas for PBMC it is 113.25 µM (Fig. 10).

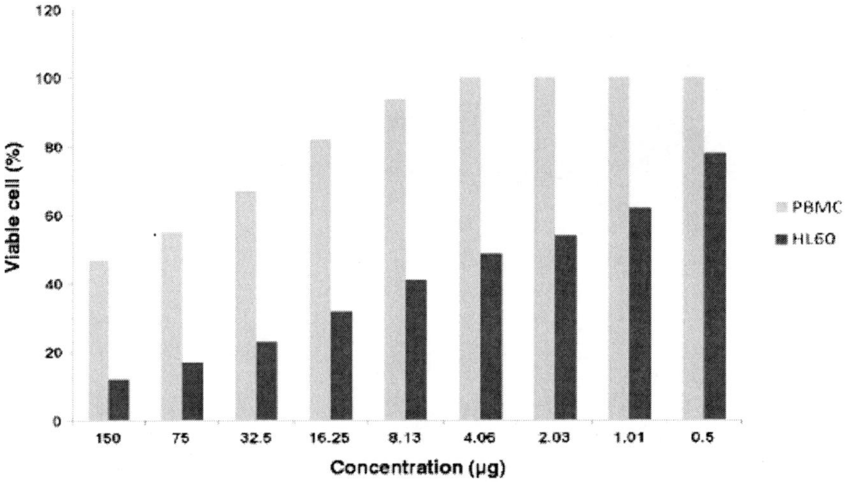

Figure 10. Differential cytotoxic effects of *C. guianensis*-synthesized gold nanoparticles on cancerous HL60 cells and PBMC from a representative experiment is presented, $n = 3$

Despite the widespread use of gold nanoparticles, there are only few studies to determine the cytotoxic effects of biologically synthesized gold nanoparticles, particularly in the context of apoptosis. MTT assay was used to appraise the effect of gold nanoparticles on proliferation of HL-60 cells. This is the first study to evaluate *C. guianensis*-based gold nanoparticles' cytotoxicity against cancer cell lines. Thus we hypothesize that cell killing could be the possible mechanism induced by the cytotoxic effect of biosynthesized gold nanoparticles.

Nanotechnology has attracted a great interest in recent years due to its expected impact on many areas such as energy, medicine, and electronics. The development of new materials with nanometer size including nanoparticles, nanotubes, nanowires, etc., is the major activity. Among all, nanoparticles with the unique properties in chemistry, optics, electronics, and magnetics have led to an increasing interest in their synthesis.

Much of the existing research in the development of anticancer therapeutics from the plants has been focused on investigating the molecular mechanism by which an agent induces cytotoxicity and apoptosis in cancer cells. This study provides valuable insight in developing nanotherapeutics against dreadful cancer.

Investigation suggests that ethnopharmacological approach on the production of gold nanoparticles will greatly facilitate on the creation of an important symbiosis between nanoscience and medical science.

4 CONCLUSIONS

The results addressed herein disclose anticancer activity of gold nanoparticles synthesized using aqueous flower extract of *C. guianensis*. It is reasonable to infer that the pharmacological properties of *C. guianensis* provide the anticancer activity of newly formed gold nanoparticles. Interestingly, it has been demonstrated that the functionalization of gold nanoparticles as anticancer nanomaterial has been achieved without doping of molecules.

ACKNOWLEDGMENT

G.S and R.G thank the INSPIRE—Department of Science and Technology, New Delhi, for financial assistance.

REFERENCES

1. Aizpurua J, Hanarp P, Sutherland DS, Kall M, Bryant GW, Garcia de Abajo FJ (2003) Optical properties of gold nanorings. Phys Rev Lett 90:057401-1–057401-4

2. Alivisatos AP (1996) Perspectives on the physical chemistry of semiconductor nanocrystals. J Phys Chem 100:13226–13239

3. Ankamwar B, Chaudhary M, Sastry M (2005) Gold nanotriangles biologically synthesized using tamarind leaf extract and potential application in vapor sensing. Synth React Inorg Met Org Nano Metal Chem 35:19–26

4. Canadian Cancer Society–National Cancer Institute of Canada (2005) Canadian Cancer Statistics 2005, Toronto, Canada, April, ISSN: 0835–2976

5. Chandran SP, Chaudhary M, Pasricha R, Ahmad A, Sastry M (2006) Synthesis of gold nanotriangles and silver nanoparticles using Aloe vera plant extract. Biotechnol Prog 22:577–583

6. Chen JC, Lu KW, Lee JH, Yeh CC, Chung JG (2009a) Gypenosides induced apoptosis in human colon cancer cells through the mitochondria-dependent pathways and activation of caspase-3. Anticancer Res 26:4313–4326

7. Chen JC, Lu KW, Tsai ML, Hsu SC, Kuo CL, Yang JS, Hsia TC, Yu CS, Chou ST, Kao MC, Chung JG, Wood WG (2009b) Gypenosides induced G0/G1 arrest via CHk2 and apoptosis through endoplasmic reticulum stress and mitochondria-dependent pathways in human tongue cancer SCC-4 cells. Oral Oncol 45:273–283

8. Crumbliss AL, Perine SC, Stonehuerner J, Tubergen KR, Zhao J, Henkens RW, O'Daly JP (1992) Colloidal gold as biocompatible immobilization matrix suitable for the fabrication of enzyme electrodes by electrodeposition. Biotechnol Bioeng 40:483–490

9. Deshpande R, Bedre MD, Basavaraja S, Sawle B, Manjunath SY, Venkataraman A (2010) Rapid biosynthesis of irregular shaped gold nanoparticles from maccrated aqueous extracellular dried clove buds (Sygyium aromaticum) solution. Colloids Surf B: Biointerfaces 79:235–240

10. El-Sayed IH, Huang X, El-Sayed MA (2006) Selective laser photo-thermal therapy of epithelial carcinoma using anti-EGFR antibody conjugated gold nanoparticles. Cancer Lett 239(1):129–135

11. Garrett MD, Workman P (1999) Discovering novel chemotherapeutic drugs for the third millennium. Eur J Cancer 35(14):2010–2030

12. Geetha M, Saluja AK, Shankar MB, Mehta RS (2004) Analgesic and anti inflammatory activity of Couroupita guianensis Aubl. J Natural Remedies 4(1):52–55

13. Ghoreishi SM, Behpour M, Khayatkashni M (2011) Green synthesis of silver and gold nanoparticles using Rosa

damasceneand its primary application in electrochemistry. Physica E 44:97–104

14. Govindaraju K, Khaleel Basha S, Ganesh Kumar VG, Singaravelu G (2008) Silver, gold and bimetallic nanoparticles production using single-cell protein (Spirulina platensis) Geitler. J Mater Sci 43:5115–5123

15. Hashmi ASK, Hutchings GJ (2006) Gold catalysis. Angew Chem Int Ed 45:7896–7936

16. Huang J, Li Q, Sun D, Lu Y, Su Y, Yang X, Wang H, Shao W, He N, Hong J, Chen C (2007a) Biosynthesis of silver and gold nanoparticles by using novel sun-dried Cinnamomum camphora leaves. Nanotechnol 18:105104–105114

17. Huang XH, Jain PK, El-Sayed IH, El-Sayed MA (2007b) Gold nanoparticles: interesting optical properties and recent applications in cancer diagnostic and therapy. Nanomedicine 2:681–693

18. Jin RC, Cao YW, Mirkin CA, Kelly KL, Schatz GC, Zheng JG (2001) Photoinduced conversion of silver nanospheres to nanoprisms. Science 294:1901–1903

19. Khaleel Basha S, Govindaraju K, Manikandan R, Ahn J, Bae EY, Singaravelu G (2010) Phytochemical mediated gold nanoparticles and their PTP 1B inhibitory activity. Colloids Surf B: Biointerfaces 75:405–409

20. Lu HF, Lai TY, Hsia TC, Tang YJ, Yang JS, Chiang JH, Lu CC, Liu CM, Wang HL, Chung JG (2010) Danthron induces DNA damage and inhibits DNA repair gene expressions in GBM 8401 human brain glioblastoma multiforms cells. Neurochem Res 35:1105–1110

21. Mirkin CA, Letsinger RL, Mucic RC, Storhoff JJA (1996) DNA-based method for rationally assembling nanoparticles into macroscopic materials. Nature 382:607–609

22. Philip D (2010) Green synthesis of gold and silver nanoparticles using Hibiscus rosa sinensis. Physica E 42:1417–1424

23. Premnathan M, Nakashima H, Kathiresan K, Rajendran N, Yamamoto N (1996) In vitro anti human immunodeficiency virus activity of mangrove plants. Ind J Med Res 103:278–281

24. Rao CNR, Cheetham AK (2001) Science and technology of nanomaterials: current state and future prospects. J Mater Chem. 11:2887–2894

25. Robert J, Jarry C (2003) Multidrug resistance reversal agents. J Med Chem 46(23):4805–4817

26. Sen IK, Maity K, Islam SS (2012) Green synthesis of gold nanoparticles using a glucan of an edible mushroom and study of catalytic activity. Carbohydrate Polymer. doi:10.1016/j.carbpol.08.058

27. Shankar SS, Rai A, Ahmed A, Sastry M (2005) Controlling the optical properties of lemon grass extract synthesized gold nanotriangles and potential application in infrared-absorbing optical coatings. Chem Mater 17:566–572

28. Shankar S, Rai A, Ahmed A, Sastry M (2004) Rapid synthesis of Au, Ag, and bimetallic Au core-Ag shell nanoparticles using Neem (Azadirachta indica) leaf broth. J Colloid Interf Sci 275:496–502

29. Singaravelu G, Arockiyamari J, Ganesh Kumar V, Govindaraju K (2007) A novel extracellular synthesis of monodisperse gold nanoparticles using marine alga Sargassum wightii Greville. Colloids Surfaces B: Biointerf 57:97–101

30. Smitha SL, Philip D, Gopchandran KG (2009) Green synthesis of gold nanoparticles using Cinnamom zeylanicum leaf broth. Spectrochim Acta, Part A Mol Biomol Spec 74:735–739

31. Sun Y, Xia Y (2002) shape-controlled synthesis of gold and silver nanoparticles. Science 298:2176–2179

32. Wu YL, Li YN, Liu P, Gardner S, Ong BS (2006) Studies of gold nanoparticles as precursors to printed conductive features for thin-film transistors. Chem Mater 18:4627–4632

Chapter 10

Preparation and Characterization of Biocompatible Polymer Particles as Potential Nanocarriers for Inhalation Therapy

Katarzyna Jabłczyńska, Magdalena Janczewska, Aleksandra Kulikowska, andTomasz R. Sosnowski

Faculty of Chemical and Process Engineering, Warsaw University of Technology, Waryńskiego 1, 00-645 Warsaw, Poland

ABSTRACT

Aim. Investigation of the possibility of manufacturing biocompatible polymer particles which have the required properties for pulmonary delivery via inhalation and simultaneously act as vehicles of nanotherapeutics.Methods. Nanostructures were obtained from biocompatible polysaccharides by successive oxidation and reactive coiling in the aqueous phase. The resultant nanosuspensions of PAD (polyaldehyde dextran) and DACMC (dialdehyde carbomethylcellulose) were used as precursors in spray drying production of powders at variable process conditions. The resultant dry microparticles were characterized by SEM observations, and their properties related to delivery by inhalation were determined by laser diffraction spectrometry following the dispersion in the commercial inhaler. Finally, the possibility of the reconstitution of nanosuspensions by powders rehydration was evaluated. Results. Synthesized nanoparticles had size of 120–170 nm. Microparticles after drying had size of 0.5–5 µm and different surface morphology. Aerosolized particles obtained from powder dispersion in the inhaler had the volumetric median diameter of ~2 and ~1 μm for PAD and DACMC, respectively. Hydration of powders led to restoring the nanosuspensions with the average particle size similar to the precursor. Conclusions. PAD and DACMC can be used to obtain nanostructures which, after processing, take a form suitable for effective delivery to the lungs via inhalation.

1. INTRODUCTION

Biocompatible and biodegradable polymeric particles are widely used as drug carriers [1–4]. Encapsulation of drug in polymer particles allows for prolonged release of medicines in the target area which means that drugs become available directly in the desired site (so they do not cause side effects) and their activity is extended in time. Typically, drug release is achieved due to polymer swelling or erosion [5]. In addition, the release rate can be "tuned" using the responsive systems; that is, it can be triggered by pH, temperature, radiation, magnetic field, and so forth [6, 7]. In such cases polymer-based carriers become the specialized and effective tool of medical treatment. Simultaneously, the controlled release allows minimizing local toxic effects of potent drugs [4].

Nanoparticles gained a lot of interest as potential vehicles of therapeutics because of several unique and beneficial features. Owing to the small area for opsonin binding, they are capable of avoiding the phagocytosis so the drug bioavailability is increased as compared to larger carriers [5]. Simultaneously, the size of nanoparticles makes them suitable to penetrate to the tumors via more leaky walls of the blood vessels (so called, EPR effect) and for this reason they are preferable carriers of anticancer therapeutics [8, 9].

The common route of delivery of drugs formed as micro- and nanoparticles is intravenous injection; however pulmonary drug delivery by inhalation becomes prospective [10–12]. It is beneficial particularly in the treatment of disorders localized within the respiratory system where diseased areas can be accessed from the outer side (i.e., via the air). Unfortunately, nanoparticles cannot be efficiently delivered by inhalation due to their poor aerosolization properties and relatively ineffective deposition in the bronchial tree and the alveoli. According to the existing knowledge based simultaneously on in vivo measurements and model calculations, the most suitable aerodynamic size of aerosol particles which assures their good penetration to the lower airways of the respiratory system is limited to 1–5 μm [12–14]. Thus, delivery of nanodrugs or nanocarriers into the lungs requires an application of additional vehicles of nanostructures in form of microsized objects which can be inhaled and effectively deposited in the respiratory system [10, 15, 16].

Typical polymers considered for use in pulmonary drug delivery are natural polysaccharides such as carrageenans, chitosan, gelatin, and hyaluronic acid, but also certain biocompatible synthetic compounds such as poly(lactic) acid, PLA; oligo(lactic) acid polymers, poly(vinyl) alcohol, PVA; and also some copolymers (e.g., poly(lactic-co-glycolide acid): PLGA) [5]. Other biocompatible polymers may be also proposed as the field is still open for innovation [17]. Such compounds can be used as carriers of drugs which are incorporated in the dissolving matrix. One of the key problems in the application of respirable drug carriers is their preparation as a formulation suitable for use with inhalers. Among several available methods of production of stable dry particles [18], spray drying (SD) became popular as a single-step and affordable process [19]. Other advantages of this technique are easy scaling up, good control over product quality (mainly: particle size and morphology), and the possibility of production of multicomponent particles [20–22].

In this paper we focus on the preparation of inhalable microparticles which can be used as vehicles for nanosized polymeric particles for delivery to the respiratory system. To achieve that aim we propose the multistep research approach which consists of the follwoing:(1)preparation of nanoparticles by oxidized dextran and carboxymethyl-cellulose (both compounds are known to be biocompatible [23, 24], and this property should be retained after oxidation as they are always partially oxidized in the native state),(2)preparation of microparticles by SD starting from the nanosuspensions obtained in step ,(3)characterization of the microparticles (powders) in respect of their aerosolization properties to confirm suitability for pulmonary drug delivery,(4)testing the possibility of reconstitution of nanostructures after powder hydration.

2. MATERIALS AND METHODS

2.1. Nanoparticles Preparation and Size Determination

The following chemicals have been used in the synthesis of nanoparticles: dextran (MW = 70 kDa, donated by Institute of Animal Physiology and Nutrition, Polish Academy of Sciences, Jablonna, Poland), Aqualon sodium carboxymethylcellulose (MW = 90 kDA, Hercules Inc., USA), dodecylamine hydrochloride, benzylamine, sodium periodate (Sigma Aldrich, Poland), and alanine (POCh, Poland).

Each of two polysaccharides was oxidized in aqueous phase with sodium periodate according to procedure described by Mu et al. [25]. Degree of oxidation after the completion of the reaction was determined by hydroxylamine hydrochloride titration method [26], and it was 5% in the case of polyaldehyde dextran (PAD) and 15% in case of dialdehyde carboxymethylcellulose (DACMC). Folding of polymer chains was achieved by linking hydrophobic amines to the aldehyde groups: dodecylamine hydrochloride in the case of PAD and benzylamine in the case of DACMC. Other aldehyde groups were substituted by alanine. These reactions allowed obtaining nanoparticles which were then purified by 30 min dialysis done in tubular membranes made of regenerated cellulose (MWCO 14 000, Carl Roth GmbH + Co. KG, Germany) against water purified with the reverse osmosis. The outer liquid was agitated with the magnetic stirrer (150 rpm). The size of obtained nanostructures was determined at room temperature by nanoparticle tracking analysis (NTA) using Nanosight LM10-HS device (Malvern Instruments, UK). Each nanosuspension (approximate concentration: 20 mg/mL) was diluted 100-fold with water before the measurements. Analyses were triplicated and the gathered data were averaged.

2.2. Powder Production and Characterization

Dry powder was produced with the standard spray drying method (SD) using Mini Spray Dryer B-290 (Büchi, Switzerland) operated in the open mode. Some details of the technique and the apparatus are given elsewhere [22]. The aqueous nanosuspensions (approximate concentration: PAD: 6% and DACMC: 2%) were pumped to the pneumatic nozzle with the volumetric rate of 3 mL/min and dispersed by compressed air (flow rate: 14 dm^3/min). The powders formed due to evaporation of water from droplets on contact with hot air (inlet temperature, = 100, 150, or 200°C) were separated in the high performance glass cyclone. Two process parameters were adjusted: the flow rate and the inlet temperature of the drying air . These parameters were selected as decisive based on our previous studies related to use of spray drying for preparing of inhalable powders [20, 22]. Experimental settings of the drying are listed in Table 1. Collected powders were inspected visually using scanning electron microscope (SEM, model TM1000, Hitachi, Japan) after coating with 20 nm layer of gold (K550x Sputter Coater, Quorum Technologies, UK).

Table 1: Processing conditions of spray drying: different flow rates and temperatures of the drying air.

	$Q = 20\ m^3/hr$		
Designation	Exp. 1	Exp. 2	Exp. 3
T_{in} [°C]	100	150	200
T_{out} [°C]	~45	~57	~68
	$Q = 35\ m^3/hr$		
Designation	Exp. 4	Exp. 5	Exp. 6
T_{in} [°C]	100	150	200
T_{out} [°C]	~55	~85	~100

2.3. Aerosol Properties of Powders

Powder aerosolization was tested using the commercially available capsule inhaler (Cyclohaler, Adamed, Poland). Before each experiment capsules were loaded with approximately 10 mg powder aliquots. Volumetric particle size distribution was determined with the laser diffraction aerosol spectrometer (Spraytec, Malvern Instruments, UK) additionally equipped with the dedicated inhalation chamber, Figure 1. Aerosol was created by the airflow drawn through the inhaler at the rate of 100 dm^3/min which is the typical value obtained during medical inhalations with this type of inhaling device. The aerosol cloud was introduced into the inhalation chamber via the standard inlet tube (so called: USP, i.e., United States Pharmacopeia, inlet [27]). The cloud was automatically sensed by the optical system allowing determining the particle size distribution (measuring period: 0.5 s, sampling rate: 1 kHz). Based on the complete, time-averaged size distributions, two essential factors were evaluated and compared: the volumetric median diameter (VMD = Dv50) and the percentage of particles smaller than 4.7 μm (so called, fine particle fraction: FPF). Both parameters are the essential quality indicators of aerosol produced by the inhalation drug delivery systems [12].

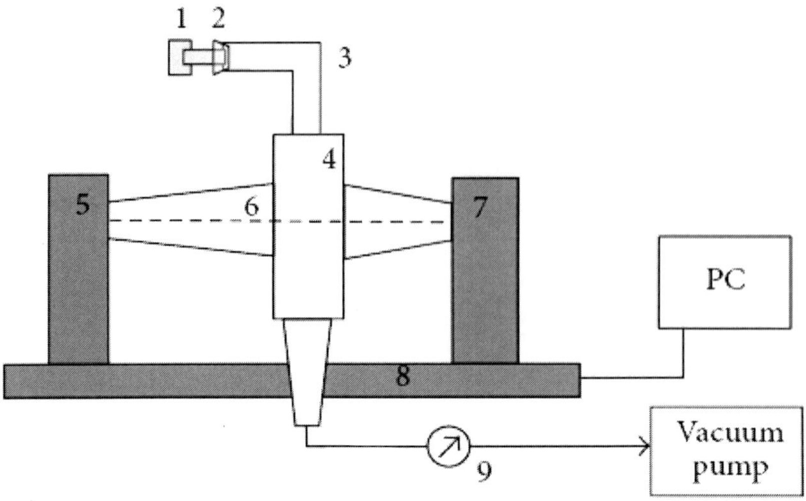

Figure 1: The experimental set-up for determination of particle size distribution of aerosolized powder: 1: inhaler, 2: adapter, 3: USP inlet, 4: inhalation chamber, 5: laser emitter of Spraytec spectrometer, 6: laser beam, 7: laser detector of Spraytec spectrometer, 8: optical bench, and 9: valve and air flowmeter.

It should be noted here that laser diffraction allows to find the distribution based on particles volume which is, in general, not equivalent to the one based on the aerodynamic size (e.g., measured by cascade impactors [27]). By definition, aerodynamic particle diameter equals

$$d_{ae} = d_p \sqrt{\frac{\rho_p}{\xi \rho_w}}, \quad (1)$$

where is the equivalent geometric diameter of the particle, density of particle material, density of water, and the dynamic shape factor [16]. Divergence between both diameters becomes important only for highly porous particles (like those studied by Tsapis et al. [15]) or particles with very irregular shape (needles, fibers, fractal-like aggregates, and plates:). For particles with virtually spherical shape () and density comparable to water, it can be claimed that both diameters are practically equivalent. This assumption remains also valid for particles studied in this work.

2.4. Nanoparticle Reconstitution after Powder Rehydration

In order to check if nanocolloids can be restored after rehydration of dry particles, the powders (20 mg aliquots) were mixed with water (1 mL) and gently agitated by magnetic ministirrer for 30 minutes at room temperature (agitation speed: 300 min^{-1}). Determination of particle size distribution in the suspension was done by the same methodology as for the initial assessment, that is, by NTA.

3. RESULTS AND DISCUSSION

Total concentration of PAD and DACMC synthesized nanoparticles in the samples used in NTA analyses was in the range of 10^8 particles/mL. The examples of size distributions obtained by NTA measurements for both types of nanoparticles are presented in Figure 2. The nanoparticles were polydisperse with the average particle size: 168.5 ± 16.6 nm and the count mode: 107 ± 1.9 nm in case of PAD and the average size: 118.0 ± 0.7 nm and the count mode: 96.0 ± 0.5 nm in case of DACMC. For PAD particles it is seen that the distribution is characterized by the main maximum corresponding to the modal value and the additional local peak which probably shows aggregates. To better describe the size distribution we introduce the span, which can be determined according to the formula:

$$S = \frac{D_{90} - D_{10}}{D_{50}}, \quad (2)$$

where denotes the th percentile of the cumulative distribution. Span values provide data regarding the width (polydispersity) of the particle size distribution. The calculated values of were 1.16 ± 0.04 and 1.06 ± 0.02 for PAD and DCMC nanoparticles, respectively (these data are shown in Figure 8(b)—“sample 0”).

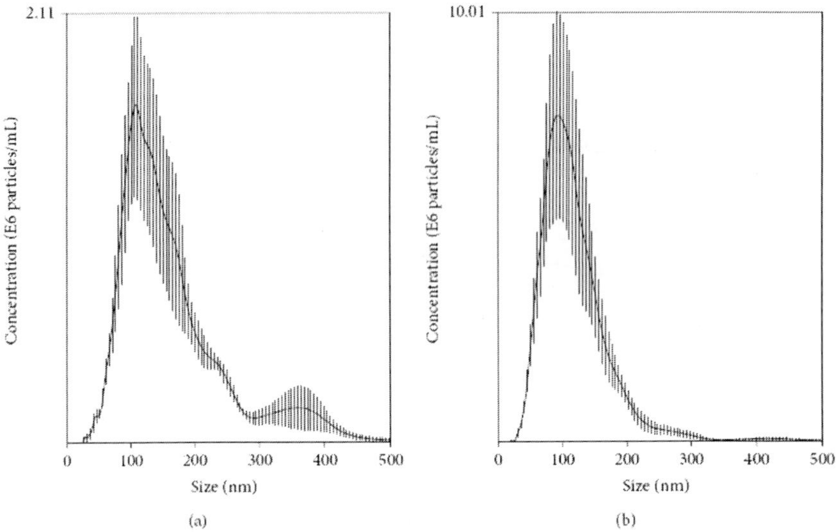

Figure 2: Examples of size distribution of PAD (a) and DACMC (b) nanoparticles.

SEM pictures of powders obtained by drying of nanosuspensions of polymeric nanoparticles are presented in Figures 3 and 4. These pictures are presented to illustrate the average geometrical size and morphology of dried material (no statistical analysis of particle sizes was done based on SEM measurements). In case of PAD (Figure3), powder particles are typically characterized by wrinkled surface and the degree of corrugation increases when the drying becomes faster. At the low flow rate of the drying air with = 100°C–150°C (= 20 m^3/hr), some spherical and smooth particles can be found as indicated by arrows in Figure 3.

Such particles are formed when drying process is slow enough to allow the uniform evaporation of water from droplets. Higher drying temperatures and increased airflow rates are responsible for the formation of particles with a corrugated surface.

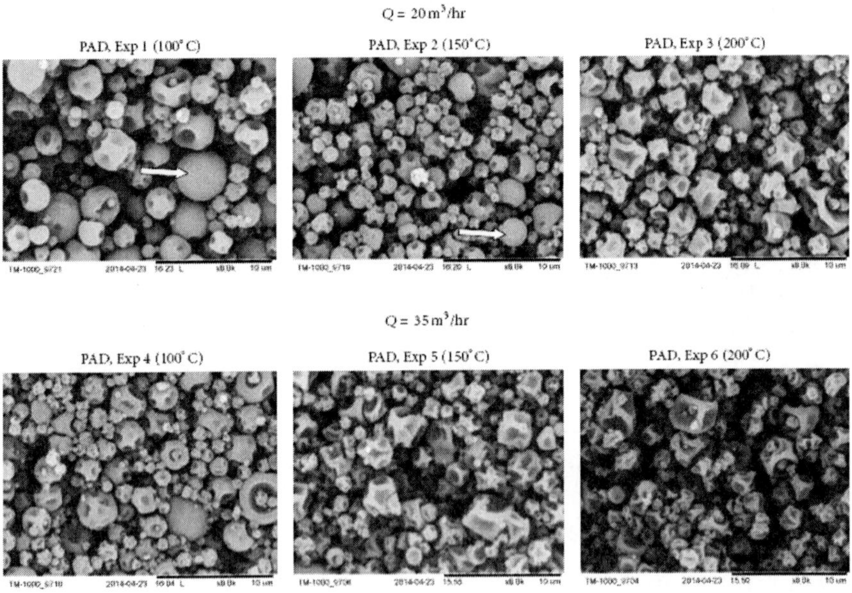

Figure 3: SEM pictures of powders obtained by spray drying of PAD nanosuspensions. Arrows indicate spherical particles with a smooth surface.

At very high drying rates (Exps 3, 5, and 6), powder particles are highly deformed and crumpled. This effect is due to the surface collapse when the outer solid crust (shell) is formed over the liquid content of the inner core of the droplet as suggested by other authors [28]. In such case, water evaporates through the crust leaving empty spaces behind so the crust becomes wrinkled as it collapses to fill these spaces, Figure 5(a).

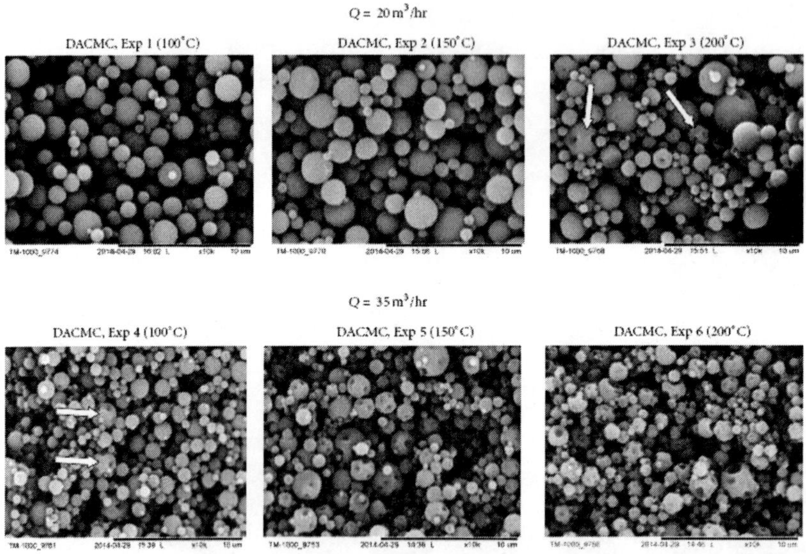

Figure 4: SEM pictures of powders obtained by spray drying of DACMC nanosuspensions. Arrows indicate deformed particles with a wrinkled surface.

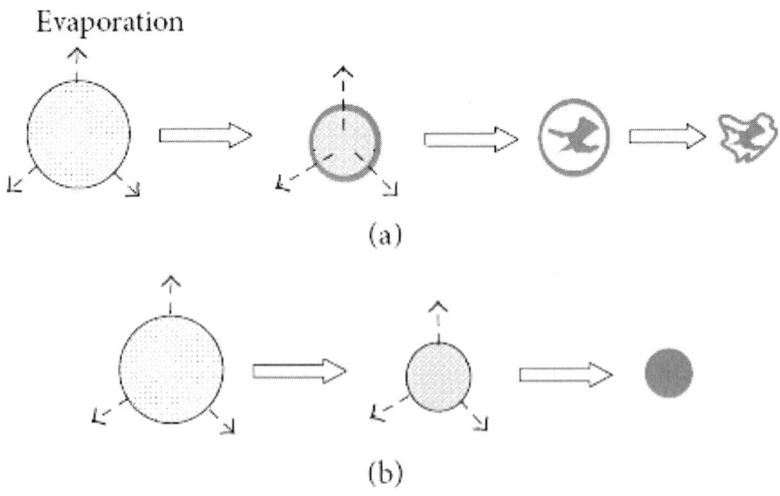

Figure 5: Hypothetical steps during formation of particles during drying: (a) at high drying rates formation of crust and evaporation of water from the inner liquid core leads to a deformed particle; (b) for low drying rate and/or lower concentration of the nanosuspension, droplets evaporate uniformly and the spherical particles are formed.

Based on the presented SEM pictures it can be found that the range of particle size is similar independently of the drying rate. Evidently, particles are not of equal size due to the polydispersity of the sprayed droplets. All particles are in the range of 0.5–5 μm, which is appropriate for powders designed for pulmonary delivery via inhalation.

In case of DACMC powders shown in Figure 4 the trend of changes in surface morphology is less apparent than the one observed for PAD particles.

At the lower flow rate of drying air (= 20 m^3/hr) particles are formed as spherical and smooth. Some deformations of the surface are observed only at the highest drying temperature (200°C) as indicated by arrow in this figure. When the flow rate of drying air increases, irregularities on particle surface become visible already at = 100°C. Particle corrugation is predominant at the highest drying rate but it is still much less remarkable when compared to PAD powders. It is expected that due to a lower concentration of the nanoparticles in the droplet, the mechanisms of drying is similar to the one shown in Figure 5(b), where the outer shell is not formed. It can be seen that DACMC particles are polydisperse and their size is typically below 3 μm. Higher flow rates of the drying air allows to obtain smaller particles.

Size distribution of particles dispersed in the air are compared in Figures 6 and 7, with a focus on two parameters: volumetric median diameter (VMD = Dv50) and the fraction of particles smaller than 4.7 μm (fine particle fraction: FPF). As mentioned earlier, both the median diameter and the FPF are the most important parameters for the evaluation of aerosol suitability for drug delivery via the inhalative route [12].

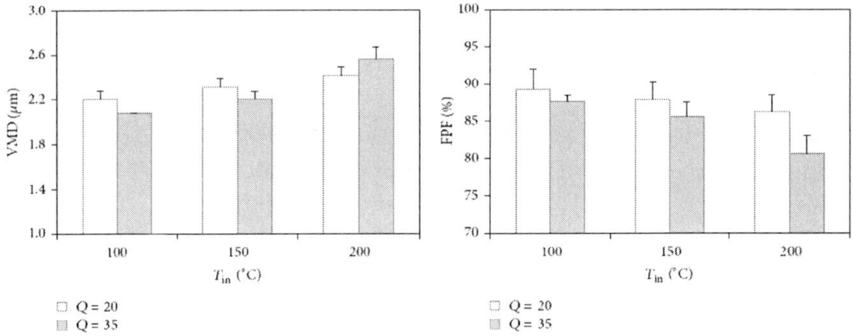

Figure 6: Volumetric median diameter (VMD) and fraction of fine particles (FPF) for PAD microparticles as a function of the temperature and the flow rate of the drying air (m^3/hr). Error bars denote the standard deviation.

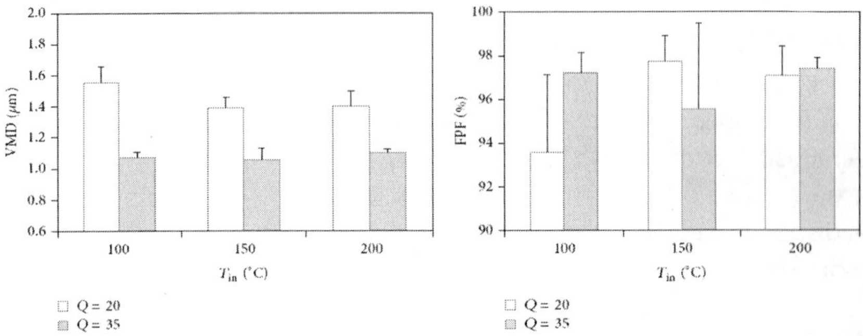

Figure 7: Volumetric median diameter (VMD) and fraction of fine particles (FPF) for DACMC microparticles as a function of the temperature and the flow rate of the drying air (m^3/hr). Error bars denote the standard deviation.

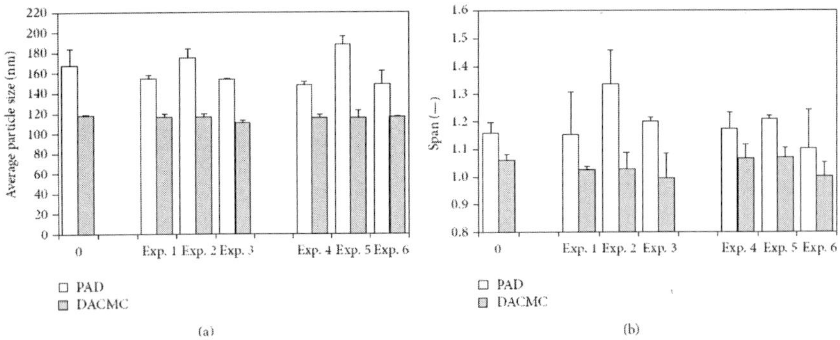

Figure 8: Average size (a) and span of the distribution (b) for nanoparticles obtained after reconstitution of spray dried powders with water at room temperature. Sample "0" denotes the original nanosuspensions (precursors). Error bars indicate the standard deviations.

The comparison shows that DACMC particles are at average almost twice smaller than PAD particles (VMD 1.1–1.5 μm and 2–2.6 μm, resp.) and the average size (VMD) of aerosol particles noticeably depends on drying conditions. Smaller size of DACMC particles results from the lower concentration of the precursor nanosuspension than in the case of PAD. In spite of the discussed differences in size, both types of powders may be considered as very good candidates for carriers of inhaled drugs. Fine particle fraction (FPF) is always higher than 80%, suggesting the possibility to deliver almost all the powder emitted from the inhaler into the distal parts of the respiratory system.

The average size of aerosolized PAD particles increases with the drying rate (higher flow and higher temperature of the hot air) which is related to the observed particle deformations. This effect can be explained in two ways as follows.(1)Since a spherical particle has the lowest volume, so deformation of particle with the given mass always leads to a higher volumetric size.(2)Particles with corrugated surface can be more difficult to disperse into single particles (due to interlocking effect [29]), so the observed distribution of particle size in the aerosol corresponds not to individual particles but rather to some aggregates which had not been dispersed in the inhaler. Referring to SEM pictures of produced PAD powders (Figure 3) it is seen that some small particles (<1 μm) are located in the cavities of larger particles. If such structures are not broken apart by the aerodynamic interactions, the relative amount of small particles in the aerosol will be decreased, and it will result in the higher average particle size (VMD).

The situation is different in case of DACMC particles for which the surface deformation caused by drying is weaker. Formation of the external crust can be delayed in this case due to the lower polymer concentration and lower liquid viscosity, so the particle shape almost always remains spherical according to the mechanism shown in Figure 5(b). Some surface defects are observed mainly at the high drying rates. It is found that powders obtained at higher flow rates of the drying air are aerosolized to smaller particles than the ones obtained at the lower airflow rate (Figure 7). The reason for that is not fully clear but the effect may be related to the structural changes of the DACMC nanostructures during the loss of water due to evaporation, which can be dependent on the drying rate.

Finally, the size distribution of nanoparticles reconstituted following the addition of water is compared in Figure 8(a). In general, it is seen that the nanostructure of colloids is restored after hydration of spray dried powders. This observation confirms that material processing during SD does not destroy the initial properties of tested polymers including the capability of self-organization (such as coiling/folding) in the aqueous environment. A scatter of the average particle size observed for PAD nanoparticles in Figure 8(a) cannot be reasonably linked to the drying conditions since the maximum can be found at the moderate inlet air temperatures (= 150°C).

Considering the values of span (2) presented in Figure 8(b), which give more information on the size distribution, it can be concluded that polydispersity of PAD nanoparticles is always higher than the one of DACMC. Particles processed by drying at 150°C and rehydration show wider distribution (= 1.2–1.35 after drying as compared to = 1.15 for the precursor). On the other hand, reconstituted nanosuspensions obtained from particles processed at both lower and higher drying temperatures are either less or equally polydisperse as the precursor.

4. CONCLUSIONS

Presented investigations demonstrate the following.(i)Nanostructures of biocompatible polymers PAD and DACMC with the average size of 120–170 nm can be obtained by a relatively simple chemical procedure in aqueous environment.(ii)Obtained nanoparticles can be conveniently and effectively converted into dry powders using spray drying technique from aqueous suspensions without any additives.(iii)Selected parameters of SD process, such as inlet temperature and flow rate of drying air (both determining the drying rate), are essential for surface morphology of produced powder particles.(iv)The resulting powders of both polymers have the adequate properties to be delivered to the lungs via inhalation using a simple and inexpensive capsule-type inhaler available on the market.(v)After powders reconstitution in water, the initial nanostructures are restored, giving the opportunity to study their suitability as potential drug carriers acting in the sites of deposition of inhaled microparticles.

The proposed methodology forms the general framework for the production of drug-loaded polymeric nanoparticles for pulmonary delivery via inhalative route as micrometric powders. In contrast to the earlier concepts (as the one presented by Tsapis et al. [15]), we use aqueous nanocolloids formed by self-organizing biocompatible polymeric particles which then are dried without any special chemical additives and foreign structures. Further studies focused on the application of the proposed platform for embedding individual drugs intended for treatment of pulmonary diseases using nanosized polymeric carriers are underway.

CONFLICT OF INTERESTS

The authors declare that there is no conflict of interests regarding the publication of this paper.

ACKNOWLEDGMENTS

The work is financed by statutory activity of the Faculty of Chemical and Process Engineering, Warsaw University of Technology. The input of

Katarzyna Jabłczyńska and Tomasz R. Sosnowski is related to their participation in the COST Action MP1106 "Smart and green interfaces: from single bubbles and drops to industrial, environmental and biomedical applications."

REFERENCES

1. E. Fattal, H. Hillaireau, S. Mura, J. Nicolas, and N. Tsapis, "Targeted delivery using biodegradable polymeric nanoparticles," in Fundamentals and Applications of Controlled Drug Delivery, J. Siepmann, R. A. Siegel, and M. J. Rathbone, Eds., pp. 255–288, CRS & Springer, New York, NY, USA, 2012.

2. J. Panyam and V. Labhasetwar, "Biodegradable nanoparticles for drug and gene delivery to cells and tissue," Advanced Drug Delivery Reviews, vol. 55, no. 3, pp. 329–347, 2003.

3. F. Danhier, E. Ansorena, J. M. Silva, R. Coco, A. Le Breton, and V. Préat, "PLGA-based nanoparticles: an overview of biomedical applications," Journal of Controlled Release, vol. 161, no. 2, pp. 505–522, 2012.

4. H. M. Mansour, M. Sohn, A. Al-Ghananeem, and P. P. DeLuca, "Materials for pharmaceutical dosage forms: molecular pharmaceutics and controlled release drug delivery aspects," International Journal of Molecular Sciences, vol. 11, no. 9, pp. 3298–3322, 2010.

5. P. Sheth and P. B. Myrdal, "Polymers for pulmonary drug delivery," in Controlled Pulmonary Drug Delivery, H. D. C. Smyth and A. J. Hickey, Eds., pp. 265–282, Controlled Release Society & Springer, New York, NY, USA, 2011.

6. J. Wei, X.-J. Ju, X.-Y. Zou et al., "Multi-stimuli-responsive microcapsules for adjustable controlled-release," Advanced Functional Materials, vol. 24, no. 22, pp. 3312–3323, 2014.

7. Y. Lu, W. Sun, and Z. Gu, "Stimuli-responsive nanomaterials for therapeutic protein delivery," Journal of Controlled Release, vol. 194, pp. 1–19, 2014.

8. J. Fang, H. Nakamura, and H. Maeda, "The EPR effect: unique features of tumor blood vessels for drug delivery, factors involved, and limitations and augmentation of the effect," Advanced Drug Delivery Reviews, vol. 63, no. 3, pp. 136–151, 2011.

9. S. Acharya and S. K. Sahoo, "PLGA nanoparticles containing various anticancer agents and tumour delivery by EPR effect," Advanced Drug Delivery Reviews, vol. 63, no. 3, pp. 170–183, 2011.

10. W. Yang, J. I. Peters, and R. O. Williams III, "Inhaled nanoparticles—A current review," International Journal of Pharmaceutics, vol. 356, no. 1-2, pp. 239–247, 2008.

11. J. C. Sung, B. L. Pulliam, and D. A. Edwards, "Nanoparticles for drug delivery to the lungs," Trends in Biotechnology, vol. 25, no. 12, pp. 563–570, 2007.

12. S. Newman, Respiratory Drug Delivery: Essential Theory and Practice, RDD Online/VCU, Richmond, VA, USA, 2009.

13. H. Bisgaard, C. O'Callaghan, and G. C. Smaldone, Eds., Drug Delivery to the Lungs, Marcel Dekker, New York, NY, USA, 2002.

14. T. R. Sosnowski, A. Moskal, and L. Gradoń, "Dynamics of oropharyngeal aerosol transport and deposition with the realistic flow pattern," Inhalation Toxicology, vol. 18, no. 10, pp. 773–780, 2006.

15. N. Tsapis, D. Bennett, B. Jackson, D. A. Weitz, and D. A. Edwards, "Trojan particles: large porous carriers of nanoparticles for drug delivery," Proceedings of the National Academy of Sciences of the United States of America, vol. 99, no. 19, pp. 12001–12005, 2002.

16. T. R. Sosnowski, "Nanosized and nanostructured particles in pulmonary drug delivery," Journal of Nanoscience and Nanotechnology, vol. 15, no. 5, pp. 3476–3487, 2015.

17. H. M. Mansour, Y.-S. Rhee, and X. Wu, "Nanomedicine in pulmonary delivery," International Journal of Nanomedicine, vol. 4, pp. 299–319, 2009.

18. L. Gradoń and T. R. Sosnowski, "Formation of particles for dry powder inhalers," Advanced Powder Technology, vol. 25, no. 1, pp. 43–55, 2014.

19. R. Vehring, "Expert review: pharmaceutical particle engineering via spray drying," Pharmaceutical Research, vol. 25, no. 5, pp. 999–1022, 2008.

20. K. Kramek-Romanowska, M. Odziomek, T. R. Sosnowski, and L. Gradoń, "Effects of process variables on the properties of spray-dried mannitol and mannitol/disodium cromoglycate powders suitable for drug delivery by inhalation," Industrial and Engineering Chemistry Research, vol. 50, no. 24, pp. 13922–13931, 2011.

21. A. B. D. Nandiyanto and K. Okuyama, "Progress in developing spray-drying methods for the production of controlled morphology particles: from the nanometer to submicrometer size ranges," Advanced Powder Technology, vol. 22, no. 1, pp. 1–19, 2011.

22. M. Odziomek, T. R. Sosnowski, and L. Gradoń, "Conception, preparation and properties of functional carrier particles for pulmonary drug delivery," International Journal of Pharmaceutics, vol. 433, no. 1-2, pp. 51–59, 2012.

23. J. Maia, M. B. Evangelista, H. Gil, and L. Ferreira, "Dextran-based materials for biomedical applications," in Carbohydrates Applications in Medicine, M. H. Gil, Ed., pp. 31–53, Research Signpost, Kerala, India, 2014.

24. L. Jiang, Y. Li, L. Zhang, and X. Wang, "Preparation and characterization of a novel composite containing carboxymethyl cellulose used for bone repair," Materials Science and Engineering C, vol. 29, no. 1, pp. 193–198, 2009.

25. C. Mu, J. Guo, X. Li, W. Lin, and D. Li, "Preparation and properties of dialdehyde carboxymethyl cellulose crosslinked gelatin edible films," Food Hydrocolloids, vol. 27, no. 1, pp. 22–29, 2012.

26. H. Zhao and N. D. Heindel, "Determination of degree of substitution of formyl groups in polyaldehyde dextran by the

hydroxylamine hydrochloride method," Pharmaceutical Research, vol. 8, no. 3, pp. 400–402, 1991.

27. USP General Chapters, USP LTHEXA601> Aerosols, Nasal Sprays, Metered-Dose Inhalers, and Dry Powder Inhalers, USP 32-NF-27, US Pharmacopeial Convention, Rockville, Md, USA, 2009.

28. J. M. Gac and L. Gradoń, "A distributed parameter model for the spray drying of multicomponent droplets with a crust formation," Advanced Powder Technology, vol. 24, no. 1, pp. 324–330, 2013.

29. X. M. Zeng, G. P. Martin, and C. Marriott, Particulate Interactions in Dry Powder Formulations for Inhalation, CRC Press, London, UK, 2000.

Chapter 11

A Multifunctional Ribonuclease A-Conjugated Carbon Dot Cluster Nanosystem for Synchronous Cancer Imaging and Therapy

Huiyang Liu[1], Qin Wang[1], Guangxia Shen[1,3*], Chunlei Zhang[1], Chao Li[1], Weihang Ji[2], Chun Wang[3*] and Daxiang Cui[1,2*]

[1]*Institute of Nano Biomedicine and Engineering, Key Laboratory for Thin Film and Microfabrication of Ministry of Education, Department of Instrument Science and Engineering, School of Electronic Information and Engineering, Shanghai Jiao Tong University, Shanghai 200240, People's Republic of China.*

[2]*Research Institute of Translation Medicine, Shanghai Jiao Tong University, Shanghai 200240, People's Republic of China.*

[3]*Department of Biomedical Engineering, University of Minnesota (Twin Cities), Minneapolis, MN 55455, USA.*

ABSTRACT

Carbon dots exhibit great potential in applications such as molecular imaging and in vivo molecular tracking. However, how to enhance fluorescence intensity of carbon dots has become a great challenge. Herein, we report for the first time a new strategy to synthesize fluorescent carbon dots (C-dots) with high quantum yields by using ribonuclease A (RNase A) as a biomolecular templating agent under microwave irradiation. The synthesized RNase A-conjugated carbon dots (RNase A@C-dots) exhibited quantum yields of 24.20%. The fluorescent color of the RNase A@C-dots can easily be adjusted by varying the microwave reaction time and microwave power. Moreover, the emission wavelength and intensity of RNase A@C-dots displayed a marked excitation wavelength-dependent character. As the excitation wavelength alters from 300 to 500 nm, the photoluminescence (PL) peak exhibits gradually redshifts from 450 to 550 nm, and the intensity reaches its maximum at an excitation wavelength of 380 nm. Its Stokes shift is about 80 nm. Notably, the PL intensity is gradually decreasing as the pH increases, almost linearly dependent, and it reaches the maximum at a pH = 2 condition; the emission peaks also show clearly a redshift, which may be caused by the high activity and perfective dispersion of RNase A in a lower pH solution. In high pH solution, RNase A tends to form RNase A warped carbon dot nanoclusters. Cell imaging confirmed that the RNase A@C-dots could enter into the cytoplasm through cell endocytosis. 3D confocal imaging and transmission electron microscopy observation confirmed partial RNase A@C-dots located inside the nucleus. MTT and real-time cell electronic sensing (RT-CES) analysis showed that the RNase A@C-dots could effectively inhibit the growth of MGC-803 cells. Intra-tumor injection test of RNase A@C-dots showed that RNase A@C-dots could be used for imaging in vivo gastric cancer cells. In conclusion, the as-prepared RNase A@C-dots are suitable for simultaneous therapy and in vivo fluorescence imaging of nude mice loaded with gastric cancer or other tumors.

Keywords: Carbon dots RNase A MGC-803 cell line Microwave irradiation Molecular imaging MTT

BACKGROUND

Carbon dots (C-dots) are a new member of the carbon nanomaterial family after C_{60}, carbon nanotubes, and graphene and were firstly discovered by accident when researchers were trying to purify single-walled carbon nanotubes (SWCNTs) fabricated by arc discharge methods [1]. Since then, many studies concerning C-dots have been reported [2, 3, 4]. C-dots have attracted much attention due to their well-defined, nearly isotropic shapes together with their ultrafine dimensions and tunable surface functionalities. Moreover, a variety of simple, fast, and cheap synthetic routes for C-dots have been developed in the past few years including arc discharge, laser ablation, electrochemical oxidation, hydrothermal, combustion/thermal, supported synthetic, and microwave methods [4, 5,6]. Most notable superiority, however, is their potential as replacements for toxic heavy metal-based quantum dots (QDs) which are currently intensively used and are plagued by safety concerns and known environmental hazards [2, 5, 6].

C-dots have proven themselves in various applications with photoluminescence properties comparable and even superior to those of QDs [2, 3, 7], such as high photostability, tunable emission, large two-photon excitation cross section [8, 9], and non-blinking fluorescence [10]. C-dots have been successfully applied in bioimaging [11], both in vitro [8] and in vivo [12], and even showed significant utility in multiphoton imaging [9]. Moreover, beyond these apparently straightforward applications, more complicated designs aimed at multifunctional nanosystems based on C-dots have been reported. For example, Huang and his collaborators [13] have developed a new theranostic platform based on photosensitizer-conjugated carbon dots with excellent imaging and tumor-homing ability for NIR fluorescence imaging-guided photodynamic therapy. Moreover, a C-dot-based inorganic-organic nanosystem for two-photon imaging and biosensing of pH variation in living cells and tissues has also been designed by Kong's research group [14]. Almost during the same period, C-dots with PEI (polyetherimid)-passivation were used for bioimaging and as nanocarrier for gene delivery [15]. However, with the rapid progress of research and application, many defects were thoroughly exposed such as low photoluminescence intensity, short wavelength excitation, and difficulties in separation and purification, which did hinder it to further in vitro or in vivo biological applications.

Previously, preparation of surfaced-functionalized C-dots usually included three steps: synthesis of raw C-dots, passivation operations, and functionalization reactions [16]. Most C-dots prepared, if without further complicated purification, passivation, and functionality, featured quite low quantum yield (around or less than 5%) [1, 17, 18, 19,20, 21, 22] and retained very limited application potentials. So it is extremely necessary to find a simply strategy to fabricate surface-functionalized C-dots with relatively high quantum efficiency.

As to the preparation methods, they could be divided into two categories: top-down methods and bottom-up methods. The bottom-up methods usually suffer from complex processes, or expensive starting materials and severe synthetic conditions, which are unlikely to be extended significantly in the near future [23]. Alternatively, bottom-up synthetic approaches based on chemistry have been desired to achieve C-dots with fluorescence. Presently, Li et al. reported a facile hydrothermal method to prepare luminescent carbon dots (L-CDs) with high quantum yield value (44.7%) and controllable emission wavelengths and used prepared carbon dots to detect toxic Be^{2+} ions [6].

To date, microwave pyrolysis approach, as one family member of bottom-up synthesis methods, has been developed and widely used for its simplicity, cost/time-efficiency, environmental friendliness, easiness to scale up, and more importantly convenience to realize synthesis, passivation, and functionalization reactions simultaneously through only one synthesis step [4, 24].

Herein, we report for the first time a green synthesis route, only one synthesis step followed by limited and simple purification, without further passivation and surface functionality to prepare ribonuclease A-conjugated C-dot nanoclusters (RNase A@C-dots). It is well known that RNase A is a low molecular weight protein (approximately 124 residues, approximately 13.7 kDa, pI = 9.4) with a globular conformation (2.2 nm × 2.8 nm × 3.2 nm) [25]. The protein has proved to be thermally stable [26], even under microwave heating for a couple of minutes [27]. In addition, RNase A has been confirmed to be able to inhibit the growth of cancer cells as a result of its enzymatic activity of degrading cellular RNA and has been proven to be effective in clinical trials as a chemotherapeutic agent [28, 29]. In our previous work, we used RNase A as a biomolecular templating agent to synthesize CdTe QD nanoclusters [27]. Meanwhile, through chemical bonding of the targeting RGD peptide on the RNase A@CdTe QD cluster surface, we constructed multifunctional biological nanoprobes which shows the efficiency of the nanosystem for synchronous in vitro targeted cancer imaging and therapy [27]. Inspired by the achievements of previous studies and concerned with the shortcomings along with the accomplishments, we proposed the synthesis of RNase A@C-dots via a one-step microwave-assisted method using citric acid as carbon precursor and RNase A as an assisting agent. The method greatly simplified the synthesis processes, conveniently realized the improvement of the photoluminescence intensity, and largely retained the activity of RNase A for potential therapeutic applications. Prepared RNase A@C-dots exhibited multifunctional properties and were successfully employed for tumor fluorescence imaging and therapy.

METHODS

Materials

Bovine pancreatic ribonuclease A (RNase A) and polyethylene glycol (PEG_{2000N}) were purchased from Sigma-Aldrich Chemical Co. (St. Louis, MO, USA). Citric acid (CA, analytical grade) was bought from Shanghai Chemical Reagent Co., Ltd. (Shanghai, China). 3-[4,5-Dimethylthiazol-2yl]-2,5-diphenylterazolium bromide (MTT) was obtained from Invitrogen Corporation (Carlsbad, CA, USA). MGC-803 cell lines were obtained from the Cell Bank of Type Culture Collection of Chinese Academy of Sciences. Cell culture products and reagents, unless pointed out, were all purchased from Gibco (Invitrogen Corporation, Carlsbad, CA, USA). All chemical reagents were used without further purification. All solutions were made with purified water (with a low electroconductivity of 18.2 MΩ cm).

Synthesis of RNase A@C-dots, C-dot, and C-dots-NH_2 (C-dot surface modified by PEG_{2000N})

For the synthesis of RNase A@C-dots, 2 g citric acid and 0.15 g RNase A were diluted in 10 ml water within a 25-ml glass bottle and put under ultrasonic for 1 to 2 min to form a uniform solution. Then, the transparent solution was put into a domestic microwave oven (700 W) for 3 to 5 min. After cooling to room temperature, the obtained brown C-dot solution was dialyzed against pure water with a dialysis membrane (molecular weight cutoff (MWCO) of 1,000) for 2 days to remove unreacted citric acid. Finally, the dry C-dot composite was freeze-dried in vacuum, weighed, and dissolved in ultrapure water with a fixed concentration.

In control experiments, citric acid without RNase A was treated with the same procedure and the final product was named C-dots. Then, to modify the surface of C-dots with PEG_{2000N}, the mixture solution of C-dots and PEG_{2000N}(mass ratio, C-dots/PEG_{2000N} =1:20) was refluxed with nitrogen gas protection at 120°C for 72 h. Then, the mixture was shifted into a dialysis membrane (MWCO of 3,000) against pure water to remove surplus PEG_{2000N}.

Characterization

To determine the size and morphology, RNase A@C-dots were characterized by high-resolution transmission electron microscopy (HR-TEM, JEM-2100 F, 200 kV, JEOL Ltd., Tokyo, Japan). The samples for TEM/HR-TEM were made by simply dropping aqueous solution of the C-dots onto a 300-mesh copper grid casted with a carbon film. UV–Vis absorption spectra of the C-dots were measured with a Varian Cary 50 spectrophotometer (Varian Inc., Palo Alto, CA, USA). Fluorescence excitation and emission spectra of RNase A@C-dots were recorded on a Hitachi FL-4600 spectrofluorimeter (Hitachi Ltd., Tokyo, Japan). Zeta potential of RNase A@C-dots was measured on a Nicomp 380 ZLS zeta potential/particle sizer (PSS. Nicomp, Santa Barbara, CA, USA). X-ray photoelectron spectroscopy (XPS) was obtained at room temperature by a Kratos Axis Ultra spectrometer (AXIS-Ultra DLD, Kratos Analytical Ltd., Tokyo, Japan) using a monochromated Al Kα (1486.6 eV) source at 15 kV. Fourier transform infrared (FTIR) spectra were obtained on a Nicolet 6700 spectrometer (Thermo Electron Corporation, Madison, WI, USA). The samples for FTIR measurement were prepared by grinding the dried C-dots with KBr together and then compressed into thin pellets. X-ray diffraction (XRD) profiles of the C-dot powders were recorded on a D/MAX 2600 PC (Rigaku, Tokyo, Japan) equipped with graphite monochromatized Cu Kα (λ = 0.15405 nm) radiation at a scanning speed of 4°/min in the range from 10° to 60°. Time-resolved fluorescence intensity decay of RNase A@C-dots was performed on a LifeSpec II (Lifetime only, Edinburgh Instruments, Livingston, UK). The sample was excited by 380-nm laser, and the decay was measured in a time scale of 0.024410 ns/channel.

Quantum yield measurement

To assess the quantum yield of RNase A@C-dots, quinine sulfate in 0.1 M H_2SO_4 (quantum yield, 54%) was used as a reference fluorescence reagent. The final results were calculated according to Equation 1 below:

$$\Phi_{\text{sample}} = \frac{A_{\text{std}}}{A_{\text{sample}}} \times \frac{F_{\text{sample}}}{F_{\text{std}}} \times \frac{n^2_{\text{sample}}}{n^2_{\text{std}}} \times \Phi_{\text{std}} \quad (1)$$

where Φ_{std} is the known quantum yield of the standard compound, F_{sample} and F_{std} stand for the integrated fluorescence intensity of the sample and the standard compound in the emission region from 380 to 700 nm, $A_{std}$and A_{sample} are the absorbance of the standard compound and the sample at the excitation wavelength (360 nm), and n is the refractive index of solvent (for water, the refractive index is 1.33).

To minimize the reabsorption effects, UV absorbance intensities of the samples and standard compound should never exceed 0.1 at the excitation wavelength. Photoluminescence (PL) emission spectra of all the sample solutions were measured at the excitation wavelength of 360 nm. The integrated fluorescence intensity is the area under the PL curve in the wavelength from 380 to 700 nm.

Cell culture, cell viability assay, and time-dependent cell response profiling

The human gastric cancer cell line MGC-803 cell was maintained at 37°C (5% CO_2) in Dulbecco's modified Eagle's medium (DMEM, HyClone, Thermo Fisher Scientific, Waltham, MA, USA) supplemented with 10% (*v*/*v*) fetal bovine serum (Gibco), 100 U/ml penicillin, and 1 mg/ml streptomycin.

For MTT assay, MGC-803 cells were seeded in a 96-well plate (Corning Costar, Corning, NY, USA) with a density of 5×10^3 cells/well with 10% fetal bovine serum and then cultured overnight. After culturing, those cells were incubated with C-dots of various concentrations for 24 h. Following the incubation, the supernatant was removed and the cells were washed once with 0.01 M PBS. Then 150 μl DMEM and 15 μl MTT stock solution (5 mg/ml in PBS, pH 7.4) were added to each well, and after this, the cells were allowed to incubate for 4 h at 37°C. Finally, after removing the culture medium, 150 μl DMSO was added to dissolve the Formosan crystals. The optical density (OD) was measured at 570 nm on a standard microplate reader (Scientific Multiskan MK3, Thermo Fisher Scientific, Waltham, MA, USA). The cell viability was calculated according to the following formula: Cell viability = (OD of the experimental sample/OD of the control group) × 100%. The cell viability of control groups was denoted as 100%.

The time-dependent cell response profiles were performed using a real-time cell electronic sensing (RT-CES) system. Firstly, 100 μl of media was added to 16-well E-plates to record background readings, and then, 100 μl of cell suspension (containing about 5,000 cells) was added. Secondly, the cells in the E-plates were allowed to incubate at room temperature for 30 min. After the incubation, the E-plates were put on the reader in the incubator to continuously record the electric impedance which is reflected by cell index. After 20 to 24 h, the RNase A@C-dots and C-dots of certain concentration were added into the E-plates to mix with cells. For comparison, each plate also contained wells added with RNase A and wells with cells alone in the media in addition to media-only wells. The cells were monitored every 2 min for the first 1 h after the addition of C-dots and RNase A to get the short-term response and for every 30 min from 1 h after C-dot addition to about 48 h to record the long-term response.

Laser scanning confocal microscopy imaging in vitro

For fluorescence imaging with RNase A@C-dots, MGC-803 cells were first plated on 14-mm glass coverslips and allowed to adhere for 24 h at 37°C. Second, the cells were co-incubated with 120 μM RNase A@C-dots for 24 h. Then, the cells were washed with phosphate buffered (PBS) solution to remove unbound nanoparticles. Finally, the cells were fixed with 4% paraformaldehyde, and the nuclei of the cells were stained with 4′,6-diamidino-2-phenylindole (DAPI) (0.5 mg/ml in PBS).

Confocal fluorescence 2D or 3D imaging was performed on a TCS SP5 confocal laser scanning microscope (Leica Microsystems, Mannheim, Germany) with an objective lens (×63). In our experiment, we used a 408-nm excitation wavelength laser. Optical sections were averaged three times to reduce noise.

RNase A@C-dots for in vivo fluorescence imaging

Male 4-week-old athymic nude mice were purchased from Shanghai Slac Laboratory Animal Co. Ltd (Shanghai, China). All experiments that involve animal use were performed in compliance with the relevant laws and institutional guidelines. All animal experiments were approved by the Institutional Animal Care and Use Committee of Shanghai Jiao Tong University (No. SYXK2007-0025). For the establishment of the tumor model, MGC-803 cells were resuspended in PBS, and 2×10^6 cells per site were subcutaneously injected. The tumor nodules had reached a volume of 0.1 to 0.3 cm^3 approximately 3 weeks post-injection. For in vivo fluorescence tumor imaging experiments, 100 µl (5 mg/ml) RNase A@C-dot aqueous solution was intratumorally injected into the MGC-803 tumor-bearing mice. Time-course fluorescent images (excitation, 500/20 nm; emission, 600/30 nm; integration time, 5 s) were acquired on a Bruker In-Vivo F PRO imaging system (Bruker, Billerica, MA, USA).

RESULTS AND DISCUSSION

Characterization and properties of RNase A@C-dots

TEM images of the as-prepared RNase A@C-dots that were trapped in the dialysis membrane (MW cutoff 1,000) are shown in Figure 1a; the size of the RNase A@C-dots varies mainly within 25 to 45 nm with relatively irregular morphologies. High-resolution TEM image (Figure 1b, the zoomed-in image of the area within the circle in Figure 1a) clearly shows that the particles are actually formed by encapsulating several C-dots within the RNase A film, so we can call them clusters. The clusters can also extremely easily disperse in pure water. In Figure 1c, the average size of C-dot that dispersed out of the dialysis membrane is about 4 nm (Figure 1f) in diameter with nice spherical morphologies (Figure 1d), and the dispersions are also excellent. Lattice spacing of approximately 0.23 nm clearly displayed in the high-resolution TEM image (Figure 1d) indicates the (100) facet of graphite [30].

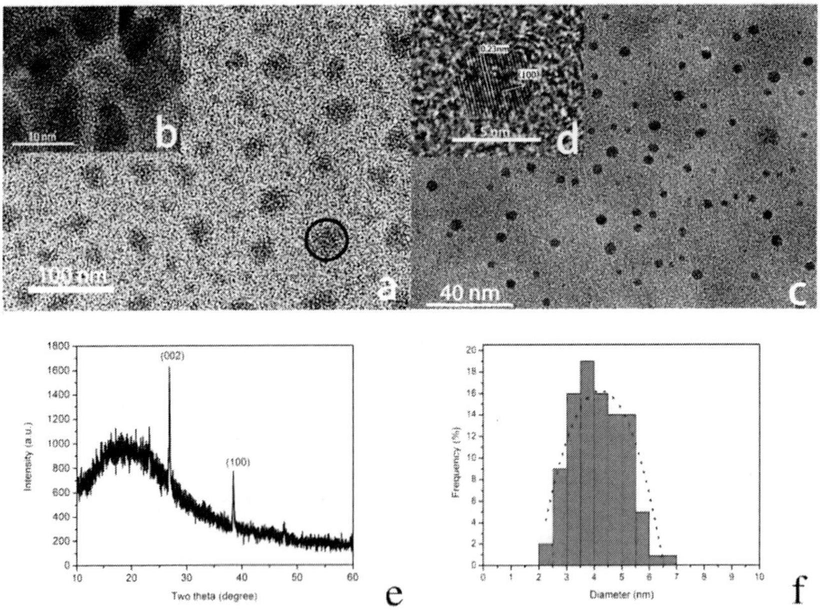

Figure 1. TEM and HR-TEM images, XRD pattern, and size distribution of RNase A@C-dots. (a) TEM image of the as-prepared RNase A@C-dots inside the dialysis membrane after dialyzing against pure water. One typical RNase A@C-dot cluster is labeled with a black circle. **(b)** High-resolution TEM (HR-TEM) image of one focused area within the black circle. **(c)** TEM image of the C-dots outside the dialysis membrane. **(d)** HR-TEM image of one single C-dot. **(e)** XRD pattern of RNase A@C-dots. **(f)** Size distribution of C-dots.

We can reasonably conclude that during the reaction process accelerated by microwave heating, RNase A capped the different numbers of C-dots that cause the different sizes of particles. When dialyzing against pure water, the smaller single particles diffused out of the dialysis membrane (MW cutoff 1,000), while the larger sized clusters remained inside the membrane. So we can collect two kinds of the relative uniform particles. In our experiments, we use the RNase A@C-dot clusters that are retained in the dialysis membrane except for special description.

As shown in Figure 1e, the XRD pattern of the RNase A@C-dot clusters has two distinctly sharp peaks at 2ϑ of approximately 27° ($d = 0.33$ nm) and approximately 39° ($d = 0.23$ nm) which can be attributed to (002) and (100) facets of graphite [30]. Notably, there is a broad peak at 2ϑ of around 20° ($d = 0.42$ nm) which is probably the reflection of the (002) facet of graphite; however, the larger interlayer spacing of 0.42 nm compared to that of bulk graphite which is about 0.33 nm might have resulted from the poor crystallization [31].

The UV–Vis absorption spectra (Figure 2a, black line) of the RNase A@C-dots feature a typical absorbance of C-dots which shows strong optical absorption in the UV region with a tail extending out into the visible range [8]. On the other hand, the absorbance peak of the pure RNase A is at approximately 275 nm as shown in Figure 2a (red line). Compared with UV–Vis absorbance peaks of C-dots (prepared by microwave synthesis using citric acid as a carbon precursor without RNase A) and the pure RNase A, there are clearly differences in UV–Vis absorption spectra. First, the absorbance peak of the C-dots (Additional file 1: Figure S2a) is at approximately 240 nm which has resulted from π-π^* transition [32], while in the absorbance spectrum of RNase A@C-dots (Figure 2a, black line), the peak shifts to approximately 260 nm which may be caused by the increasing size of RNase A@C-dots as a cluster and the synergy of RNase A and C-dots. In the TEM image of C-dots, it has shown clearly that the RNase A@C-dots are actually clusters with several C-dots capped by RNase A films. The RNase A itself did not distinctly change its UV–Vis absorption character before and after microwave treatment for 4 min (see Additional file 1: Figure S1). Second, there is a noticeable absorbance increase of RNase A@C-dots from 300 to 450 nm compared to that of C-dots which is very likely to benefit from the surface passivation by RNase A [24].

Dramatic changes have been reflected in their PL properties. The PL spectrum of RNase A@C-dots (Figure 2b) shows a clear λ_{ex} dependence of both emission wavelength and intensity just as we have reported before [8]. Specifically, as the excitation wavelength changes from 300 to 500 nm in a 20-nm increment, the PL peak shifted from 450 to 550 nm, while the intensity increases before the excitation wavelength reaches 380 nm and then gradually decreases followed by increase of excitation wavelength. However, in the PL spectra of C-dots (Additional file 1: Figure S2b), we cannot find that there is no a typical λ_{ex} dependence character. When the excitation wavelength changes from 280 to 440 nm, the PL intensity at around 480 nm varies

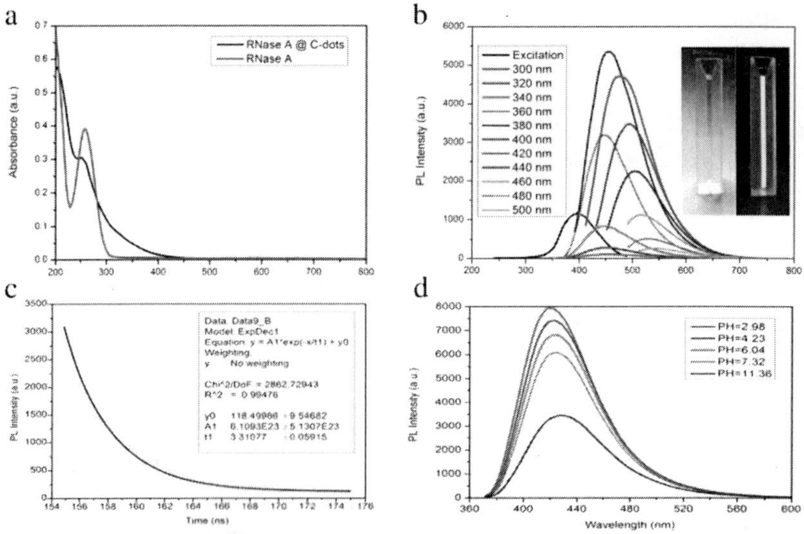

Figure 2. UV–Vis absorption and PL spectra and fluorescence decay profile of RNase A@C-dots. (a) UV–Vis absorption of the as-prepared RNase A@C-dots (black line) and RNase A treated by microwave for 4 min (red line). **(b)** PL spectra of the as-prepared RNase A@C-dots at excitation from 300 to 500 nm in 20-nm increment. Inset: image of the as-prepared RNase A@C-dot dispersion under visible light (left) and UV light (right). **(c)** Fluorescence decay profile (λ_{ex} = 380 nm, λ_{em} = 450 nm) of the as-prepared RNase A@C-dots. **(d)** The effect of the solution pH value over the fluorescence (λ_{ex} = 360 nm) of the as-prepared RNase A@C-dots.

and hits its maximum at an excitation wavelength of 380 nm. But the emission wavelength does not change its location. Moreover, before the excitation wavelength reaches 380 nm, there is more than one emission peak in the PL spectra with only one peak around 480 nm remaining when excited at 390 nm and longer wavelength. Furthermore, photoluminescence excitation (PLE) spectra of RNase A@C-dots (Figure 2b) have only one peak located at around 390 nm, while the PLE spectra of C-dots (Additional file 1: Figure S2b) owns two with an additional one around 290 nm.

The existence of RNase A has not only changed the features and locations of PL spectra but also enhanced the intensity of photoluminescence. When excited at 360 nm, the intensity of RNase

A@C-dots is about 30 times the intensity of C-dots (Additional file 1: Figure S2c). As to quantum yield, Table 1 shows that the quantum yield of the RNase A@C-dots is 24.20% which is dramatically higher than the 0.87% yield of C-dots. Even after having been passivated with PEG_{2000} which is widely accepted as an efficient way to improve the quantum yield of C-dots [8], the quantum yield of C-dots is 4.33%, still much lower than that of the RNase A@C-dots.

Table 1 Related photoluminescent quantum yield (PLQY) of RNase A@C-dots, C-dots, and C-dots-PEG $_{2000}$ (C-dots passivated by PEG $_{2000}$)

Sample	RNase A@C-dots	C-dots	C-dots-PEG_{2000}
PLQY [%]	24.20	0.87	4.33

Luminescence decay (Figure 2c) has an average excited-state lifetime of 3.3 ns for emission at 450 nm with an excitation wavelength of 380 nm which is comparable to those reported [2, 23]. The relatively short lifetime might as well suggest the radioactive recombination of the excitation contributing to the fluorescence [23].

The FTIR spectrum (Figure 3d) shows the presence of (C = O) (1,719 cm^{-1}), (O-H) (3,425 cm^{-1}), (C-N) (1,209 cm^{-1}), and (N-H) (2,994 cm^{-1}) which directly indicates Rnase A coated C-dot surface. This can also be confirmed by the X-ray photoelectron spectroscopy (XPS) of RNase A@C-dots (as shown in Figure 3a,b,c). Moreover, the high-resolution N 1 s spectrum of the RNase A@C-dots (Figure 3c) has clear signs of both amide N (399.3 eV, C-N) and doping N (400.4 eV, O = C-NH-) atoms. The XPS (Additional file 1: Figure S3) of the C-dots only shows the signals of -COOH and -OH, and neither amide N nor doping N is detected. So we may speculate that the RNase A might have played double roles in the microwave-assisted synthesis process: N doping and surface passivation. They are responsible for the enhanced PL intensity of RNase A@C-dots [33].

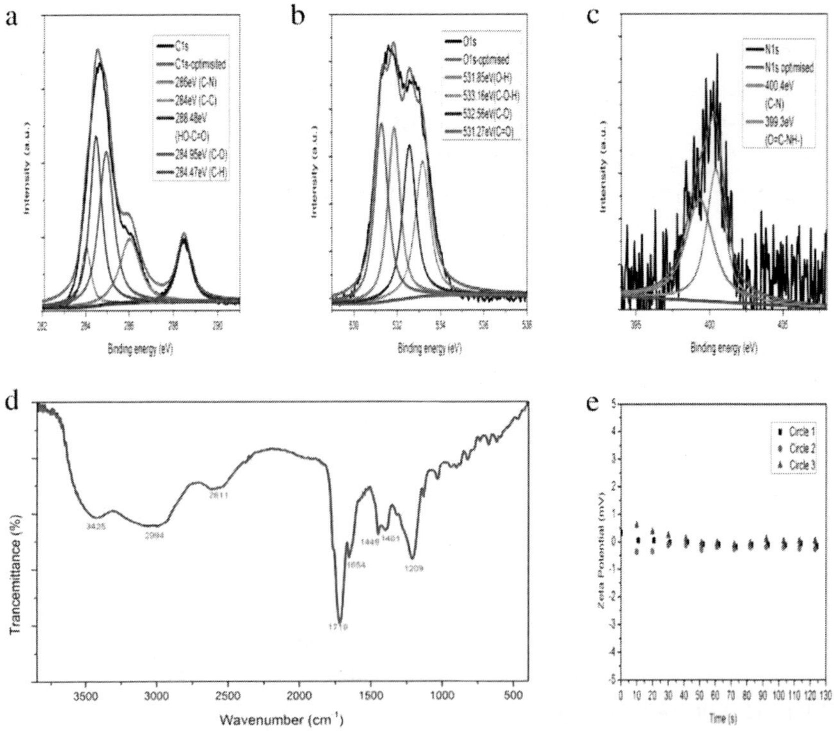

Figure 3. XPS and FTIR spectra and zeta potential. (a) XPS C 1 s spectrum. **(b)** XPS O 1 s spectrum. **(c)** XPS N 1 s of RNase A@C-dots. **(d)** FTIR spectra of RNase A@C-dots. **(e)** Zeta potential of RNase A@C-dots.

The average zeta potential of C-dots (Figure 3e) is 0.02 mV, slightly beyond zero. Considering the fact that cells are with positive charges, a zeta potential of no less than zero is definitely favorable in cell labeling and imaging. (The influence of microwave condition on PL of carbon dots was also investigated, as shown in Additional file 1: Figure S5).

Effects of pH on PL properties of RNase A@C-dots

Although the mechanism of PL properties of C-dots is still unclear and debatable, there is solid evidence of lower quantum efficiency of C-dots that is caused by the fast recombination of excitations located at surface energy traps [8]. Therefore, after modifying the surface of C-dots using different surface passivation reagents, the PL properties of the C-dots can be significantly improved [7, 8, 34]. In this work, we firstly introduce the bioactive enzyme RNase A to synthesize C-dots by one-step micro-assisted synthesis method. The mechanism of the PL enhancement could be explained by following two reasons: Firstly, we propose that the electron-donating effect which resulted from the abundant amino acid groups on the surface of RNase A, especially those amino acids with benzene rings, might contribute a lot to the much enhanced PL intensity of the C-dots. To test our assumption, we select tryptophan and thenylalanine as replacements of RNase A to synthesize C-dots in the same conditions. As shown in Additional file1: Figure S5b, both tryptophan and thenylalanine can greatly enhance the PL intensity. Secondly, we think that in the microware heating reaction, RNase A acts as a N doping reagent that causes the PL enhancement of the C-dots. The data of IR and XPS can also support the point.

In the biological application, pH is a very important factor that we firstly take into consideration. Herein, the influence of pH values over the PL of the RNase A@C-dot clusters is indicated in Figure 2d. The fact that pH values could affect the PL intensity has been seen in quite a few studies [10, 21, 32, 35]. Generally, PL intensity reaches its maximum at a certain pH values, 4.5 [35] or 7 [21]. At the same time, a slight redshift in the emission peak was identified with the increase of pH value [35]. Interestingly, the pH value played a unique role upon the PL of RNase A@C-dots. There was a noticeable redshift in the emission peak when the pH went from 2.98 to 11.36. However, the PL intensity decreases continuously as pH values increase. Specifically, the C-dots lost about 25% of its PL intensity when the pH increases from 2.98 to 7.32 and retain only 40% of its intensity when the pH value comes to 11.36. We speculate that at the lower pH condition, the RNase A coating on the surface of C-dots keeps a high activity and the RNase A-modified C-dots remain monodispersed in the water solution. Although the underlying origin is still vague, the fact that the C-dots keep its PL intensity at a relatively high level, going through the pH value from very acidic to neutral, shows promising advantages in biological applications.

Laser scanning confocal microscopy imaging in vitro

Figure 4 shows the 2D images of MGC-803 cells labeled with RNase A@C-dots. After co-incubation with RNase A@C-dots, MGC-803 cells show bright green color over the entire cell upon excitation at 405 nm.

The nuclei marked by PI, when excited at 536 nm, featured strong red fluorescence. A merge image clearly shows that the RNase A@C-dots can enter the cell via the endocytic route. Moreover, we can also find that in up to 10% cells, there are clearly green dots existing in the nucleus. Meanwhile, a 3D confocal imaging (Figure 5) of the cell clearly reveals that the RNase A@C-dots have entered the cell, while the carbon dots reported before [7] were mostly in the cytoplasm and membrane, with only minor penetration into the cell nucleus. Until now, we can give an explanation for the transportation into the nucleus. It may be caused by the small size of RNase A@C-dots which enables perfect dispersion or assists protein (derived from RNase A) action.

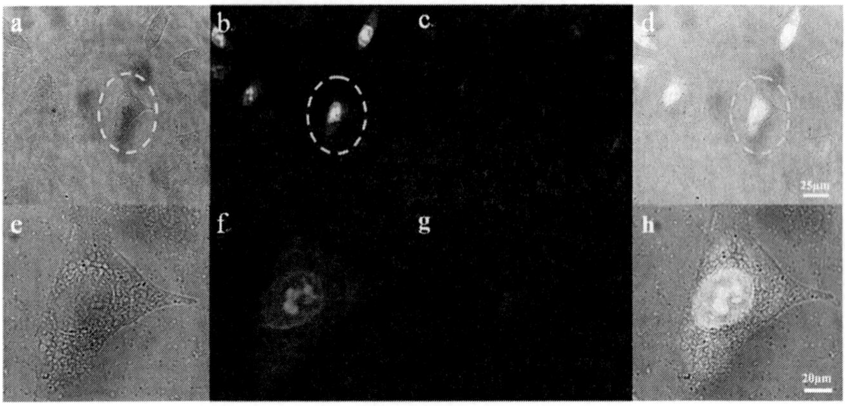

Figure 4. Laser scanning confocal microscopy images of MGC-803 cells. **(a)** Picture of MGC-803 cells under white light. **(b)**Picture of MGC-803 cells under excitation at 405 nm. **(c)** Picture of MGC-803 cells under excitation at 536 nm. **(d)**Overlapping picture of MGC-803 cells under excitation at 405 and 536 nm. **(e)** Amplified picture of a single MGC-803 cell under white light. **(f)** Amplified picture of a single MGC-803 cell under excitation at 405 nm. **(g)** Amplified picture of a single MGC-803 cell under excitation at 536 nm. **(h)** Overlapping picture of a single MGC-803 cell under excitation at 405 and 536 nm.

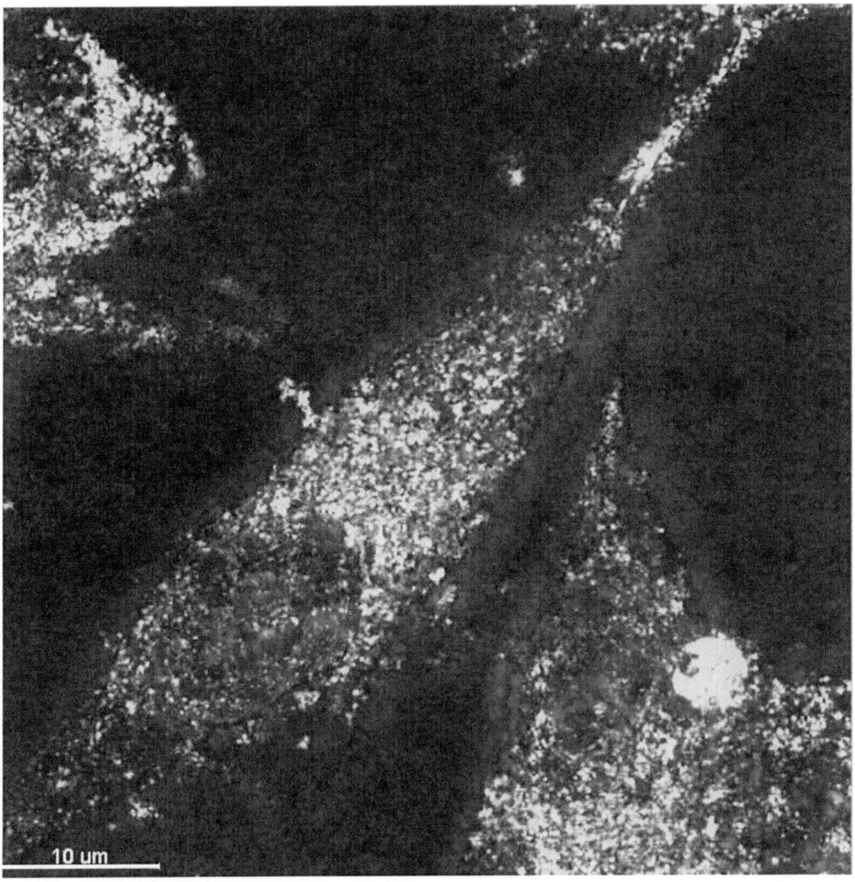

Figure 5. Laser scanning confocal microscopy images (3D mode) of MGC-803 cells.

Cytotoxicity assay by MTT and real-time cell electronic sensing

To test the potential of the RNase A@C-dots in cancer therapy, MTT assay was used to determine the cytotoxicity profile. The different concentrations of RNase A@C-dots were incubated with MGC-803 cells, respectively, for 24 h at 37°C. In control experiments, we select RNase A and C-dots to carry out accordingly the same procedure and keep equal contents of bare C-dots with RNase A@C-dot solution. The results (Figure 6a) show clearly that RNase A alone could restrain the cancerous cells due to the ribonuclease-mediated toxicity [27]. Moreover, the ability of RNase A in inhibiting the cancerous cells exhibits a content-dependent character with a relatively low cell viability (61%) at higher concentration (300 µg/ml) and a high one at lower concentration (36.5 µg/ml). Noting the fact that the bare C-dots demonstrate no cytotoxicity (cell viability 92.7%) even at the highest concentration (3,000 µg/ml), we could conclude reasonably that the low cell viability (68.5%) which resulted from C-dot treated at the same concentration comes not from the bare C-dots but from RNase A on the surface via its ribonuclease-mediated toxicity. So, by MTT assay, we have validated the potential of the RNase A@C-dots in cancer therapy.

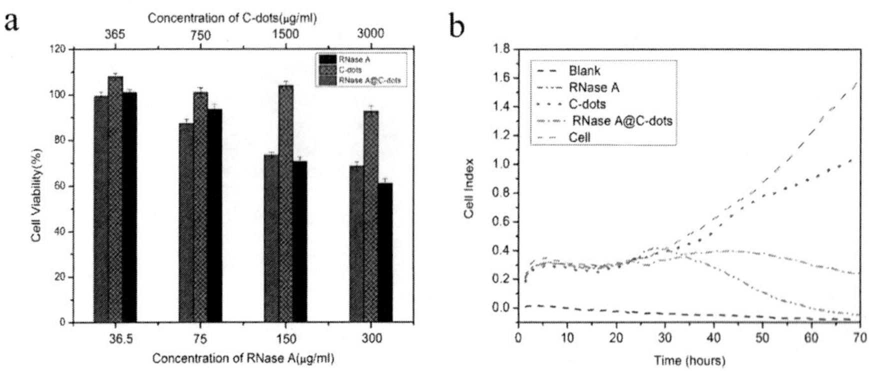

Figure 6. Cytotoxicity assay results. (a) MTT assay determined cytotoxicity profile of RNase A, C-dots, and RNase A@C-dots after 24 h incubation with MGC-803 cells at varied concentrations (sample size $N = 3$). **(b)** Dynamic monitoring cytotoxic response of MGC803 cells to RNase A, C-dots, and RNase A@C-dots.

While MTT assay only gave the information of cytotoxicity at fixed time points, the time-dependent cell response profiling was performed using real-time cell electronic sensing (RT-CES). Without cell labeling, the RT-CES assay directly reflected changes in cell biological status including cell viability, cell number, morphology, and adhesion [36]. Briefly, increasing in cell adhesion or cell spread will result in a larger cell/electrode contact area which is presented by a larger cell index (CI) value, while on the other hand, toxicity induced cells can round up leading to a smaller CI [37]. In good accordance with the MTT, RNase A (150 µg/ml) or RNase A@C-dots with the same RNase A concentration (150 µg/ml) were used based on the results of MTT assay. RNase A alone can inhibit and kill cancerous cells with a final CI value very close to zero (Figure 6b), and RNase A@C-dots also show competent ability in killing cancer cells with a CI value of around 0.2 compared to 1.8 of cells alone. In fact, RNase A and C-dots featured some differences concerning their performances. After adding of RNase A, the CI value increased a little bit in the first 4 h and then decreased continuously, while the adding of RNase A@C-dots resulted in a nearly unchanged CI value until about 50 h and then a decrease in CI value until the end. We suggest that this might have resulted from the difference of migration rate. In order to inhibit the cancerous cells, RNase A must enter cells and mount to a certain concentration. Suffering from a lower migration rate, it takes more time for RNase A@C-dots to concentrate into the cells compared to RNase A. As expected, RNase A@C-dots could hardly be considered as toxic as the CI value kept increasing at the beginning of nearly 50 h. However, after 50 h, the CI value became lower than that of the control group. This may be caused by the concentration accumulative effect of RNase A@C-dots in the cells which could have an impact over the status of the cells within an acceptable range. So it is proven that the RNase A@C-dots could kill cancerous cells with its ribonuclease-mediated toxicity from surface-doped RNase A, and not C-dots itself. However, the dose of the RNase A or RNase A@C-dots is a key factor to have an effect on the therapy, and the specific mechanism is still unclear and further study is necessary.

RNase A@C-dots for in vivo imaging of gastric cancer

As shown in Figure 7, obvious luminescence signal could be observed in the tumor after intratumoral injection. The RNase A@C-dots resulted in high contrast images and could be easily distinguished from the background. The luminescence intensity shows a clear time-dependent characteristic. Twelve hours after injection, the luminescence intensity had been dramatically decreased. This could probably be explained by the ability of carbon dots to pass the glomerulus and be excreted by urine [38].

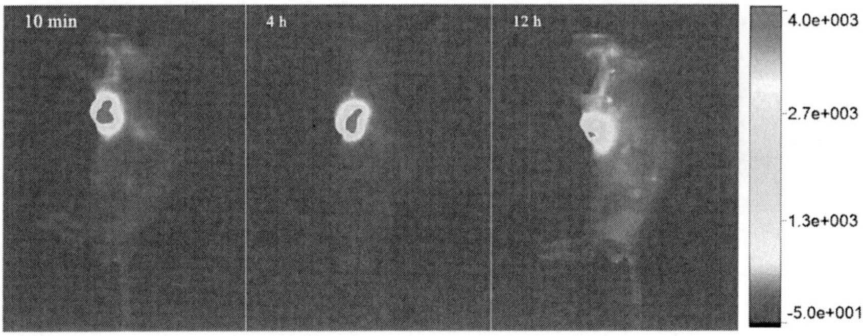

Figure 7. Representative in vivo fluorescence images of MGC-803 tumor-bearing mouse. After intratumoral injection with RNase A@C-dots after 10 min, 4 h and 12 h.

CONCLUSIONS

In summary, we have synthesized the multifunctional RNase A@C-dots particles by one-step microwave method using the biological molecule of RNase A as an assistant reagent. The RNase A@C-dots show much enhanced fluorescence intensity in contrast to bare C-dots. The quantum yield is nearly 30 times higher reaching 24.20% instead of 0.87% with a narrow Stokes shift only of approximately 80 nm. The RNase A@C-dots could not only penetrate the cell membrane but can also enter the nuclei of cells efficiently. Moreover, the RNase A@C-dots also show potential ability in inhibiting and killing cancer cells. Hopefully, the RNase A@C-dots could be used in nanodiagnostics and nanotherapeutics in the feature. But before that, the detailed mechanism which still remains vague behind the interactions between the C-dots and cancer cells should be fully understood.

ACKNOWLEDGEMENTS

This work is supported by the National Key Basic Research Program (973 Project) (No. 2011CB933100), National Natural Scientific Fund (Nos. 81225010, 81327002, 31100717 and 31170961), 863 project of China (2012AA022703), Shanghai Science and Technology Fund (Nos. 13NM1401500 and 11 nm0504200), and Shanghai Jiao Tong University Innovation Fund for Postgraduates (No. AE340011).

COMPETING INTERESTS

The authors declare that they have no competing interests.

AUTHORS' CONTRIBUTIONS

LH carried out the preparation and characterization of RNase A@C-dots and drafted the manuscript. WQ finished the MTT test. ZC finished the gastric cancer-bearing animal model preparation. LC and JW finished the RNase A@C-dots intratumor injection and imaging experiment. SG, WC, and CD designed and coordinated all the experiments. All authors read and approved the final manuscript.

REFERENCES

1. Xu X, Ray R, Gu Y, Ploehn HJ, Gearheart L, Raker K, Scrivens WA: Electrophoretic analysis and purification of fluorescent single-walled carbon nanotube fragments. *J Am Chem Soc* 2004, 126: 12736–12737.

2. Baker SN, Baker GA: Luminescent carbon nanodots: emergent nanolights. *Angew Chem Int Ed* 2010, 49: 6726–6744.

3. Li H, Kang Z, Liu Y, Lee S-T: Carbon nanodots: synthesis, properties and applications. *J Mater Chem* 2012, 22: 24230–24253.

4. Xu M, Li Z, Zhu X, Hu N, Wei H, Yang Z, Zhang Y: Hydrothermal/solvothermal synthesis of graphene quantum dots and their biological applications. *Nano Biomed Eng* 2013, 5: 65–71.

5. Wang K, Gao Z, Gao G, Wo Y, Wang Y, Shen G, Cui D: Systematic safety evaluation on photoluminescent carbon dots.*Nanoscale Res Lett* 2013, 8: 1–9.

6. Li X, Zhang S, Kulinich SA, Liu Y, Zeng H: Engineering surface states of carbon dots to achieve controllable luminescence for

solid-luminescent composites and sensitive Be2$^+$ detection. *Sci Rep* 2014, 4: 4976.

7. Sun Y-P, Luo PG, Sahu S, Yang S-T, Sonkar SK, Wang J, Wang H, Lecory GE, Cao L, Sun Y: Carbon "quantum" dots for optical bioimaging. *J Mater Chem B* 2012, 1: 2116–2127.

8. Sun Y-P, Zhou B, Lin Y, Wang W, Fernando KS, Pathak P, Meziani MJ, Harruff BA, Wang X, Wang H, Luo PG, Yang H, Kose ME, Chen B, Veca LM, Xie S: Quantum-sized carbon dots for bright and colorful photoluminescence. *J Am Chem Soc*2006, 128: 7756–7757.

9. Cao L, Wang X, Meziani MJ, Lu F, Wang H, Luo PG, Lin Y, Harruff BA, Veca LM, Murray D, Xie S, Sun Y: Carbon dots for multiphoton bioimaging. *J Am Chem Soc* 2007, 129: 11318–11319.

10. Liu R, Wu D, Liu S, Koynov K, Knoll W, Li Q: An aqueous route to multicolor photoluminescent carbon dots using silica spheres as carriers. *AngewChem Int Ed* 2009, 48: 4598–4601.

11. Shen B: Systems molecular imaging: right around the corner. *Nano Biomed Eng* 2014, 6: 1–6.

12. Yang S-T, Cao L, Luo PG, Lu F, Wang X, Wang H, Meziani MJ, Liu Y, Qi G, Sun Y: Carbon dots for optical imaging in vivo.*J Am Chem Soc* 2009, 131: 11308–11309.

13. Huang P, Lin J, Wang X, Wang Z, Zhang C, He M, Wang K, Chen F, Li Z, Shen G, Cui D, Chen X: Light–triggered theranostics based on photosensitizer–conjugated carbon dots for simultaneous enhanced–fluorescence imaging and photodynamic therapy. *Adv Mater* 2012, 24: 5104–5110.

14. Kong B, Zhu A, Ding C, Zhao X, Li B, Tian Y: Carbon dot–based inorganic–organic nanosystem for two–photon imaging and biosensing of pH variation in living cells and tissues. *Adv Mater* 2012, 24: 5844–5848.

15. Liu C, Zhang P, Zhai X, Tian F, Li W, Yang J, Liu Y, Wang H, Wang W, Liu W: Nano-carrier for gene delivery and bioimaging based

on carbon dots with PEI-passivation enhanced fluorescence. *Biomaterials* 2012, 33: 3604–3613.

16. da Silva J, Goncalves HMR: Analytical and bioanalytical applications of carbon dots. *Trac-Trends Anal Chem* 2011, 30: 1327–1336.

17. Zhou J, Booker C, Li R, Zhou X, Sham T-K, Sun X, Ding Z: An electrochemical avenue to blue luminescent nanocrystals from multiwalled carbon nanotubes (MWCNTs). *J Am Chem Soc* 2007, 129: 744–745.

18. Hu S-L, Niu K-Y, Sun J, Yang J, Zhao N-Q, Du X-W: One-step synthesis of fluorescent carbon nanoparticles by laser irradiation. *J Mater Chem* 2009, 19: 484–488.

19. Pan D, Zhang J, Li Z, Wu M: Hydrothermal route for cutting graphene sheets into blue–luminescent graphene quantum dots. *Adv Mater* 2010, 22: 734–738.

20. Yifeng E, Bai L, Fan L, Han M, Zhang X, Yang S: Electrochemically generated fluorescent fullerene[60] nanoparticles as a new and viable bioimaging platform. *J Mater Chem* 2011, 21: 819–823.

21. Liu H, Ye T, Mao C: Fluorescent carbon nanoparticles derived from candle soot. *Angew Chem Int Ed* 2007, 46: 6473–6475.

22. Bourlinos AB, Stassinopoulos A, Anglos D, Zboril R, Karakassides M, Giannelis EP: Surface functionalized carbogenic quantum dots. *Small* 2008, 4: 455–458.

23. Zhu H, Wang X, Li Y, Wang Z, Yang F, Yang X: Microwave synthesis of fluorescent carbon nanoparticles with electrochemiluminescence properties. *Chem Commun* 2009, 5: 118–5120.

24. Peng H, Travas-Sejdic J: Simple aqueous solution route to luminescent carbogenic dots from carbohydrates. *Chem Mater*2009, 21: 5563–5565.

25. Bernstein FC, Koetzle TF, Williams GJ, Meyer EF Jr, Brice MD, Rodgers JR, Kennard O, Shimanouchi T, Tasumi M: The protein

data bank: a computer-based archival file for macromolecular structures. *J MolBiol* 1977, 112: 535–542.

26. Raines RT: Ribonuclease A. *Chem Rev* 1998, 98: 1045–1066.

27. Kong Y, Chen J, Gao F, Li W, Xu X, Pandoli O, Yang H, Ji J, Cui D: A multifunctional ribonuclease–a–conjugated CdTe quantum dot cluster nanosystem for synchronous cancer imaging and therapy. *Small* 2010, 6: 2367–2373.

28. Reddi K, Holland JF: Elevated serum ribonuclease in patients with pancreatic cancer. *Proc Natl Acad Sci* 1976, 73: 2308–2310.

29. Leland PA, Schultz LW, Kim B-M, Raines RT: Ribonuclease A variants with potent cytotoxic activity. *Proc Natl Acad Sci*1998, 95: 10407–10412.

30. Lu J, Yang J-x, Wang J, Lim A, Wang S, Loh KP: One-pot synthesis of fluorescent carbon nanoribbons, nanoparticles, and graphene by the exfoliation of graphite in ionic liquids. *ACS Nano* 2009, 3: 2367–2375.

31. Zhang J, Shen W, Pan D, Zhang Z, Fang Y, Wu M: Controlled synthesis of green and blue luminescent carbon nanoparticles with high yields by the carbonization of sucrose. *New J Chem* 2010, 34: 591–593.

32. Pan D, Zhang J, Li Z, Wu C, Yan X, Wu M: Observation of pH-, solvent-, spin-, and excitation-dependent blue photoluminescence from carbon nanoparticles. *Chem Commun* 2010, 46: 3681–3683.

33. Zhai X, Zhang P, Liu C, Bai T, Li W, Dai L, Liu W: Highly luminescent carbon nanodots by microwave-assisted pyrolysis.*Chem Commun* 2012, 48: 7955–7957.

34. Tian L, Ghosh D, Chen W, Pradhan S, Chang X, Chen S: Nanosized carbon particles from natural gas soot. *Chem Mater*2009, 21: 2803–2809.

35. Zhao Q-L, Zhang Z-L, Huang B-H, Peng J, Zhang M, Pang D-W: Facile preparation of low cytotoxicity fluorescent carbon

nanocrystals by electrooxidation of graphite. *Chem Commun* 2008, 5116–5118.

36. Xing JZ, Zhu L, Jackson JA, Gabos S, Sun X-J, Wang X-b, Xu X: Dynamic monitoring of cytotoxicity on microelectronic sensors. *Chem Res Toxicol* 2005, 18: 154–161.

37. Xing JZ, Zhu L, Gabos S, Xie L: Microelectronic cell sensor assay for detection of cytotoxicity and prediction of acute toxicity. *Toxicol Vitro* 2006, 20: 995–1004.

38. Tao H, Yang K, Ma Z, Wan J, Zhang Y, Kang Z, Liu Z: In vivo NIR fluorescence imaging, biodistribution, and toxicology of photoluminescent carbon dots produced from carbon nanotubes and graphite. *Small* 2012, 8: 281–290.

Chapter 12

Inhibiting the Growth of Pancreatic Adenocarcinoma In Vitro andIn Vivo through Targeted Treatment with Designer Gold Nanotherapeutics

Rachel A. Kudgus[1], Annamaria Szabolcs[1], Jameel Ahmad Khan[1], Chad A. Walden[2], Joel M. Reid[2], J. David Robertson[3], Resham Bhattacharya[1], Priyabrata Mukherjee[1,2,4*]

[1] *Department of Biochemistry and Molecular Biology, College of Medicine, Mayo Clinic, Rochester, Minnesota, United States of America,*

[2] *Department of Physiology and Biomedical Engineering, College of Medicine, Mayo Clinic, Rochester, Minnesota, United States of America,*

[3] *Department of Chemistry and University of Missouri Research Reactor, University of Missouri, Columbia, Missouri, United States of America,*

[4] *Mayo Clinic Cancer Center, College of Medicine, Mayo Clinic, Rochester, Minnesota, United States of America*

ABSTRACT

Background

Pancreatic cancer is one of the deadliest of all human malignancies with limited options for therapy. Here, we report the development of an optimized targeted drug delivery system to inhibit advanced stage pancreatic tumor growth in an orthotopic mouse model.

Method/Principal Findings

Targeting specificity *in vitro* was confirmed by preincubation of the pancreatic cancer cells with C225 as well as Nitrobenzylthioinosine (NBMPR - nucleoside transporter (NT) inhibitor). Upon nanoconjugation functional activity of gemcitabine was retained as tested using a thymidine incorporation assay. Significant stability of the nanoconjugates was maintained, with only 12% release of gemcitabine over a 24-hour period in mouse plasma. Finally, an *in vivo* study demonstrated the inhibition of tumor growth through targeted delivery of a low dose of gemcitabine in an orthotopic model of pancreatic cancer, mimicking an advanced stage of the disease.

Conclusion

We demonstrated in this study that the gold nanoparticle-based therapeutic containing gemcitabine inhibited tumor growth in an advanced stage of the disease in an orthotopic model of pancreatic cancer. Future work would focus on understanding the pharmacokinetics and combining active targeting with passive targeting to further improve the therapeutic efficacy and increase survival.

INTRODUCTION

Pancreatic cancer is the fourth leading cause of cancer deaths in America [1]. It continues to have a less than 5% survival rate over 5 years, with a median survival of only six months [2],[3]. Pancreatic cancer is an aggressive and illusive cancer that is typically diagnosed at the late stages of the disease where surgical intervention is no longer an option and traditional chemotherapeutics have minimal therapeutic effects.

Gemcitabine is the standard of care for pancreatic cancer treatment [4]–[8]. The therapeutic efficacy of gemcitabine is governed by the triple phosphorylation within the cell by deoxycytidine kinase (dCK) to an active form; followed by subsequent intercalation into the DNA of the cell leading to the inhibition of DNA synthesis and hence, inhibition of cellular proliferation [9], [10]. Despite this being the current protocol, gemcitabine continues to have a modest beneficial outcome on its own in a clinical setting [11], [12]. There have been a number of combination therapies that utilize gemcitabine and other drugs or antibodies in an attempt to enhance the therapeutic effects of the gemcitabine, but all have shown dismal outcomes [4],[13]–[17].

Nanotechnology has the potential to overcome the limitations in current cancer therapeutic options [18]–[23]. The adverse effects of chemotherapies are an enormous problem in the current treatment of cancer in general, causing systemic toxicity leading to severe side effects. The utilization of monoclonal antibodies conjugated to gold nanoparticles has proven to be effective in targeting cancer cells with an over expression of EGFR (epidermal growth factor receptor) [24], [25]. Gold nanoparticles have been shown to be biologically viable and highly adaptable for conjugation with nearly any compound having an amine or thiol functionality utilizing Au-SH, Au-NH_2 interactions [18], [26]–[30].

In this study we utilized cetuximab, an anti-EGFR monoclonal antibody, as a targeting agent. Cetuximab was approved by the FDA for the treatment of colorectal cancer, as well as head and neck cancer in 2004 [31]–[38]. Our group previously reported the effective targeting of EGFR-overexpressing pancreatic cancer cells both *in vitro* and *in vivo* with gold nanoparticles conjugated with C225 as a targeting agent [24]. Utilizing these findings we now incorporated gemcitabine in the nanoformulation to create an optimized targeted drug delivery vehicle to inhibit the growth of pancreatic cancer cells simulating an advanced stage of the disease in an orthotopic model.

The aim of this current study was to develop a gold nanoparticle-based therapeutic with enhanced efficacy to inhibit pancreatic cancer growth in an advanced stage of the disease. The designer therapeutic introduced in this paper is a novel approach to increasing the efficacy of gemcitabine, or any chemotherapy, with the utilization of a targeted delivery system that employs gold nanoparticles as the delivery vehicle. This study was aimed to evaluate the *in vitro* and *in vivo* anti-tumor effect of a gold nanoparticle based targeted drug delivery system that inhibits pancreatic tumor growth in an advanced stage of the disease.

MATERIALS AND METHODS

Materials

Tetrachloroauric acid trihydrate and sodium borohydride were from Sigma-Aldrich, St. Louis, MO. ^{3}H-thymidine was from Perkin-Elmer, (Waltham, MA). Media and PBS was purchased from Mediatech (Manassas, VA). Scintillation cocktail was purchased from Fisher Scientific.

Synthesis and Characterization of Au-antibody and Au-antibody-gemcitabine Nanoconjugates

The core gold nanoparticles (GNPs) were synthesized by reduction of 1200 ml of 0.1 mM tetrachloroauric acid trihydrate ($HAuCl_4$) solution with 600 ml of a freshly prepared aqueous solution containing 51.6 mg of sodium borohydride ($NaBH_4$) under vigorous and constant stirring, overnight at ambient temperature. Upon addition of the sodium borohydride, the pale yellow solution becomes orange and then turns to a wine red color within minutes. The GNPs were characterized by UV-visible spectrometry, scanning from 400–800 nm and transmission electron microscopy (TEM) after drop-coating 10 μl of the sample on a 400 mesh carbon-coated copper grid followed by side blotting. The size of the nanoparticles was determined from analysis of the TEM images and Dynamic Light Scattering (DLS) (Malvern Zetasizer Nano ZS). Zeta potential measurements were done using a clear zeta disposable capillary (Malvern DTS1061).

The GNP-antibody conjugates (AC4 and AI4) were synthesized by mixing 4 μg/ml of antibody (C225 or IgG, respectively) with the core GNP solution as previously reported. Cetuximab (C225) was purchased as a solution of 2 mg/ml (Erbitux™ Injection, ImClone Inc and Bristol-Myers Squibb Co.) and whole molecule human IgG was purchased as a solution of 10.0–11.2 mg/ml (Jackson Immuno Research Laboratories, Inc.). After dilution in 1 ml of water each antibody was added dropwise to the GNP solutions. These solutions were stirred vigorously at ambient temperature for 1 hr. One half of these solutions were centrifuged at 20,000 rpm in a Beckman Ultracentrifuge in a 50.2 Ti rotor to separate AC4 and AI4 nanoconjugates from unconjugated antibody.

The other half of the solution was subjected to further conjugation with various concentrations of gemcitabine (Eli Lilly, Indianapolis, IN) to generate ACG4X and AIG4X (X = 1, 2, 4, 6 and 8 µg/ml). These solutions were also stirred vigorously at ambient temperature for 1 hr and then centrifuged at 20,000 rpm in a Beckman Ultracentrifuge in a 50.2 Ti rotor to separate ACG4X and AIG4X from unbound antibody and gemcitabine. All conjugates formed a loose pellet at the bottom of the centrifuge tube and were collected after careful aspiration of the supernatant. The gold concentration of the nanoconjugates was determined from absorbances obtained by UV-visible spectrometry (SpectraMax M5e) at 500 nm (A_{500}) and 800 nm (A_{800}), taken before and after centrifugation and by instrumental neutron activation analysis (INAA). The antibody loading was previously determined [24] and the gemcitabine concentration in the nanoconjugates was determined through high-performance liquid chromatography (HPLC) analysis of the supernatant and subtracted from the total µg added to determine the bound concentration as previously reported [25]. The size and hydrodynamic diameter of the nanoparticle conjugates was determined from analysis of the TEM images and DLS, respectively. Zeta potential measurements were done using a clear zeta disposable capillary (Malvern DTS1061).

The stability of the ACG4X and AIG4X conjugates was tested against 150 mM sodium chloride (NaCl) solution. The absorbance spectrum was taken for all nanoconjugates before and after incubation with NaCl solution for 15 minutes.

Release Study

The release profile of gemcitabine in different biological fluids was characterized following incubation of 100 µl of nanoconjugates having a gemcitabine concentration of 24.4 µg/ml with 100 µl of PBS or mouse plasma and incubated for different time periods. For a control, nanoconjugates were incubated in water, this sample was used to determine the baseline (free) gemcitabine concentration at the zero time point. The samples were centrifuged at 100,000 g for 1 hr and the supernatants were collected. The concentration of gemcitabine in the supernatants was determined by HPLC analysis. The total concentration of gemcitabine at different time points was plotted after subtracting the baseline concentration.

Cell Culture

Pancreatic cancer cell lines: AsPC-1, PANC-1 and MiaPaca-2 were grown in RPMI and Dulbecco's Modified Eagles medium (Gibco). All media was supplemented with 10% fetal bovine serum (Gibco) and 1% antibiotics (Penicillin/Streptomycin) and the cell lines were maintained at 37°C, in a humidified atmosphere under 20% O_2 and 5% CO_2.

^{3}H-thymidine Incorporation Assay

For each cell line, (3×10^4) cells were seeded in 24-well culture plates in their respective media and allowed to incubate overnight (16 hrs). After incubation for 2 hrs with ACG44, AIG44 and no gold controls at 0.1, 1 and 10 μM concentrations of gemcitabine cells were washed with PBS to remove unbound nanoconjugates and replaced with fresh media followed by additional incubation for another 48 hrs. At the end of 48-hr incubation the experiment, the media in the wells was replaced with ^{3}H-thymidine containing media (1 μCi/mL) and incubated for an additional 4 hrs at 37°C and processed for the assay as described previously [39]. Experiments were repeated at least three times, in triplicate each time, averages and standard deviations are reported.

In vitro Targeting Studies

To determine the effect of serum components on the targeting efficacy of the nanoconjugates, we preincubated AC4, AI4, ACG44 and AIG44 in RPMI containing fetal bovine serum for 15 mins. After incubation we studied cellular uptake in AsPC-1 cells in 100 mm tissue culture dishes. Both preincubated and as synthesized nanoconjugates were added to the cells in separate culture dishes and incubated at 37°C for 2 hrs. After the treatment the media was removed and the cells were washed once with PBS to remove excess nanoconjugates and trypsinized to obtain a cell pellet for gold content determination by INAA.

Inhibitor Studies

Cells were pre-treated with either C225 or NBMPR (Nitrobenzylthioinosine) to determine the specificity of uptake of ACG44 and AIG44 nanoconjugates. AsPC-1 cells were grown in 100 mm tissue culture dishes and pre-treated with either 50 µg/mL of C225 or 100 nM NBMPR for 1 hr followed by the addition of 2 µg/mL ACG44 and AIG44, respectively. After 2 hrs, the culture medium was removed, the plates were washed once with PBS to remove any unbound nanoconjugates and cells were trypsinized to obtain a cell pellet to determine gold content by INAA.

Measurement of Gold Content by Instrumental Neutron Activation Analysis (INAA)

Samples were analyzed by instrumental neutron activation analysis at the University of Missouri Research Reactor Center as previously described [24], [25], [40]–[43]. Briefly, cell pellets/tissues were prepared by weighing the samples into high-density polyethylene irradiation vials and lyophilized to a dry weight. Solution samples were prepared by gravimetrically transferring 100 µl to an irradiation vial followed by lyophilization. All samples were loaded in polyethylene transfer "rabbits" in sets of nine and irradiated for 90 sec in a thermal flux density of approximately 5×10^{13} n cm^{-2} s^{-1}. The samples were then allowed to decay for 24 to 48 hrs and counted on a high-purity germanium detector for 3600 sec at a sample-to-detector distance of approximately 5 cm. The mass of gold in each sample was quantified by measuring 411.8 keV gamma ray from the β^- decay of ^{198}Au ($t_{1/2} = 2.7$ days). The area of this peak was determined by the Genie ESP spectroscopy package from Canberra. A minimum of six geometrically equivalent comparator standards were also run. The standards were prepared by aliquoting approximately 0.1 (n = 3) and 0.01 (n = 3) µg of gold from a (10.0±0.5) µg/mL certified standard solution (High-Purity Standards) in the polyethylene irradiation vials, and were used with each sample set.

Transmission Electron Microscopy (TEM)

TEM samples (cell pellets and tissues) were fixed in trumps solution and processed as previously described [24]. Micrographs were taken on a TECNAI 12 operating at 120 KV.

Animal Handling and in vivo Tumor Uptake

Male athymic nude mice (NCr-nu; 4–6 weeks old) were purchased from the National Cancer Institute-Frederick Cancer Research and Development Center (Frederick, MD). All mice were housed and maintained under specific pathogen-free conditions in facilities approved by the American Association for Accreditation of Laboratory Animal Care and in accordance with current regulations and standards of the U.S. Department of Agriculture, U.S. Department of Health and Human Services, and NIH. All studies were approved and supervised by the Mayo Clinic Institutional Animal Care and Use Committee.

For the generation of orthotopic pancreatic tumor models, before injection, tumor cells were washed twice with PBS, lifted with 0.25% trypsin, centrifuged for 5 minutes, and reconstituted in PBS. AsPC-1 cells (1.5×10^6) were implanted into the pancreas of nude mice. The mice were imaged non-invasively every week under isoflurane anesthesia using a Xenogen-IVIS-cooled CCD optical system (Xenogen-IVIS) as previously described [24]. Seven days after tumor cell implantation, the mice were randomized into 6 groups (n = 5). All nanoconjugates were normalized to a gold concentration of 450 μg/mouse (1.8 mg/kg of gemcitabine) and injected i. p. thrice for week one and twice for weeks two and three. The mice were sacrificed on day 28 and the tumors, kidneys, liver, lungs, spleen, pancreas and blood were collected and analyzed for gold content through INAA.

Immunohistochemistry

Tumor samples were fixed in 4% paraformaldehyde and stained for hemotoxylin and eosin (H&E) and Ki-67. The percentage of Ki-67 positive cells in 5 high-powered fields at 20X was determined through visual inspection and counting.

Statistical Analysis

Statistical analysis was done by a two-tailed student t-test and a value of $P<0.05$ was considered to be significant.

RESULTS AND DISCUSSION

Synthesis and Characterization of Gold Nanoparticles and Nanoconjugates

Physicochemical characterization of the unmodified GNPs and the nanoconjugates were performed by UV-visible spectroscopy (UV-vis), transmission electron microscopy (TEM), dynamic light scattering (DLS) and zeta potential (ζ-Potential) measurements.

The UV-visible spectrum of unmodified GNPs exhibits a characteristic surface plasmon resonance (SPR) band of spherical gold nanoparticle at 512 nm as previously reported [24],[25]. Addition of an anti-EGFR antibody cetuximab (C225), or its non-targeted counterpart immunoglobulin G (IgG) at a concentration of 4 µg/ml to the GNP solution increases the absorbance of the solution with a simultaneous red shift in the λ_{max} value from 512 nm of unmodified GNP to 518 nm for Au-C225 (AC4) and Au-IgG (AI4) conjugates [24], [25], respectively. Such a red shift in the SPR band suggests binding of C225 and IgG to the GNP surface as previously reported [24], [44]. The rationale for selecting a concentration of 4 µg/ml of C225/IgG was based on our previous report where we demonstrated that the AC4 conjugates have the highest ability to target EGFR-overexpressing pancreatic cancer cells both *in vitro* and *in vivo* in an orthotopic pancreatic cancer model [24]. Based on this information, we next designed a targeted drug delivery system with the incorporation of gemcitabine (Gem) on the AC4 and AI4 nanoconjugates. The addition of different concentrations of gemcitabine (1, 2, 4, 6, and 8 µg/ml) to the AC4 and AI4 solutions caused a further red-shift in the λ_{max} from 518 nm to 520 nm for the ACGs and AIGs, suggesting binding of gemcitabine to the available reactive surface on the gold nanoparticle (Figures S1A,B).

Stability of the nanoconjugates in 150 mM sodium chloride (NaCl) further supports the binding of both C225/IgG and gemcitabine on the GNPs. It is evident from Figure 1A and B that the addition of 150 mM NaCl to unmodified GNPs shifted the λ_{max} from 512 nm to 562 nm with a strong decrease in absorbance, suggesting significant aggregation of uncovered GNPs by NaCl in the absence of surface protection by C225/IgG and Gem. However, the addition of NaCl to the ACGs and AIGs did not alter the absorbance and λ_{max} value, thereby confirming the stabilization of GNPs by conjugation with C225/IgG and gemcitabine.

TEM analysis further confirms the absence of aggregation as well as the formation of ~5 nm spherical nanoparticles (Figure 1C, D). Dynamic light scattering and zeta potential results were used to further characterize the hydrodynamic diameter (HD) as well as the charge of the particles at each step of conjugation (Table 1 and Table S1).

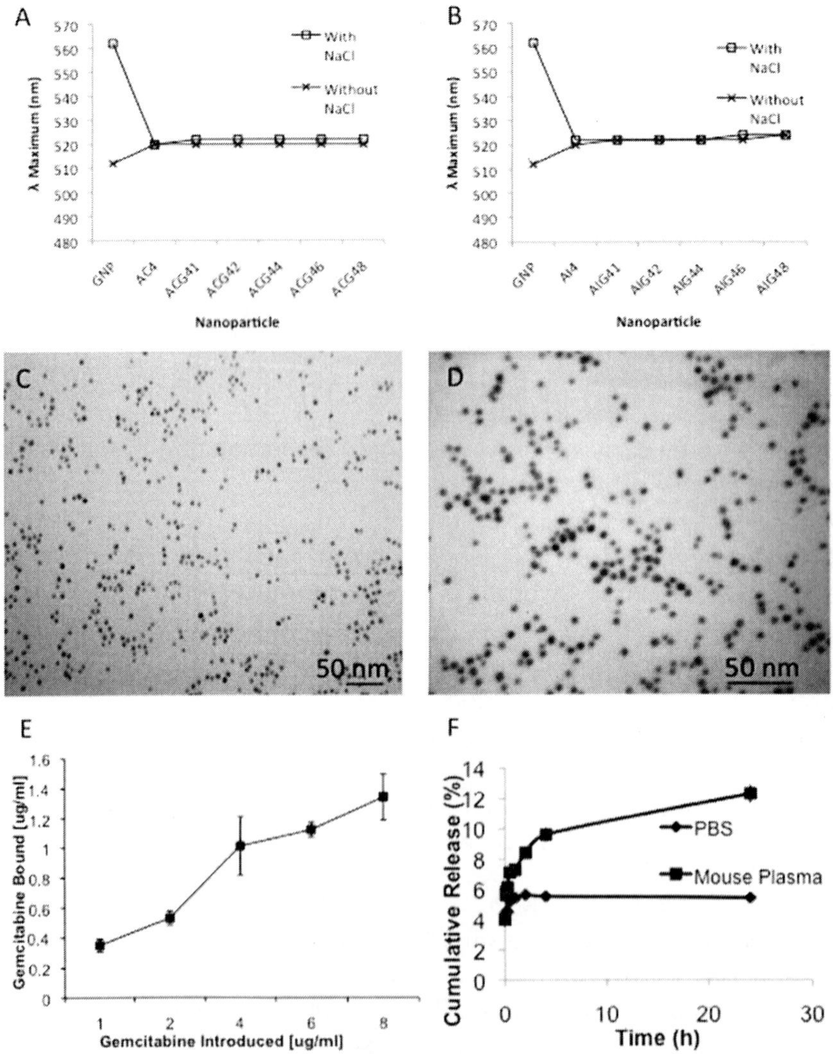

Figure 1. Physicochemical characterization of gold nanoconjugates.

Figure 1A and 1B describes the changes in the λ_{max} value of GNP and different ACG44 and AIG44 nanoconjugates, respectively, with/without incubation with NaCl for 15 minutes. Figure 1C and 1D exhibits the transmission electron micrographs (TEM) of ACG44 and AIG44 nanoconjugates, drop coated after synthesis without alteration.Figure 1E describes the amount of gemcitabine bound to AC4 nanoconjugates analyzed by HPLC; the x-axis shows the µg/ml used to synthesize the conjugates and the y-axis represents the µg/ml bound to the particle. Figure 1F describes the release of gemcitabine from ACG44 nanoconjugates when incubated in PBS and mouse plasma over time.

Table 1. Dynamic Light Scattering and Zeta Potential Measurements of GNP (the core particle), ACG44 and AIG44.

Sample	DLS (d.nm)	Zeta Potential (mV)
GNP*	5.3	−29.6
ACG44	32.09	−20.2
AIG44	88.95	−20.6

A MELVERN Zetasizer Nano ZS instrument was used to measure both the DLS and ζ-Potentials of all the nanoconjugates. The average of 5 independent runs is presented in Table 1. As expected, the HD increases from 5 nm for the unmodified GNP, to approximately 38 nm for AC4 and 56 nm for AI4, further demonstrating the binding of C225 and IgG to GNP. The addition of gemcitabine, at all concentrations does not alter the HD of the nanoconjugates; this observation was expected due to the small molecule size of gemcitabine. The ζ-potential measurements also followed a similar trend; as expected, the GNP was most negative, with an average of approximately −30 mV. The ζ-Potential starts to become less negative with the addition of C225 and IgG due to the antibody binding. In turn, there is a minor increase in ζ-potential with the addition of gemcitabine. These results clearly suggest the binding of C225/IgG and gemcitabine to the nanoparticle to form ACGs and AIGs.

Quantifying the Gemcitabine Loading on AC4 and AI4

Using varying concentrations of ^{125}I-labeled C225 and IgG we previously demonstrated that nearly 90% of 4 μg/ml antibody was bound to the GNP [24]. To determine the loading of gemcitabine on AC4 and AI4, gemcitabine was added to the antibody covered particles in various concentrations (X = 1, 2, 4, 6 and 8 μg/ml) under vigorous stirring at room temperature. After one hour, the nanoconjugates containing gemcitabine were purified by ultracentrifugation. The ACG4X and AIG4X pellets were collected at the bottom of the centrifuge tubes and the supernatant, containing the unbound gemcitabine was analyzed using HPLC. The bound fraction was calculated by subtracting the concentration of gemcitabine present in the supernatant from the original concentration introduced during the nanofabrication process. The concentration of bound gemcitabine increases from approximately 0.4 to 1 μg/ml for the ACG4X particles with the introduction of 1–4 μg/ml (Figure 1E). However, the addition of 6 and 8 μg/ml of gemcitabine does not significantly increase the amount gemcitabine in the nanoconjugate. Therefore, the optimum conjugation reaction with the highest percent yield for gemcitabine bound to the particle was determined to be 4 μg/ml. As expected, the AIG4X particles showed a similar trend for gemcitabine binding (data not shown). Subsequently, the ACG44 and AIG44 nanoconjugates were employed for all further experiments.

The ACG44 and AIG44 nanoconjugates were synthesized using the AC4 and AI4 solutions, respectively, as described in the materials and methods section. This synthesis was possible due to the spontaneous binding of the antibodies through their cysteine/lysine residues utilizing the Au-S/Au-NH_2 bond as previously described [24]. It has been well described in the literature that interactions of proteins, antibodies and small molecules with gold could be due to electrostatics, covalent bonding or hydrophobic interactions. The addition of gemcitabine exploits the Au-NH_2 binding through the amine moiety on gemcitabine to the gold particle surface. Our previous data suggests the initial binding is due to electrostatics and then covalent, investigated with XPS and TGA analysis and previously reported by our group [25],[45].

Mechanism and Targeting Efficacy of ACG44 and AIG44 in vitro

Studies were performed to ascertain the targeting efficacy of C225 and the functional activity of gemcitabine in the nanoconjugated form against various pancreatic cancer cell lines *in vitro*. The targeting experiments were performed in two ways to address the role of serum components on targeting efficacy; (i) the nanoconjugates were preincubated with cell growth media for 15 minutes before adding to the cells in tissue culture dishes; (ii) as synthesized nanoconjugates were directly added to the cells in tissue culture dishes. It is evident from theFigure 2A and Figure S2 that the addition of C225/IgG increases the absorbance of the GNPs followed by a red shift in the λ_{max}. Subsequent addition of gemcitabine further shifts the λ_{max}while simultaneously increasing the absorbance, suggesting binding of both the components to the GNPs. Interestingly, preincubation with cell growth media decreases the absorbance of all the nanoconjugates probably due to the formation of a protein corona around the GNPs [46]. Additionally, TEM analysis showed efficient intracellular uptake of the ACG44 nanoconjugates in AsPC-1 cells (Figure 2B) and no significant aggregation of the particles in the presence of serum was observed (Figure S3) further supporting the formation of protein-corona after pre-incubation with the serum.

Figure 2A depicts the absorbance spectrums of GNP, AC4 and ACG44 before and after pre-incubation with serum either 15 minutes at room temperature or 2 hrs at 37°C.Figure 2B and 2D are transmission electron microscopy images of the *in vitro* uptake of ACG44 and AIG44 in AsPC-1 cells, respectively. Figure 2C describes the effect of pre-incubation with serum on the cellular uptake of the nanoconjugates into AsPC-1 cells analyzed for gold content utilizing INAA. Figure 2E also depicts INAA analysis of cellular uptake of ACG44 and AIG44 in AsPC-1 cells, both with/without pre-incubation with C225 or NBMPR to demonstrate possible uptake mechanisms. Figure 2F shows the anti-proliferative effect of ACG44, AIG44 and CG44 on AsPC-1 cells determined through ^{3}H-thymidine incorporation.

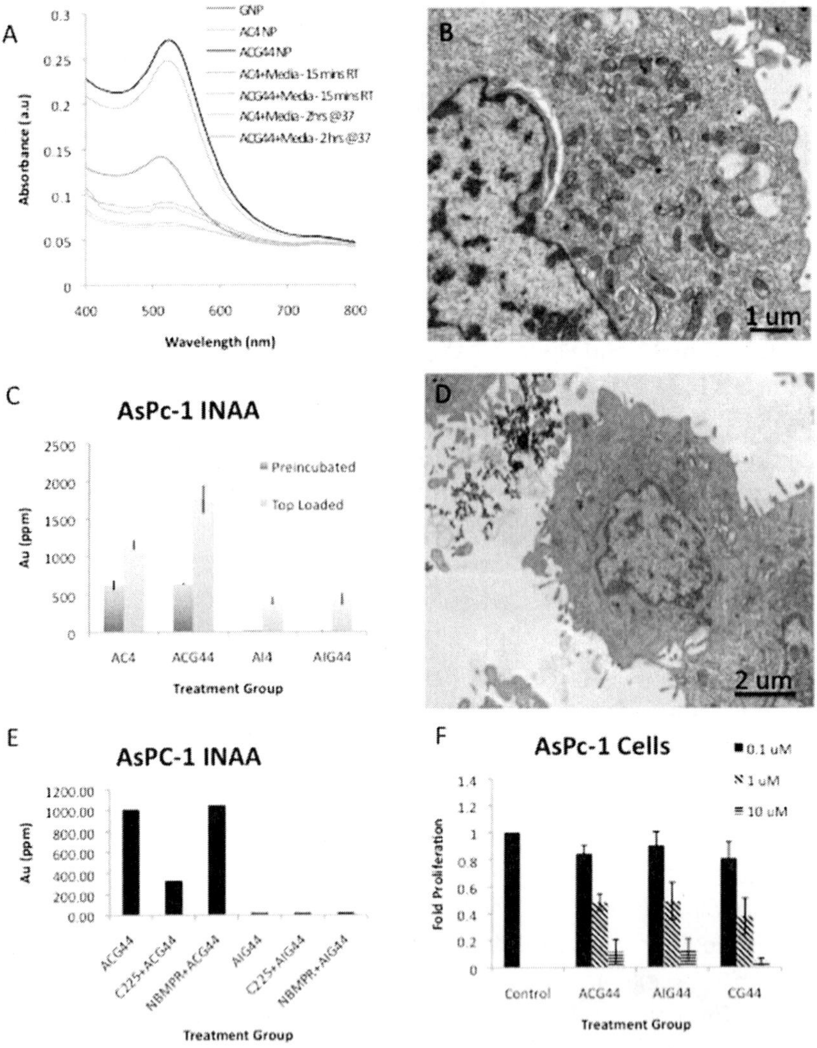

Figure 2. Role of pre-incubation with serum, C225 and NBMPR on targeting efficacy of gold nanoconjugates and their *in vitro* biological function.

The effect of preincubation on the intracellular uptake of different nanoconjugates (AC4, ACG44, AI4 and AIG44) with AsPC-1 cells *in vitro* was determined. Uptake efficiency was determined by measuring the gold content in the cell pellet through INAA analysis (Figure 2C). It is evident from the Figure that AC4 and ACG44 are far more effective in targeting AsPC-1 cells than AI4 and AIG44. It is also interesting to note that cellular uptake of ACG44 is higher than AC4. This enhanced uptake of ACG44 could be due to the presence of gemcitabine, mediating uptake through nucleoside transporters (NTs), or due to an alternative path because of the available reactive surface area on gold nanoparticles. The non-specific uptake appears to be minimized after preincubation, which could be due to the coating of serum components on the available gold surface. Non-specific uptake of AI4 and AIG44 was completely inhibited by preincubation with the cell growth media. These data clearly suggest that C225 retains its specific targeting ability to EGFR-expressing cancer cells *in vitro*. The ability of C225 in the nanoconjugated form to effectively target EGFR over-expressing AsPC-1 cells was further confirmed by preincubation with C225. Preincubating AsPC-1 cells with C225 greatly diminished the uptake of ACG44, whereas there was no intracellular uptake of AIG44. These results further confirm that the endocytosis of ACG44 is via the EGFR pathway. Similarly, no difference in intracellular uptake was observed when cells were pre-treated with a nucleoside transporter blocker (NBMPR) [47]–[49], suggesting the absence of nucleoside transporter mediated uptake of the nanoconjugates (Figure 2E).

Testing Functional Activity of Gemcitabine in the Nanoconjugated Form with Various Pancreatic Cancer Cell Lines in vitro

We utilized three different pancreatic cancer cell lines, AsPC-1, PANC-1 and MiaPaca-2, all having variable EGFR expression, to test whether the activity of gemcitabine had been retained in the nanoconjugated form. It is evident from the Figures that ACG44, AIG44 and CG44 (a no gold control containing gemcitabine and C225) substantially inhibited proliferation of pancreatic cancer cells in a concentration dependent manner as determined by ^{3}H-thymidine assays. It is also apparent from the Figure that maximum inhibition of AsPC-1 cells was observed at the highest dose of both ACG44 and AIG44, which is comparable to the same dose of C225 and gemcitabine in the no gold control, CG44. A similar trend was observed with PANC-1 and MiaPaca-2 cells (Figure 2F and Figure S4). These results clearly demonstrate that gemcitabine retains its functional activity in the nanoconjugated form.

Stability of the Nanoconjugates in Biological Fluids

It is important to test the stability of the nanoconjugates in biological fluids before *in vivo*applications. The stability of the nanoconjugates in terms of gemcitabine release was performed in phosphate buffered saline (PBS) and in mouse plasma. It is evident from theFigure 1F that the ACG44 nanoconjugates are very stable both in PBS (only 5% of bound gemcitabine is released over a period of 24 hrs) as well as in mouse plasma (~12% of gemcitabine released over a period of 24 hrs). Furthermore, for future clinical application it is important to determine the stability of the nanoconjugates after long-term storage. To address this concern, we flash froze the nanoconjugates in liquid nitrogen and lyophilized them to a powder form. The powder was easily reconstituted in water, with no noticeable aggregation observed upon visual inspection. The solution was then tested for functional efficacy to inhibit the proliferation of AsPC-1 cells. Similar inhibition in proliferation of pancreatic cancer cells was observed by the reconstituted nanoconjugates, confirming the stability of the nanoconjugates under long-term storage conditions (Figure S5).

Therapeutic Efficacy of the Nanoconjugates to Inhibit Tumor Growth in an Orthotopic Model of Pancreatic Cancer

To test the therapeutic efficacy of the nanoconjugates to inhibit tumor growth *in vivo*, we generated an orthotopic model of pancreatic cancer by implanting 2×10^6 AsPC-1 cells directly into the pancreas of 4–6 week old nude male mice. To simulate an advanced stage of the disease, tumors were allowed to grow for 7 days before initiation of the treatment (Figure 3A). One week after the tumor cell implantation, the mice were imaged non-invasively through bioluminescence for tumor growth and randomized into 6 groups (n =5) before initiation of the treatment. The animals were injected in the intraperitoneal (i.p.) cavity thrice a week for the first week and twice for the next two weeks with 450 μg of gold nanoconjugates, 1.8 mg/kg of gemcitabine. The tumor progression was monitored non-invasively once a week with bioluminescence imaging as discussed above (Figure 3B). Bioluminescence measurements clearly demonstrate a significant reduction of tumor growth in ACG44 group as compared to the other groups. As expected, AC4 and AI4 had the least effect on decreasing the tumor growth while the AIG44 and CG44 groups had a moderate response due to the presence of gemcitabine. These observations were further confirmed by directly measuring tumor weight and volume after sacrificing the mice at the end of the experiment (Figure 3C and D). The ACG44 group showed the tightest cluster of data points as well as the highest therapeutic effect of all groups with an average tumor mass of 0.3 grams and tumor volume of 275 cm^3(0.55 g and 940 cm^3 for the PBS group). Likewise, this therapeutic effect was also shown in the tumor gold content for the ACG44 group (Figure 3E). Further TEM analysis confirmed the uptake of ACG44 into the tumor tissue (Figure 3F), also show AIG44 internalization in Figure S7. Additionally, the biodistribution of gold in the liver, lungs, kidneys and spleen was also analyzed with INAA (Figure S6). As expected, the organs with the greatest uptake of gold were the spleen and the liver in all of the treatment groups. These results were further confirmed at the molecular level by quantifying the number of proliferating cells in different treatment groups using hematoxilin-eosin (H&E) and Ki-67 staining (Figure 4). Figure 4 exhibits H&E and Ki-67 for tumor tissue from the PBS (4A and B) and ACG44 groups (Figure 4C and D), respectively. The number of cancer cells as demonstrated by H&E staining are far less in ACG44 group than in the control PBS group. Furthermore, the number of proliferating cell nuclei as demonstrated by Ki-67 staining, is significantly decreased (~60%) in the ACG44 group as opposed to the control PBS group (Figure 4E). Interestingly, treatment with ACG44 also revealed the presence of gold nanoparticles in the form of black specs inside the tumor tissue, suggesting better tumor penetration with the ACG44 nanoconjugates compared to the other groups. Additionally, it is evident from Figure 4 that the number of Ki-67 positive cells is greatly diminished surrounding the nanoparticles, suggesting a better therapeutic effect correlating with proximity to the nanoparticles. Taken together, these data indicate that the targeted delivery of a low dose of gemcitabine via gold nanoparticles can significantly inhibit the tumor growth in an advanced model of orthotopic pancreatic cancer *in vivo*.

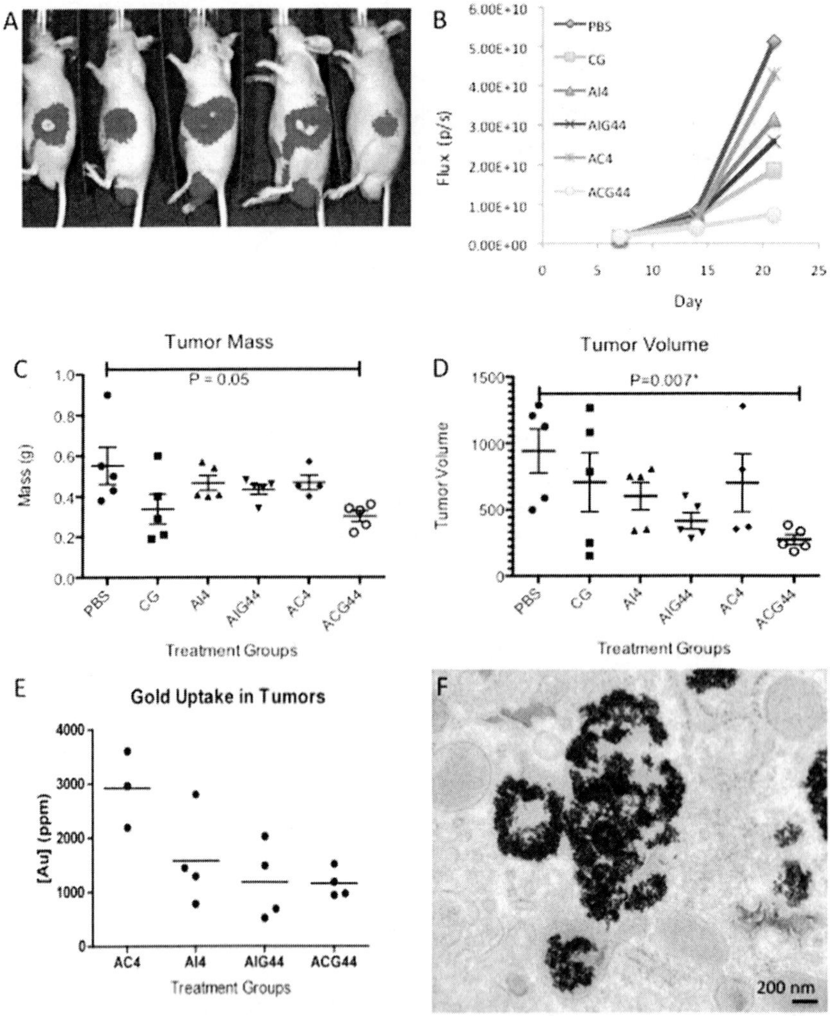

Figure 3. *In vivo* effects of gold nanoconjugates in an orthotopic model of pancreatic cancer.

Figure 3A shows a representative bioluminescence image of 5 mice, 7 days after orthotopic implantation of AsPC-1 cells into the pancreas. Figure 3B is flux quantification from the bioluminescence imaging taken every 7 days. Figure 3C, 3D and 3E all show scatter plots of tumor analysis of each animal per group, post study termination. Figure 3C shows tumor mass, 3D shows tumor volume determined through caliper measurements and 3E shows total gold uptake in each tumor determined by INAA. Figure 3F is a TEM micrograph showing ACG44 conjugates in a cross section of tumor tissue.

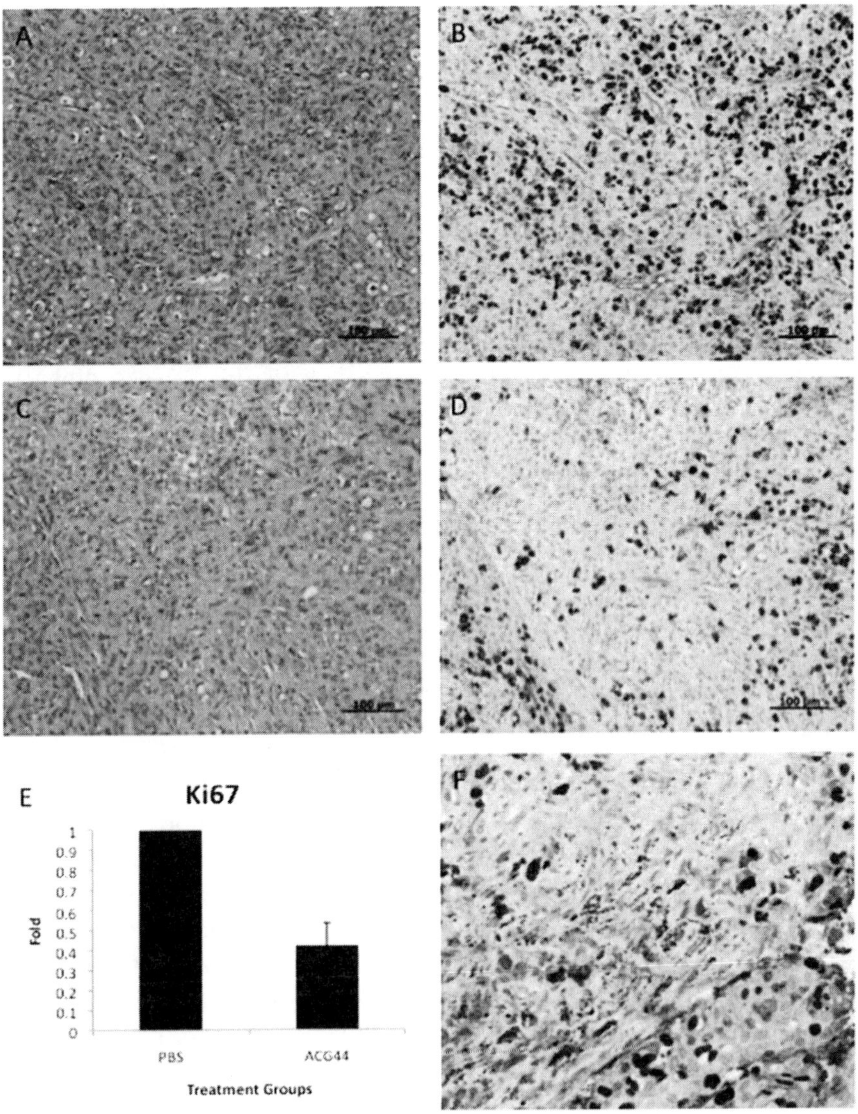

Figure 4. Immunohistochemistry Analysis of Tumors from the PBS and ACG44 groups.

Figure 4A and 4B show representative images of H&E and Ki-67 stained tumor tissues, respectively, from the PBS treated group whereas Figure 4C and 4D show images of H&E and Ki-67 staining of tumor tissue from the ACG44 treated group. All images were taken with 20× magnification. Figure 4E is quantification of the Ki-67 positive proliferative nuclei shown in Figures 4B and 4D. Figure 4F is a tumor image of Ki-67 staining from the ACG44 treated group, taken at 100 X to show gold accumulation (black spots) at a high magnification.

DISCUSSION

Pancreatic cancer is one of the deadliest among human malignancies with no effective therapies currently available [11], [15]. Pancreatic cancer is typically detected in the late stage of the disease and the overall survival from this late diagnosis is commonly just a few months[1]. Surgery is the only option when detected early and gemcitabine is the front line chemotherapy for the advanced stage of the disease. However, chemotherapy with gemcitabine has only a limited therapeutic effect due to severe dose limiting toxicity. Thus, the overall survival is only 5–6 months. For this reason, effective therapeutic strategies are urgently required to combat this deadly disease. Therefore, any approach that will reduce the systemic toxicity and increase the efficacy of gemcitabine will have a significant impact on the therapeutic management of pancreatic cancer.

It has been recently recognized that nanotechnology has great potential to improve the quality of lives of cancer patients [22], [50], [51]. Major areas where nanotechnology can impact significantly in cancer are; i) Detection/diagnosis; (ii) Imaging and (iii) Therapeutics [52], [53]. Specifically, targeted drug delivery could significantly impact the therapeutic management of cancer by increasing the efficacy and reducing systemic toxicity of many chemotherapeutics. Development of a nanoparticle formulation to effectively target tumors is an area of active investigation. Among the inorganic nanomaterials, gold nanoparticles have generated considerable interest in various biomedical applications including targeting [27]. Several advantages that GNPs have over other nanomaterials are; (i) ease of synthesis; (ii) ease of characterization due to the presence of the SPR band; (iii) ease in binding of biomolecules such as peptides, proteins and antibodies exploiting the gold-thiol, gold-amine interactions and most importantly, (iv) biocompatibility compared to other inorganic nanomaterials currently being investigated [30], [54]–[57]. Previously we demonstrated that the targeted delivery of a low dose of gemcitabine using cetuximab bound to a gold nanoparticle in a "2 in 1" fashion resulted in significant inhibition of tumor growth at an early stage of an orthotopic model of pancreatic cancer [25]. EGFR is overexpressed in a number of human malignancies. The FDA approved cetuximab, an anti-EGFR antibody, for the use alone or in combination therapies to treat various malignancies. Therefore, the successful development of a targeted drug delivery system containing C225, gemcitabine and gold nanoparticles could be widely applicable to a variety of malignancies including pancreatic cancer. Recently, we defined the design criteria to effectively target pancreatic cancer cells in an orthotopic model of pancreatic cancer *in vivo*[24]. Based on this prior work, we report here the design of an optimized targeted drug delivery system that inhibits pancreatic tumor growth in an advanced stage of the disease in an orthotopic model.

The binding of C225 and gemcitabine to the gold nanoconjugates was demonstrated by an increase in absorbance and a red shift of the absorption maxima in the SPR band of gold nanoparticles. These findings were further confirmed by stability testing in 150 mM NaCl. Uncovered nanoparticles undergo rapid aggregation in the presence of high salt concentration. However, such aggregation is prevented through surface coverage of the gold nanoparticles by a combination of cetuximab and gemcitabine.

Gemcitabine, being a purine nucleoside requires nucleoside transporters, such as human equilibrative nucleoside transporters (hENT) or concentrative nucleoside transporters (hCNT) for intracellular uptake [58]–[61]. Therefore, ACG44 may be taken up by the cells either via EGFR endocytosis through active targeting with C225 or via nucleoside transporters (NTs). In general, nanoconjugates having C225 exhibit much higher cellular uptake compared to nanoconjugates having the non-targeting antibody, IgG. Furthermore, preincubating pancreatic cancer cells that overexpress EGFR, such as AsPC-1, with C225 significantly reduces the uptake of ACG44 nanoconjugates, while the uptake of AIG44 remains unaffected. Additionally, treatment with a NT inhibitor, NBMPR, does not reduce the uptake of either of the nanoconjugates. Together, these results support the conclusion that

ACG44 enters into the cells through EGFR mediated endocytosis and that NTs do not contribute significantly to the uptake of the nanoconjugates. These findings could prove beneficial in combating gemcitabine resistance in cancer cells with a low expression of NTs. It is also important to note that preincubating the nanoconjugates in serum, decreases the uptake of both AC4 and ACG44, suggesting the adsorption of serum proteins blocks the available reactive surface on the gold particle and thereby increases the specificity of targeting. Likewise, preincubation of AI4 and AIG44 in serum reduced the intracellular uptake, presumably by blocking the available surface area on the gold particle that is involved in non-specific uptake. The fact that AI4 and AIG44 uptake is reduced to a non-detectable level, further confirms the targeting specificity of AC4 and ACG44.

Stability of the nanoconjugates under the physiological salt concentrations (150 mM NaCl) and in biological fluids (PBS and mouse plasma) demonstrates the suitability of these nanoconjugates for *in vivo* use. Only 12% of gemcitabine was released over a 24 hr period in mouse plasma. Previously, we demonstrated a similar amount of C225 released under various physiological environments [24].

Finally, the efficacy of the nanoconjugates *in vivo* in an aggressive orthotopic model of pancreatic cancer was demonstrated. It is important to note here, that treatments in many studies are typically initiated in this model on day 3 or 4 after tumor cell implantation in the pancreas. However, to simulate an advanced stage of the disease, we allowed the tumor cells to grow in the pancreas for 7 days before initiating the treatment. Typically, all the animals would die in a model like this within 3–4 weeks of implantation. However, our *in vivo* data clearly demonstrate that a low dose of gemcitabine delivered in a targeted fashion significantly reduced the tumor growth in this advanced stage model. This study highlights the potential of a gold nanoparticle based targeted drug delivery system to inhibit tumor growth in a orthotopic model of pancreatic cancer in advanced stage of the disease.

CONCLUSION

In conclusion, we demonstrated that a low dose of gemcitabine delivered in the form of a targeted drug delivery system inhibits tumor growth in an advanced stage of an orthotopic model of pancreatic cancer. Using different cellular uptake path inhibitors we demonstrated that the uptake of the nanoconjugates is specific to the EGFR pathway. We also demonstrated significant stability of the nanoconjugates under different biological environments, as well as long-term stability of the nanoconjugates after lyophilization and storage. The potential impact of this study to inhibit pancreatic tumor growth at the advanced stage is significant, as no therapy is currently available for this deadly disease. Future work will focus on further improving the therapeutic efficacy, understanding the pharmacokinetics and combining active targeting with passive targeting.

AUTHOR CONTRIBUTIONS

Conceived and designed the experiments: RB JMR PM. Performed the experiments: RK AS JAK JDR CW. Analyzed the data: RK AS JAK JDR CW RB JMR PM. Contributed reagents/materials/analysis tools: JMR JDR. Wrote the paper: RK AS JAK JDR CW RB JMR PM.

REFERENCES

1. Jemal A, Siegel R, Xu J, Ward E (2010) Cancer statistics, 2010. CA Cancer J Clin 60: 277–300.

2. Shore S, Vimalachandran D, Raraty MG, Ghaneh P (2004) Cancer in the elderly: pancreatic cancer. Surg Oncol 13: 201–210.

3. Maitra A, Hruban RH (2008) Pancreatic cancer. Annu Rev Pathol 3: 157–188.

4. Burris HA 3rd, Moore MJ, Andersen J, Green MR, Rothenberg ML, et al (1997) Improvements in survival and clinical benefit with gemcitabine as first-line therapy for patients with advanced pancreas cancer: a randomized trial. J Clin Oncol 15: 2403–2413.

5. Burris H, Storniolo AM (1997) Assessing clinical benefit in the treatment of pancreas cancer: gemcitabine compared to 5-fluorouracil. Eur J Cancer 33 Suppl 1S18–22.

6. Rathos MJ, Joshi K, Khanwalkar H, Manohar SM, Joshi KS (2012) Molecular evidence for increased antitumor activity of gemcitabine in combination with a cyclin-dependent kinase inhibitor, P276-00 in pancreatic cancers. J Transl Med 10: 161.

7. Wong A, Soo RA, Yong WP, Innocenti F (2009) Clinical pharmacology and pharmacogenetics of gemcitabine. Drug Metab Rev 41: 77–88.

8. Bayraktar S, Bayraktar UD, Rocha-Lima CM (2010) Recent developments in palliative chemotherapy for locally advanced and metastatic pancreas cancer. World J Gastroenterol 16: 673–682.

9. Plunkett W, Huang P, Xu YZ, Heinemann V, Grunewald R, et al. (1995) Gemcitabine: metabolism, mechanisms of action, and self-potentiation. Semin Oncol 22: 3–10.

10. Hidalgo M (2010) Pancreatic cancer. N Engl J Med 362: 1605–1617.

11. Kleeff J, Michalski C, Friess H, Buchler MW (2006) Pancreatic cancer: from bench to 5-year survival. Pancreas 33: 111–118.

12. Philip PA (2010) Novel targets for pancreatic cancer therapy. Surg Oncol Clin N Am 19: 419–429.

13. Moore MJ, Goldstein D, Hamm J, Figer A, Hecht JR, et al. (2007) Erlotinib plus gemcitabine compared with gemcitabine alone in patients with advanced pancreatic cancer: a phase III trial of the National Cancer Institute of Canada Clinical Trials Group. J Clin Oncol 25: 1960–1966.

14. Conroy T, Desseigne F, Ychou M, Bouche O, Guimbaud R, et al. (2011) FOLFIRINOX versus gemcitabine for metastatic pancreatic cancer. N Engl J Med 364: 1817–1825.

15. Philip PA, Benedetti J, Corless CL, Wong R, O'Reilly EM, et al. (2010) Phase III study comparing gemcitabine plus cetuximab

versus gemcitabine in patients with advanced pancreatic adenocarcinoma: Southwest Oncology Group-directed intergroup trial S0205. J Clin Oncol 28: 3605–3610.

16. Kindler HL, Niedzwiecki D, Hollis D, Sutherland S, Schrag D, et al. (2010) Gemcitabine plus bevacizumab compared with gemcitabine plus placebo in patients with advanced pancreatic cancer: phase III trial of the Cancer and Leukemia Group B (CALGB 80303). J Clin Oncol 28: 3617–3622.

17. Bramhall SR, Schulz J, Nemunaitis J, Brown PD, Baillet M, et al. (2002) A double-blind placebo-controlled, randomised study comparing gemcitabine and marimastat with gemcitabine and placebo as first line therapy in patients with advanced pancreatic cancer. Br J Cancer 87: 161–167.

18. Paciotti GF, Myer L, Weinreich D, Goia D, Pavel N, et al. (2004) Colloidal gold: a novel nanoparticle vector for tumor directed drug delivery. Drug Deliv 11: 169–183.

19. Dreaden EC, Alkilany AM, Huang X, Murphy CJ, El-Sayed MA (2012) The golden age: gold nanoparticles for biomedicine. Chem Soc Rev 41: 2740–2779.

20. Brigger I, Dubernet C, Couvreur P (2012) Nanoparticles in cancer therapy and diagnosis. Adv Drug Deliv Rev.

21. Saha K, Bajaj A, Duncan B, Rotello VM (2011) Beauty is skin deep: a surface monolayer perspective on nanoparticle interactions with cells and bio-macromolecules. Small 7: 1903–1918.

22. 22.Kudgus RA, Bhattacharya R, Mukherjee P (2011) Cancer nanotechnology: emerging role of gold nanoconjugates. Anticancer Agents Med Chem 11: 965–973.

23. Arvizo RR, Bhattacharyya S, Kudgus RA, Giri K, Bhattacharya R, et al. (2012) Intrinsic therapeutic applications of noble metal nanoparticles: past, present and future. Chem Soc Rev 41: 2943–2970.

24. Khan JA, Kudgus RA, Szabolcs A, Dutta S, Wang E, et al. (2011) Designing nanoconjugates to effectively target pancreatic cancer cells in vitro and in vivo. Plos One 6: e20347.

25. Patra CR, Bhattacharya R, Wang E, Katarya A, Lau JS, et al. (2008) Targeted delivery of gemcitabine to pancreatic adenocarcinoma using cetuximab as a targeting agent. Cancer Res 68: 1970–1978.

26. Qian X, Peng XH, Ansari DO, Yin-Goen Q, Chen GZ, et al. (2008) In vivo tumor targeting and spectroscopic detection with surface-enhanced Raman nanoparticle tags. Nat Biotechnol 26: 83–90.

27. Perrault SD, Walkey C, Jennings T, Fischer HC, Chan WC (2009) Mediating tumor targeting efficiency of nanoparticles through design. Nano Lett 9: 1909–1915.

28. Han G, Ghosh P, Rotello VM (2007) Functionalized gold nanoparticles for drug delivery. Nanomedicine (Lond) 2: 113–123.

29. Khan JA, Pillai B, Das TK, Singh Y, Maiti S (2007) Molecular effects of uptake of gold nanoparticles in HeLa cells. Chembiochem 8: 1237–1240.

30. Daniel MC, Astruc D (2004) Gold nanoparticles: Assembly, supramolecular chemistry, quantum-size-related properties, and applications toward biology, catalysis, and nanotechnology. Chemical Reviews 104: 293–346.

31. Rocha-Lima CM, Soares HP, Raez LE, Singal R (2007) EGFR targeting of solid tumors. Cancer Control 14: 295–304.

32. Herbst RS, Kim ES, Harari PM (2001) IMC-C225, an anti-epidermal growth factor receptor monoclonal antibody, for treatment of head and neck cancer. Expert Opin Biol Ther 1: 719–732.

33. Kim ES, Lu C, Khuri FR, Tonda M, Glisson BS, et al. (2001) A phase II study of STEALTH cisplatin (SPI-77) in patients with advanced non-small cell lung cancer. Lung Cancer 34: 427–432.

34. Kim ES, Khuri FR, Herbst RS (2001) Epidermal growth factor receptor biology (IMC-C225). Curr Opin Oncol 13: 506–513.

35. Liao HJ, Carpenter G (2009) Cetuximab/C225-induced intracellular trafficking of epidermal growth factor receptor. Cancer Res 69: 6179–6183.

36. Li S, Schmitz KR, Jeffrey PD, Wiltzius JJ, Kussie P, et al. (2005) Structural basis for inhibition of the epidermal growth factor receptor by cetuximab. Cancer Cell 7: 301–311.

37. Orth JD, Krueger EW, Weller SG, McNiven MA (2006) A novel endocytic mechanism of epidermal growth factor receptor sequestration and internalization. Cancer Res 66: 3603–3610.

38. Schreiber AB, Libermann TA, Lax I, Yarden Y, Schlessinger J (1983) Biological role of epidermal growth factor-receptor clustering. Investigation with monoclonal anti-receptor antibodies. J Biol Chem 258: 846–853.

39. Arvizo RR, Giri K, Moyano D, Miranda OR, Madden B, et al. (2012) Identifying new therapeutic targets via modulation of protein corona formation by engineered nanoparticles. Plos One 7: e33650.

40. Arvizo RR, Rana S, Miranda OR, Bhattacharya R, Rotello VM, et al. (2011) Mechanism of anti-angiogenic property of gold nanoparticles: role of nanoparticle size and surface charge. Nanomedicine 7: 580–587.

41. Patra CR, Bhattacharya R, Mukherjee P (2010) Fabrication and functional characterization of goldnanoconjugates for potential application in ovarian cancer. J Mater Chem 20: 547–554.

42. Patra CR, Bhattacharya R, Mukhopadhyay D, Mukherjee P (2010) Fabrication of gold nanoparticles for targeted therapy in pancreatic cancer. Adv Drug Deliv Rev 62: 346–361.

43. Bhattacharya R, Mukherjee P (2008) Biological properties of “naked” metal nanoparticles. Adv Drug Deliv Rev 60: 1289–1306.

44. Mangeney C, Ferrage F, Aujard I, Marchi-Artzner V, Jullien L, et al. (2002) Synthesis and properties of water-soluble gold colloids covalently derivatized with neutral polymer monolayers. J Am Chem Soc 124: 5811–5821.

45. Mukherjee P, Bhattacharya R, Bone N, Lee YK, Patra CR, et al. (2007) Potential therapeutic application of gold nanoparticles in B-chronic lymphocytic leukemia (BCLL): enhancing apoptosis. J Nanobiotechnology 5: 4.

46. Walczyk D, Bombelli FB, Monopoli MP, Lynch I, Dawson KA (2010) What the cell "sees" in bionanoscience. J Am Chem Soc 132: 5761–5768.

47. Yao SY, Ng AM, Muzyka WR, Griffiths M, Cass CE, et al. (1997) Molecular cloning and functional characterization of nitrobenzylthioinosine (NBMPR)-sensitive (es) and NBMPR-insensitive (ei) equilibrative nucleoside transporter proteins (rENT1 and rENT2) from rat tissues. J Biol Chem 272: 28423–28430.

48. Griffiths M, Beaumont N, Yao SY, Sundaram M, Boumah CE, et al. (1997) Cloning of a human nucleoside transporter implicated in the cellular uptake of adenosine and chemotherapeutic drugs. Nat Med 3: 89–93.

49. Paproski RJ, Ng AM, Yao SY, Graham K, Young JD, et al. (2008) The role of human nucleoside transporters in uptake of 3'-deoxy-3'-fluorothymidine. Mol Pharmacol 74: 1372–1380.

50. Cobley CM, Chen J, Cho EC, Wang LV, Xia Y (2011) Gold nanostructures: a class of multifunctional materials for biomedical applications. Chem Soc Rev 40: 44–56.

51. Bhattacharyya S, Kudgus RA, Bhattacharya R, Mukherjee P (2011) Inorganic nanoparticles in cancer therapy. Pharm Res 28: 237–259.

52. Giljohann DA, Mirkin CA (2009) Drivers of biodiagnostic development. Nature 462: 461–464.

53. Sardar R, Funston AM, Mulvaney P, Murray RW (2009) Gold Nanoparticles: Past, Present, and Future. Langmuir 25: 13840–13851.

54. Ferrari M (2005) Cancer nanotechnology: opportunities and challenges. Nat Rev Cancer 5: 161–171.

55. Burda C, Chen X, Narayanan R, El-Sayed MA (2005) Chemistry and properties of nanocrystals of different shapes. Chem Rev 105: 1025–1102.

56. Bhattacharya R, Mukherjee P (2008) Biological properties of "naked" metal nanoparticles. Advanced Drug Delivery Reviews 60: 1289–1306.

57. Whitesides GM (2003) The 'right' size in nanobiotechnology. Nat Biotechnol 21: 1161–1165.

58. Mackey JR, Baldwin SA, Young JD, Cass CE (1998) Nucleoside transport and its significance for anticancer drug resistance. Drug Resist Updat 1: 310–324.

59. Mackey JR, Mani RS, Selner M, Mowles D, Young JD, et al. (1998) Functional nucleoside transporters are required for gemcitabine influx and manifestation of toxicity in cancer cell lines. Cancer Res 58: 4349–4357.

60. Young JD, Yao SY, Sun L, Cass CE, Baldwin SA (2008) Human equilibrative nucleoside transporter (ENT) family of nucleoside and nucleobase transporter proteins. Xenobiotica 38: 995–1021.

61. Giovannetti E, Del Tacca M, Mey V, Funel N, Nannizzi S, et al. (2006) Transcription analysis of human equilibrative nucleoside transporter-1 predicts survival in pancreas cancer patients treated with gemcitabine. Cancer Res 66: 3928–3935.

Index